Cancer Cell Metabolism: A Potential Target for Cancer Therapy

Dhruv Kumar
Editor

Cancer Cell Metabolism: A Potential Target for Cancer Therapy

Springer

Editor
Dhruv Kumar
Amity Institute of Molecular Medicine & Stem Cell Research (AIMMSCR)
Amity University Uttar Pradesh (AUUP)
Noida, Uttar Pradesh, India

ISBN 978-981-15-1990-1 ISBN 978-981-15-1991-8 (eBook)
https://doi.org/10.1007/978-981-15-1991-8

This Springer imprint is published by the registered company Springer Nature Singapore Pte Ltd.
The registered company address is: 152 Beach Road, #21-01/04 Gateway East, Singapore 189721, Singapore

Foreword

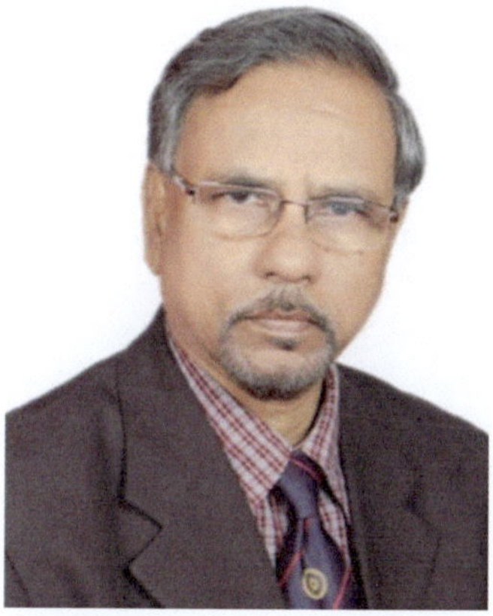

Cancer continues to be a major disease all over the world with a highest mortality rate overtaking the deaths associated with cardiovascular disease and diabetes. In fact, WHO has predicted that by 2030 every second individual will suffer from one or the other types of cancer, and it will be the prime cause of death globally. I have been working in the field of cancer since the mid-1970s and have extensively published on cancer research, specifically HPV-associated cervical cancer, head and neck cancer and breast cancer. While I work on several aspects of molecular oncology including initiation, progression, cancer biomarkers, cancer stem cells, and cancer drug discovery, I have noticed that cancer metabolism is coming in a big way and it is being considered as a hall mark of solid tumors.

I am highly impressed with the excellent job that **Dr. Dhruv Kumar** has done in highlighting abnormal energy metabolism as the central theme of the cancer in his newly edited book **Cancer Cell Metabolism: A Potential Target for Cancer Therapy**. The pivotal role of mitochondria and of aerobic glycolysis in sustaining and promoting cancer growth has been reported long back by several research groups. In 1953, the Nobel laureate, Otto Warburg demonstrated that the cancer cells perform aerobic glycolysis because of the impaired mitochondrial respiration. Cancer is generally considered as a genetic disease rather than a metabolic disease. In the last one decade, the metabolic defects in cancer cells have thought to arise as secondary consequences of genomic instability. Moreover, metabolic defects are being extensively targeted for the development of therapeutic approaches for cancer. In addition, the restriction of glucose and glutamine, which drive cancer energy metabolism, cripples the ability of cancer cells to replicate and disseminate. The gene theory has deceived us into thinking that cancer is a group of diseases. Certainly, tumors do not grow all at the same rate.

This book contains a number of key contributions that describe the molecular aspects of cancer cell metabolism, and how cancer cell metabolism can be targeted for the development of potential therapeutic approach. This book brings attention on the central issue of cancer as a metabolic disease according to Warburg's original theory. The book is unique in linking nearly all aspects of metabolic dysregulation that occur in cancer cells and tumor microenvironment. Cancer has remained incurable for many largely due to lack of clear understanding of its origin, biology, and metabolism. Hopefully, the information provided in this book will immensely improve our understanding of the disease and move the field in the right direction towards solutions and therapies, such as targeting metabolic cross talk between cancer cells and tumor microenvironment specifically through targeting cancer-associated fibroblasts.

The book is written and edited in a simple and easy-to-read language focusing mainly on cancer cell metabolism. Illustrations are clear and easy to understand. It will also be an excellent source of reference book for teachers and researchers alike.

I would like to congratulate Dr. Dhruv Kumar for his labor and love in editing this valuable book.

Bhudev Das
Amity Institute of Molecular Medicine & Stem Cell Research (AIMMSCR)
Amity University Uttar Pradesh (AUUP)
Noida, Uttar Pradesh, India

Health and Allied Sciences
Amity University Uttar Pradesh (AUUP)
Noida, Uttar Pradesh, India

Preface

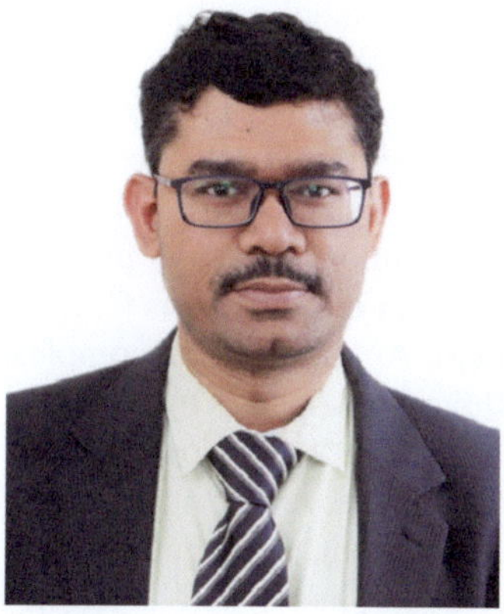

The aim of **Cancer Cell Metabolism: A Potential Target for Cancer Therapy** is to provide a comprehensive overview of recent advances in the molecular aspects of cancer cell metabolism, and how cancer cell metabolism can be targeted for the development of potential therapeutic approach. Metabolic dysregulation is a hallmark of cancer, and it is extensively targeted for the cancer therapy. I am a Cancer Biologist, trained in Bioinformatics and Translational Cancer Research. I have worked on several cancers including prostate, breast, pancreatic, and head and neck cancer. Several major findings planted the seed for this initiative. First, it became clear to me that the therapeutic action of some anticancer drugs operated largely through targeting glycolytic pathways in cancer cells. Second, that tumor microenvironment (TME) can protect cancer cells when glycolysis is limited with normal respiratory function. Finally, that cancer can be effectively managed and prevented once the metabolic cross-talk between cancer cells and TME is targeted.

The book is organized into eleven chapters, each one covering the latest developments in a specific area. The first chapter of the book introduces the readers to the recent progresses in the area of **Cancer Cell Metabolism: Solid Tumor Versus Nonsolid Tumor**. This is a central topic in cancer cell metabolism, as the metabolic regulation is totally different in solid tumors compared to non-solid tumors. The second chapter of the book is meant to give an overview of **Reprogramming of Cancer Cell Metabolism: Warburg and Reverse Warburg Hypothesis** which is a basis of metabolic reprograming in cancer cells. Sixty years ago, Otto Warburg has hypothesized that cancer cells undergo glycolysis despite the availability of adequate oxygen (aerobic glycolysis) and obtain less energy as compared to normal cells. This finding has helped many researchers to look for an alternative in treating cancer which is one of the leading causes of death today. An alternative model for cancer cell metabolism is called Reverse Warburg Effect, which provides an environment rich in energy for tumor growth. The third chapter of the book is focused on the **Molecular Aspects of Cancer Cell Metabolism: Altered Glycolysis and**

Lipid Metabolism. The metabolic alteration in pathways like glycolysis and lipid metabolism gives better chance of survival for cancer cells. Cancer cells produce lactic acid from glucose in the presence of oxygen and suppresses tricarboxylic acid (TCA) cycle. Cancer cells have the ability to perform de novo synthesis of lipids. These alteration in metabolism of cancer cells provides them multimodal advantages and differentiates them from normal cells. These altered metabolisms can be used for tracking and isolating the cancer cells from normal cell population and further can be targeted for cancer-specific treatment. The fourth and fifth chapters of the book is dedicated to the **Understanding the Metabolic Cross Talk Between Cancer Cells and Tumor Microenvironment (Cancer-Associated Fibroblasts)**. The TME is a heterogenous, complex, and dynamic setting in which both invading tumor and local stromal cells reside, co-evolve, and form a metabolic symbiosis that dictates downstream steps of cancer development and progression. Besides tumor cells, cancer-associated fibroblasts (CAFs) are the predominant cell type found in the majority of solid TME. It is recognized that cancer cells induce a metabolic phenotype in CAFs that is conducive to cancer progression. In addition, CAFs produce nutrients and metabolites, which are utilized by the tumor for energy production, proliferation, invasion, and migration. The sixth chapter of the book is focused on the **Role of Autophagy in Cancer Cell Metabolism**. Autophagy is a complex mechanism that plays a central role in maintaining cellular homeostasis by breaking down macromolecules and utilizing the metabolites as energy. This allows cells to maintain efficient ATP levels and promote cell survival by recycling macromolecules or dysfunctional organelles. Macromolecule degradation takes place in the lysosome and is identified as macroautophagy, microautophagy, or chaperone-mediated autophagy. Autophagy is also activated in response to cellular nutrient starvation as low glucose levels will cause cells to breakdown amino acids, such as glutamine. Glutaminolysis is able to support the TCA cycle and when cells undergo severe starvation they can produce adequate ATP and NADPH levels. The seventh chapter of the book is focused on the **Role of c-Met/HGF Axis in Altered Cancer Metabolism**. c-Met/HGF axis modulates glucose metabolism in cancer by altering major enzymes and transporters such as hexokinase, phosphofructokinase, lactate dehydrogenase, and glucose transporters and shifts the reliance of cancer cells on glucose rather than oxidative phosphorylation even in the presence of oxygen (Warburg phenomena). Also, c-Met/HGF axis modulates and interferes with other pathways such pentose phosphate pathway, amino acid metabolism, and TCA cycle leading to its aggressive phenotypes. The eighth chapter of the book is dedicated to the **Recent Advances in Drug Development Targeting Cancer Metabolism**. The identification and validation of cancer proteins in experiments and their atomic resolution for characterization of structural-dynamical-functional relationship is a costly, time-consuming, and more tedious process. The ninth and tenth chapters focus on **Clinical Relevance of "Biomarkers" in Cancer Metabolism and Alterations in Metabolite-Driven Gene Regulation in Cancer Metabolism**, respectively. The last chapter of the book is dedicated to the **Role of Phytochemicals in Cancer Cell Metabolism Regulation**. However, metabolomics, proteomics, and predictive in silico tools claimed well for accurately assessing the metabolic pathways, pharmacokinetics, and pharmacodynamics properties in early drug discovery stages. The generated huge amount of data from these techniques requires the development of reliable computational techniques and databases for the identification and/or prediction of cancer proteins as well as their ligands has become essential. All the recent advances in the field of cancer cell metabolism are presented in this book. This book is intended as a practical guide for researchers in both academia and industry, ranging from novice to expert level.

Finally, I would like to dedicate this book to the **millions of people who have suffered and died from the cancer**. I would like to thank all the authors who devoted part of their time to contributing a chapter to the book, and my special thanks to series editors (**Dr. Bhavik Sawhney and Mr. Selvakumar Rajendran**), publisher, and entire Springer team for their sincere assistance and support, and my family for their support and motivation. Finally, a special thanks goes to **Prof. (Dr.) Bhudev Das**, who honored us with a Foreword to this book.

Noida, India Dhruv Kumar

Contents

About the Editor

Dhruv Kumar is an Associate Professor at the Amity Institute of Molecular Medicine & Stem Cell Research (AIMMSCR), Amity University Uttar Pradesh (AUUP), Noida, Uttar Pradesh, India. His current research is focused on cancer cell metabolism, tumor microenvironment, autophagy, exosomes, mutational heterogeneity, cancer prevention, NGS, and bioinformatics.

He has received his Ph.D. in Cellular, Molecular, and Industrial Biology from the University of Bologna (UNIBO), Italy, under an Indo-Italian Government fellowship in 2012. After completing his Ph.D., he pursued postdoctoral training at the School of Medicine, University of Kansas Medical Center, Kansas City, USA. During this training, he worked towards understanding the molecular mechanism(s) of the regulation of autophagy and apoptosis in cancer stem cells (prostate, pancreatic, and breast), as well as understanding metabolic cross talk between the tumor microenvironment (cancer-associated fibroblast (CAF)) and head and neck squamous cell carcinoma (HNSCC) via HGF/c-MET and bFGF/FGFR signalling pathways.

He has published several research articles in peer-reviewed international journals including *Seninars in Cancer Biology, Annals of Oncology, Cancer Research, Scientific Reports, Genes, Radiation Research, Oncogenesis, Oncotarget, Cancer Letters, Molecular Cancer, Human Molecular Genetics, JAMA Otolaryngology, Plos One, Pharmacology & Therapeutics, Biochemical Pharmacology*, etc. and has authored and co-authored numerous books and book chapters. He is a member of many international and national scientific societies and organizations and received several prestigious national and international awards including the Senior Scientist Award, Early Career Research Award, SERB, DST-India, K-INBRE Postdoctoral Award, National Institute of General Medical Sciences, National Institute of Health, USA, Young Scientist Award, International Academy of Physical Science, Allahabad, India, Brains in Competition Award, Institute of Advanced Studies, University of Bologna, Italy, and the Indo-Italian Government Scholarship Award (Ministry of Human Resource and Development), India.

Cancer Cell Metabolism: Solid Tumor Versus Nonsolid Tumor

1

Sibi Raj, Vaishali Chandel, and Dhruv Kumar

Abstract

Metabolic regulation is considered to be one of the key hallmarks of cancer. Due to its continuous proliferation and high energy demands, cancer cells undertake increased glucose uptake as proposed by Otto Warburg, resulting in the production of enough amount of energy for their replication and survival. Totally different from the normal cell metabolism, even at aerobic conditions, cancer cells undergo glycolysis rather than oxidative phosphorylation. These glycolytic events in cancer cells elevate the expression of enzymes responsible for glucose metabolism such as hexokinase, pyruvate kinase, and lactate dehydrogenase-A. In addition, increased glucose metabolism in cancer cells leads to the formation of necessary amino acids, lipids, purines, and pyrimidine via the inter-branching biosynthetic pathways such as pentose phosphate pathway, serine biosynthesis, and glutaminolysis. Although blood cancer cells have the same way of regulating their metabolism for the survival, carbohydrate metabolism relatively is known to have very less role in the metabolic regulation in blood tumors. Lipid metabolism via the STAT-3 pathways plays a crucial role in blood tumor metabolism via oxidative phosphorylation to meet their energy demands. A deep understanding of metabolic regulation in cancer cells can pave a novel path for finding specific targets and drugs that can target the cancer cell metabolism.

Keywords

Solid tumor · Nonsolid tumor · Cancer metabolism

S. Raj · V. Chandel · D. Kumar (✉)
Amity Institute of Molecular Medicine & Stem Cell Research (AIMMSCR), Amity University Uttar Pradesh (AUUP), Noida, Uttar Pradesh, India
e-mail: dkumar13@amity.edu

D. Kumar (ed.), *Cancer Cell Metabolism: A Potential Target for Cancer Therapy*,
https://doi.org/10.1007/978-981-15-1991-8_1

1.1 Introduction

Cancer cells reprogram their pathway of nutrient acquisition and metabolic pathways to meet their survival and energetic needs. Reprogramming of metabolism in cancer cells is considered as a major hallmark of cancer (Vogelstein et al. 2004). The key question driving the research in this field is how cancer cells reprogram their metabolism which enhances their malignant properties and how to exploit metabolic targets for better treatment of cancer disease. Tumor cells reprogram their metabolism mainly to satisfy the large demand of energy flux for ATP, NADPH, NADH, and carbon skeletons (Simonnet 2002).

Otto Warburg in the 1950s had originally described the increased rate of glucose metabolism in tumor cells and production of lactate for the cancer cell survival and progression (Warburg 1956). Tumor cells mainly undergo metabolic reprogramming based on changes in the tumor environment as well as oxygen availability. Tumor cells mainly elevate the glucose and glutamine metabolism to achieve their ATP and NADPH demands (Wise et al. 2008). The elevated glycolysis not only helps the cancer cell meet the energy demands but also helps in the production of amino acids, lipids, and proteins via serine metabolism, glutamine metabolism, and lipid metabolism (Yang et al. 2016). Mitochondria is involved in major cellular processes in normal cells such as ATP production, synthesis of metabolites, triggering the production of reactive oxygen species (ROS), and apoptosis. In tumor cells, mitochondria dysfunction might play a role in the enhancement of tumor development and also decreased apoptosis and increased reactive oxidative species or drive the hypoxia-related pathways under a normoxic condition (Shapovalov et al. 2011). Glucose transporters in hepatocarcinomas, breast cancer, neuroendocrine carcinomas, lymphoblastic leukemia, and other types of several cancers are shown to be increasingly elevated (Krzeslak et al. 2012). Glycolytic genes such as hexokinase-II, pyruvate kinase, and pyruvate dehydrogenase-A were also reported to be highly upregulated in cancer cells (Denko 2008).The serine/threonine kinase Akt is one of the major constitutively activated protein kinases in cancer. Hypoxia has been reported to be the main selective force that facilitates metabolic adaptation in cancer cells (Robey et al. 2009). Recently, acidosis also has been exhibited to facilitate the metabolic reprogramming in tumor cells that lead to the inhibition of glycolysis and the use of mitochondrial oxidation as the main pathway of ATP generation (Santos et al. 2012). Although initially the Warburg effect was associated with impaired mitochondrial function, in order to reprogram metabolism in cancer cells, they need to maintain functional mitochondria ever-changing microenvironment. Various regulatory pathways are engaged in the reprogramming of tumor cell metabolism; HIF-1α and PI3K/Akt/mTOR are the most defined pathways in tumor metabolism (Lien et al. 2016). These regulatory mechanisms facilitate tumor cells to elevate the levels of various glycolytic enzymes, as well as lipogenic enzymes. Oncogenes such as c-Myc have been shown to play a role in modulating tumor metabolism (Kumar et al. 2018).

Traditionally, blood cancer has been realized to be a disease in which accumulation of slowly proliferating neoplastic lymphocytes occurs and does not undergo death due to an innate defect in their apoptotic cell death pathway machinery

(Bentley et al. 2000; Kitada et al. 2002). Aerobic glycolysis was reported in acute blood cancer and in a variety of lymphoproliferative neoplasms (Bhatt et al. 2012). Furthermore, it was reported that blood cancer cells balance their energy demands by increasing mitochondrial activity. B cell receptor activation and related pathways are thought to protect blood cancer cells from apoptosis. STAT3-driven aberrantly expressed LPL plays a major role in metabolic reprogramming by distorting the metabolism of blood cancer cell towards utilizing lipids (Rozovski et al. 2015). This event provides a sensible way to target the lipid metabolism in blood cancer cells. MiR-125 contributes to the metabolic adaptation of B lymphocytes and blood cancer cells, and its downregulation leads to a transformed state (Tili et al. 2012).

Metabolism can be defined as the complete biochemical processes that either produce or consume energy and are necessary for the survival of every living organism. Alterations in the function of master regulators of metabolism might protect cells from apoptosis-inducing pathways or initiate cellular transformation. An in-depth understanding of these processes in solid as well as nonsolid tumors will likely provide us with potential targets for therapeutic interventions in several types of tumors.

1.2 Aerobic Glycolysis

In normal cells, the majority of the glucose utilized by cells is broken down through glycolysis pathway and generates the end product pyruvate which is then transported to mitochondria, where at aerobic conditions pyruvate generates energy via the tricarboxylic acid (TCA) cycle and the electron transport chain (ETC), where mitochondrial respiration takes place. Glucose metabolism along with the oxidative phosphorylation generates 32 ATPs in normal cells (Koppenol et al. 2011). In contrast, cancer cells convert pyruvate into lactate, which is then eliminated outside the cells with the help of lactate transporters such as monocarboxylate transporters. The proliferation of cancer cells requires high amount of energy for their survival; glucose transporters such as GLUT-1 helps to consume more amount of glucose generating enough energy to meet their energy demands (Yu et al. 2017). The end product pyruvate which is derived from glucose metabolism is involved in the production of acetyl-CoA which is a precursor of fatty acid, lipid, and cholesterol synthesis. Pyruvate is similarly involved in the production of the nonessential amino acids such as aspartate and asparagine. Glucose 6-phosphate (G6P), an intermediate of glycolysis pathway which converge from glucose metabolism to the oxidative branch of the pentose phosphate pathway (PPP), results in the production of the ribose group required for the synthesis of nucleotides (Cho et al. 2018). The PPP is the pathway which produces NADPH. Furthermore, 3-phosphoglycerate (3PG) is the converging point for the production of the nonessential amino acid like serine. Tumor cells utilize the catabolized glucose via glycolysis as a key pathway for energy production. In addition, several biosynthetic molecules and NADPH are generated from glucose (Fig. 1.1).

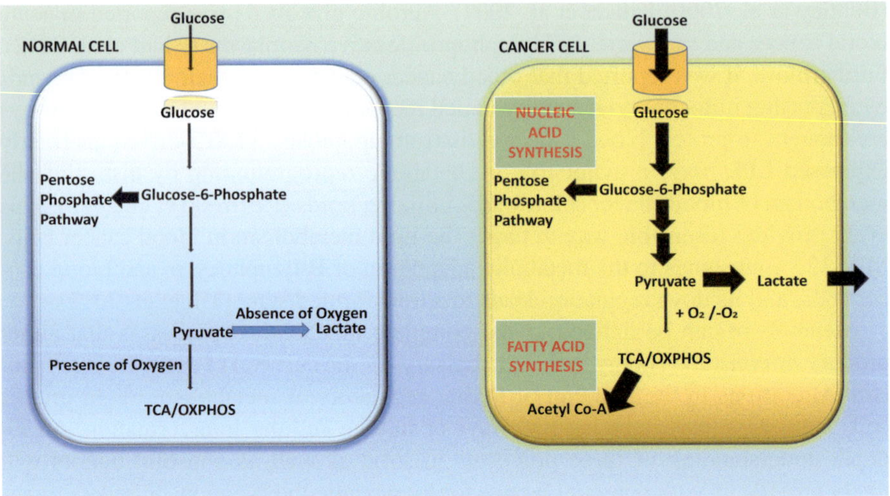

Fig. 1.1 Metabolism in normal and tumor cells. In normal cells, glucose is converted to pyruvate and subsequently followed by mitochondrial oxidation of pyruvate to carbon dioxide by entering into the TCA cycle and the oxidative phosphorylation process which produces 36 ATPs per glucose. Oxygen is necessary as it is required as the final acceptor of electrons. Under low oxygen levels, pyruvate is converted into lactate. Cancer cells convert majority of glucose to lactate irrespective of O_2 availability (the Warburg effect), and glucose metabolites are converged from energy generation to anabolic process to increase cell proliferation, at the expense of producing only two ATPs per glucose

1.3 Glutaminolysis

Glutamine is the most abundant amino acids circulating in the human body after glucose. Glutamine is important for several prominent functions in cancer cells like metabolite production, production of antioxidants for the removal of reactive oxygen species, and production of nonessential amino acids, purines, pyrimidine, and fatty acids for cellular replication and activation of cell signaling (Yang et al. 2017). Several studies have given evidence that tumor gene alteration in cancer cells reprograms glutamine metabolism. c-Myc is a proto-oncogene which transcriptionally binds to promoter regions of glutamine importers such as sodium-dependent neutral amino acid transporter type-2 and isoform of system N, resulting in elevated uptake of glutamine in cancer cells (Bhutia et al. 2016). The phosphatidyl 3-kinase/Akt/mechanistic target of rapamycin pathway is reported to be downregulated in several cancers and can influence glutamine metabolism. Glutamine can hinder cellular apoptosis to induce drug resistance. Acute glutamine deprivation in cells causes apoptosis and cell shrinkage triggered by the CD95-mediated caspase cascade. Overexpression of Bcl-2 (B cell lymphoma 2), a key mediator of the apoptotic pathway, results in a threefold increase of cellular GSH levels (Paquette et al. 2005). Increased GSH levels can then hinder apoptotic signaling induced by genotoxicity.

1.4 Serine Metabolism

One of the metabolic modulations that have been reported in cancer cells is serine metabolism. Serine acts as a central player for the synthesis of molecules such as nonessential amino acids glycine and cysteine (Combs et al. 2019). Moreover, glycine is a precursor of porphyrins and is also directly incorporated into purine nucleotide bases and into glutathione (GSH). Serine is mainly required for the synthesis of sphingolipids through the sphingosine production, and serine is a head group precursor, for phospholipids. Additionally, serine provides carbon to the one-carbon metabolic pathway, which then proceeds to the folate metabolism. The necessity of serine biosynthesis in cancer cells was suggested by Davis et al., by observing the 3-phosphoglycerate dehydrogenase activity (first catalyzing enzyme in serine biosynthesis pathway) in rat hepatoma cell lines having the fastest growth rate as well as the greatest 3-phosphoglycerate activity (Davis et al. 2004). The study by Maddocks et al. (2016) has shown that the p53 activation in the case of serine starvation blocks the nucleotide synthesis, resulting in some colorectal cancer cells to utilize less serine resources for serine-dependent pathways, enabling the survival of cells. A large number of functional metabolites that are important in cell biology are consequently associated with serine/glycine and THF-dependent one-carbon metabolism such as adenosine (AMP/ADP/ATP), S-adenosyl methionine (SAM), guanosine (GMP/GDP/GTP), nicotinamide (NAD/NADP), and glutathione (GSH/GSSG).

1.5 Fatty Acid Metabolism

Fatty acids are required by actively proliferating cancer cells for performing biological activities such as membrane development, protein modification, and bioenergetics requirements. Many proteins involved in de novo fatty acid synthesis are upregulated in cancer cells helping them to exhibit a lipogenic phenotype. Overexpression of multi-enzyme complex fatty acid synthase (FASN) is commonly observed in various tumors and often is a cause for poor prognosis (Menendez et al. 2007). The expression of many enzymes, which are involved in fatty acid synthesis, such as acetyl-CoA carboxylase (ACC) and ATP citrate lyase (ACL) is often associated with the increased FASN activity, oncogenic progression. Signaling in cancer cells facilitates both directly and indirectly to the elevation of fatty acid synthesis pathways (Mashima et al. 2009). The high expression and activity of ACL, ACC, and FASN in several cancer implicates this pathway could be involved in elevated tumor cell survival and proliferation. PI3K/Akt and MAPK signaling lead to the elevated expression of FASN and other lipogenic proteins. ACL is a direct target of Akt phosphorylation. Blocking the ACL activity in tumor cells having increased glucose metabolism contributed to the decreased proliferation and survival of cancer cells (Hatzivassiliou et al. 2005). In addition, the RNAi-mediated knockdown of ACC showed low proliferation and survival of few cancer cells. In addition to its role in fatty acid synthesis, existing literatures in the field suggests that FASN is also a metabolic oncogene. Ectopic expression of FASN in non-transformed prostrate cells deviated the cells from apoptosis, and a xenograft model injected with the transgenic FASN-expressing prostrate cells resulted in high neoplasia when compared to controls (Flavin et al. 2010). Cerulenin and C75, small molecule inhibitors of FASN, preferentially promote apoptosis of cancer cells compared to normal cells. In addition, various dietary compounds and polyphenols like catechin, epigallocatechin, and luteolin, which are naturally present, are being studied as potential inhibitors of fatty acid synthesis.

1.6 Drugs Targeting Cellular Metabolism in Solid Tumor

1.6.1 Drugs Targeting Glucose Metabolism

Various compounds have shown the ability to block the activity of various regulators involved in the glycolytic pathway. Silybin blocks the activity of GLUT transporter proteins, lonidamine blocks the activity of hexokinase, and 2-deoxyglucose acts as a competitive inhibitor of glucose metabolism. AZD3965 blocks the activity of MCT which is a glucose transporter. TLN-232 inhibits the PKM2 dimer, a small molecular inhibitor CPI-613 of pyruvate dehydrogenase and α-ketoglutarate dehydrogenase, and dichloroacetate (DCA) inhibits pyruvate dehydrogenase kinase (Zhan et al. 2011; Stuart et al. 2014; Beloueche-Babari et al. 2017; Nayak et al. 2018).

1.6.2 ROS Modulating Agents

Drugs that are involved in the inhibition of mitochondrial activity have been studied in early phase clinical trials. Drug molecules that inhibit the reactive oxygen species production include ATN-224, mangafodipir/calmangafodipir, motexafin, ARQ-501, elesclomol, arsenic trioxide, STA-4783, 2-ME, and ENMD-1198. Phenylethylisothiocyanate downregulation of glutathione, buthionine sulfoximine inhibits the GSH synthesis, and imexon depletion of GSH through thiol binding (Lowndes et al. 2008; Mehta et al. 2009; Zhou et al. 2011; Nagai et al. 2012; Shapiro et al. 2005) (Table 1.1).

1.7 Metabolism in Nonsolid Tumor

The nonsolid tumor or blood cancer is commonly known as leukemia or lymphoma. Blood cancer is a disease where slowly proliferating neoplastic cells accumulate and do not undergo death due to inherent defects in apoptotic pathways. Approximately 0.1–1.75% blood cells are reported to proliferate daily, and their metabolism is reprogrammed for their survival and proliferation (Chiorazzi et al. 2007). Chronic lymphoblastic leukemia (CLL) cells are reported to store cytoplasmic lipid vacuoles, and the CLL cell gene expression profile is shown to have increased gene expression that is commonly expressed in muscle and fat tissues.

Table 1.1 Metabolic drug targets for solid tumors under clinical trials

Drug	Target	Type of solid tumor	Status	Clinical trial no.
Silybin	Inhibitor of GLUT, EGFR	Pancreatic cancer	I	NCT00487721
Lonidamine	Hexokinase inhibitor	Breast cancer	II	NCT00435448
2-Deoxyglucose	Hexokinase phosphorylation inhibitor	Breast cancer/ prostrate cancer	I	NCT00633087
TLN-232	Pyruvate kinase M2 inhibitor	Esophageal cancer	II	NCT00735332
Dichloroacetate	Pyruvate dehydrogenase kinase	Gastric cancer	I	NCT03055143
ARQ-501	DNA damage checkpoint activator	Lung cancer	I	NCT00075933
Cisplatin	2-Deoxyglucose	Ovarian cancer	II	NCT03480971
Adriamycin	FASN	Breast cancer	II	NCT00003165
Doxorubicin	6PGD	Anaplastic thyroid cancer	I	NCT00077103
Sorafenib	GLS1	Hepatocellular carcinoma	III	NCT00105443
Cisplatin, radiation therapy	PKM2	Squamous cell carcinoma	III	NCT00262821

The metabolic pathways utilized by the blood cancer cells involve carbohydrate metabolism, altered lipid metabolism, and reactive oxygen species generation (Bilban et al. 2006).

1.7.1 Carbohydrate Metabolism

As discussed in solid tumor metabolism, glycolysis is the pathway which converts glucose to pyruvate, and is mostly seen as a key feature in cancer metabolism. In 1923, Otto Warburg reported that glucose is consumed by cancer cells in high amounts to meet their energy demands as to survive and proliferate. Bhatt et al. (2012) had reported that aerobic glycolysis was detected in acute leukemia and in a variety of lymphoproliferative neoplasms. Additionally, Kim et al. (2013) studies revealed that the total glycolytic activity was found to be a good way of prognosis in patients with diffuse large B cell lymphoma.

Contrastingly, studies by Lisker et al. (1966) had reported an impaired glucose tolerance test in patients with CLL and demonstrated that uptake of glucose is declined in blood cancer cells compared to normal B lymphocytes. Studies evaluating glucose metabolism in vivo by using the positron emission tomography and uptake of 2-Deoxy-2-[^{18}F] fluoroglucose (FDG) in CLL found a low level of ^{18}F-FDG avidity and low sensitivity of PET-FDG. Unlike in CLL, high avidity was detected in other lymphoproliferative diseases. Thus, while some degree of activity of the glucose metabolism is evident in CLL, this pathway does not seem to play a key role in CLL cells' metabolism, unlike its role in other rapidly proliferating lymphoproliferative neoplasms.

1.7.2 Oxidative Phosphorylation in Blood Cancer

Human mitochondrial DNA encodes 37 genes, 13 of which transcribe oxidative phosphorylation enzymes. Earlier reports from Clayton et al. (1967) showed that leukemia cells harbor alternate mt-DNA structures such as circular dimers, catenated dimmers, and trimmers. Otto Warburg had first reported that mitochondrial activity might be related to carcinogenesis. Recent studies report that blood cancer cells adjust to their high energy demands by elevating their mitochondrial activity. For example, Jitschin et al. (2014) found that the mitochondrial related activities like number of mitochondria, the total mitochondrial mass, mitochondrial biogenesis, mitochondrial electron transport activity, and mitochondrial membrane potential are high in blood cancer cells compared to normal B lymphocytes. These findings indicate that oxidative phosphorylation rate is high in blood cancer cells and, as a result, the levels of mitochondria-derived ROS are higher in blood cancer cells than in normal B cells. Moreover, when blood cancer cells are deprived of glucose, their mitochondrial oxidative phosphorylation is further increased.

1.7.3 Reactive Oxygen Species

B cell receptor activation and related pathways involving the JAK2/STAT-3 protect the blood cancer cells from apoptosis. High levels of ROS contribute to the impaired immune surveillance observed in patients with CLL (Rozovski et al. 2014). For example, CLL patients with high ROS levels have reduced numbers of activated $CD4^+$ cells, and exposure to an antioxidant restores T cell function. ROS-induced immune deregulation is probably mediated by modified DNA and lipids detected in CLL patients' plasma. However, the accumulation of ROS induces apoptosis, and antioxidants may protect CLL cells from apoptosis. For example, N-acetylcysteine known to block the generation of ROS protected CLL cells from apoptotic cell death.

1.7.4 Lipid Metabolism in Blood Tumor

A gene expression profile by Bilban et al. (2006) revealed that CLL cells' signature is similar to that of fat or muscle cells. Specifically, lipoprotein lipase (LPL) which is normally expressed in adipocytes and muscle cells was reported to be abnormally expressed in blood cancer cells. STAT3 is constitutively phosphorylated on serine 727 residue and activates genes that provide blood cancer cells with survival advantage. Rozovski et al. (2015) have recently reported that CLL phosphoserine STAT-3 binds and activates the promoter of lipoprotein lipase in blood cancer cells (Rozovski et al. 2014).

In newly diagnosed patients with blood cancer, increased uptake of cholesterol mediated by LPL resulted in relatively very low levels of cholesterol, high-density lipoprotein cholesterol (HDL-C), very-low-density lipoprotein cholesterol (VLDL-C), and triglycerides (Daniels et al. 2009). Lipid-mediated signaling might be disrupted in blood cancer cells. For example, the expression of sphingosine-1-phosphate receptor 1, known to induce lipid-dependent signaling, is low in blood cancer patients' lymph nodes, and upon B cell receptor inhibitor treatment, its level elevates, likely contributing to mobilization of blood cancer cells from lymph nodes to the peripheral blood (Till et al. 2015). CLL cells store lipids in cytoplasmic vacuoles and utilize the free fatty acids to generate energy through oxidative phosphorylation. Metabolomic analysis of CLL cells identified increased levels of FFAs and triglyceride degradation products, suggesting that these changes are induced by downregulation of microRNA (miR)-125 and a reciprocal increase in lipolysis-facilitating enzymes (Tili et al. 2012). Free fatty acids are substrate for oxidative phosphorylation and are also ligands for peroxisome proliferator-activated receptor (PPAR)-α. The free fatty acid PPAR-α complex acts as a transcription factor and transcribes enzyme necessary for oxidative phosphorylation. Ruby et al. (2010) had reported that PPAR-α is highly expressed in blood cancer cells and its level corresponds to the advanced stage of the disease. Thus, STAT3-driven aberrantly expressed LPL plays a major role in metabolic reprogramming by skewing the metabolism of CLL cell towards utilizing lipids. This phenomenon provides a new strategy for targeting lipid metabolism in CLL cells (Fig. 1.2).

1.8 Targeting Metabolic Pathways in Blood Cancer

In blood tumor, statins are known to be competitive inhibitors of 3-hydroxy-3-methyl glutaryl coenzyme A (HMG-CoA) reductase; they are reported to induce apoptosis by the activation of caspase-9. Metformin, an anti-diabetic drug, was found to inhibit the mitochondrial respiratory chain and subsequently mitochondrial oxidative phosphorylation. Because metformin inhibits oxidative phosphorylation in CLL cells and possesses a potential antileukemic activity, clinical trials of metformin in CLL have been initiated. Also, the PPAR-α antagonist MK886 and PK11195, a benzodiazepine that blocks mitochondrial F1F0-ATPase has been reported to target oxidative phosphorylation in blood cancer cells (Garcia-Ruiz et al. 2012; Spaner et al. 2013; Adekola et al. 2015) (Table 1.2).

1.9 Conclusion

Tumor metabolism has been a widely researched study and is significantly identified as completely different from the normal cell metabolism. Increased metabolic demands in cancer cells met by elevated glycolysis resulting in the activation of glycolytic genes such as hexokinase-II, pyruvate kinase-M2, and lactate dehydrogenase-A. Glycolysis generates intermediates for biosynthetic pathways such as

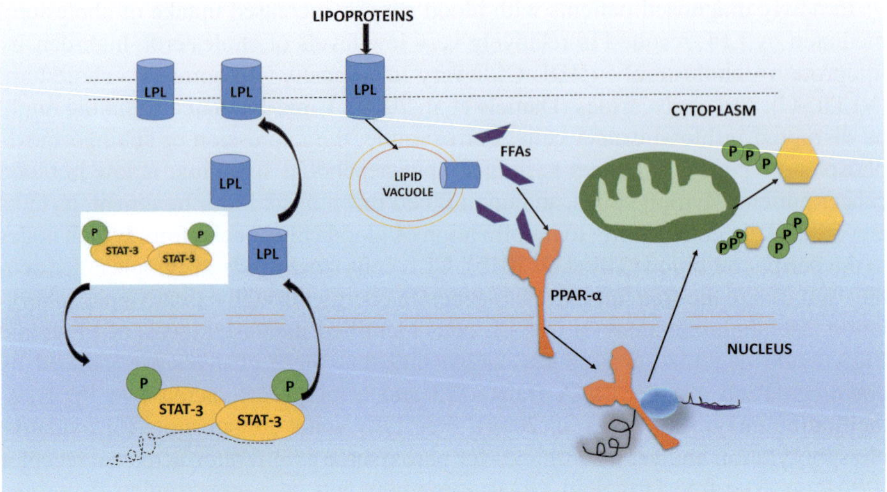

Fig. 1.2 STAT-3 is continuously proliferated in blood cancer cells on serine 427 residues. Phosphorylation of STAT-3 results in dimer formation and is transported to the nucleus which then binds to DNA and activates STAT-3 target genes. Lipoprotein lipase being a target gene for STAT-3 is abnormally expressed in blood cancer cells and maintains the cellular uptake of lipoproteins. LPL hydrolyses triglycerides that are present in lipid vacuoles into free fatty acids (FAFs). FAFs bind to PPAR-α subsequently activating the genes for oxidative phosphorylation. PPARα-target gene proteins enter the mitochondria and induce oxidative phosphorylation

Table 1.2 Metabolic drug targets for blood cancer under clinical trials

Drug	Target	Status	Clinical trial no.
Simvastatin	Competitive inhibitors of HMG-CoA reductase	I	NCT00303277
Metformin	Anti-diabetic suppressing gluconeogenesis	I	NCT02432287
MK886	Inhibition of PPARα activity	–	–
Ritonavir	Inhibits cytochrome P45—3A4 (CYP3A4)	I/II	NCT01009437
Ceramide	Inhibits GAPDH	II	NCT02834611
Daunorubicin	PFK-2	I/II	NCT03878199
Imatinib	PFK-2	–	–
Cytarabine	Mitochondrial oxidative phosphorylation	III	NCT01349972
Bortezomib	LDH-A, PDK	–	–
Carfilzomib	GLS	I	NCT01402284

pentose phosphate pathway, lipid metabolism, and serine biosynthesis pathway that serves necessary biomolecules such as amino acids, lipids, purine, and pyrimidine. The second most consumed compound after glucose in cancer cells is glutamine which helps in various fundamental functions in cancer cells like synthesis of metabolites and production of antioxidants for the removal of reactive oxygen species. Various compounds have shown the ability to inhibit various regulators involved in the glycolytic pathway and are under clinical trials. Blood cancer shows similar way of metabolic regulation, but contrastingly lipid metabolism plays certainly major role in blood tumors via the STAT-3 subsequently activating the genes for mitochondrial phosphorylation with the help of LPL and PPAR-α complexes. In addition, drugs such as simvastatin, metformin, MK8886, ritonain, and ceramide are under clinical trials which target certain metabolic intermediates in blood cancer cells. Understanding the metabolic regulation in cancer cells leads to the discovery of new drugs that target the key players in metabolism and inhibit the cancer cell proliferation and survival.

References

Adekola KUA et al (2015) Investigating and targeting chronic lymphocytic leukemia metabolism with the human immunodeficiency virus protease inhibitor ritonavir and metformin. Leuk Lymphoma 56:450

Beloueche-Babari M et al (2017) MCT1 inhibitor AZD3965 increases mitochondrial metabolism, facilitating combination therapy and noninvasive magnetic resonance spectroscopy. Cancer Res 77:5913

Bentley DP et al (2000) The apoptotic pathway: a target for therapy in chronic lymphocytic leukemia. Hematol Oncol 18:87

Bhatt AP et al (2012) Dysregulation of fatty acid synthesis and glycolysis in non-Hodgkin lymphoma. In: Proc Natl Acad Sci U S A, vol 109, p 11818

Bhutia YD et al (2016) Glutamine transporters in mammalian cells and their functions in physiology and cancer. Biochim Biophys Acta 1863(10):2531–2539

Bilban M et al (2006) Deregulated expression of fat and muscle genes in B-cell chronic lymphocytic leukemia with high lipoprotein lipase expression. Leukemia 20:1080

Chiorazzi N et al (2007) Cell proliferation and death: Forgotten features of chronic lymphocytic leukemia B cells. Best Pract Res Clin Haematol 20(3):399–413

Cho ES et al (2018) The pentose phosphate pathway as a potential target for cancer therapy. In: Biomol Ther (Seoul), vol 26, p 29

Clayton DA et al (1967) Circular dimer and catenate forms of mitochondrial DNA in human leukaemic leucocytes. Nature 216:652

Combs JA et al (2019) The non-essential amino acid cysteine becomes essential for tumor proliferation and survival. In: Cancers, vol 11. https://doi.org/10.3390/cancers11050678

Daniels TF et al (2009) Lipoproteins, cholesterol homeostasis and cardiac health. Int J Biol Sci 5(5):474–488

Davis SR et al (2004) Tracer-derived total and folate-dependent homocysteine remethylation and synthesis rates in humans indicate that serine is the main one-carbon donor. Am J Physiol Endocrinol Metab 286:E272

Denko NC (2008) Hypoxia, HIF1 and glucose metabolism in the solid tumour. Nat Rev Cancer 8(9):705–713

Flavin R et al (2010) Fatty acid synthase as a potential therapeutic target in cancer. Future Oncol 6:551

Garcia-Ruiz C et al (2012) Statins and protein prenylation in cancer cell biology and therapy. Anti Cancer Agents Med Chem 12:303

Hatzivassiliou G et al (2005) ATP citrate lyase inhibition can suppress tumor cell growth. Cancer Cell 8:311

Jitschin R et al (2014) Mitochondrial metabolism contributes to oxidative stress and reveals therapeutic targets in chronic lymphocytic leukemia. Blood 123:2663

Kim TM et al (2013) Total lesion glycolysis in positron emission tomography is a better predictor of outcome than the International Prognostic Index for patients with diffuse large B cell lymphoma. Cancer 119:1195

Kitada S et al (2002) Dysregulation of apoptosis genes in hematopoietic malignancies. Oncogene 21:3459

Koppenol WH et al (2011) Otto Warburg's contributions to current concepts of cancer metabolism. Nat Rev Cancer 11(5):325–337

Krzeslak A et al (2012) Expression of GLUT1 and GLUT3 glucose transporters in endometrial and breast cancers. Pathol Oncol Res 18:721

Kumar D et al (2018) Cancer-associated fibroblasts drive glycolysis in a targetable signaling loop implicated in head and neck squamous cell carcinoma progression. Cancer Res 78:3769

Lien EC et al (2016) Metabolic reprogramming by the PI3K-Akt-mTOR pathway in cancer. Recent Results Cancer Res 207:39–72

Lisker A et al (1966) Abnormal carbohydrate metabolism in patients with malignant blood dyscrasias. Am J Med Sci 252(3):282–288

Lowndes SA et al (2008) Phase I study of copper-binding agent ATN-224 in patients with advanced solid tumors. Clin Cancer Res 14:7526

Maddocks ODK et al (2016) Serine metabolism supports the methionine cycle and DNA/RNA methylation through de novo ATP synthesis in cancer cells. Mol Cell 61:210

Mashima T et al (2009) De novo fatty-acid synthesis and related pathways as molecular targets for cancer therapy. Br J Cancer 100:1369

Mehta MP et al (2009) Motexafin gadolinium combined with prompt whole brain radiotherapy prolongs time to neurologic progression in non-small-cell lung Cancer patients with brain metastases: results of a phase III trial. Int J Radiat Oncol Biol Phys 73:1069

Menendez J et al (2007) Fatty acid synthase and the lipogenic phenotype in cancer pathogenesis. Nat Rev Cancer 7:763

Nagai M et al (2012) The oncology drug elesclomol selectively transports copper to the mitochondria to induce oxidative stress in cancer cells. Free Radic Biol Med 52:2142

Nayak MK et al (2018) Dichloroacetate, an inhibitor of pyruvate dehydrogenase kinases, inhibits platelet aggregation and arterial thrombosis. Blood Adv 2:2029

Paquette J et al (2005) Rapid induction of the intrinsic apoptotic pathway by L-glutamine starvation. J Cell Physiol 202:912

Robey R et al (2009) Is Akt the "Warburg kinase"?-Akt-energy metabolism interactions and oncogenesis. Semin Cancer Biol 19:25

Rozovski U et al (2014) Stimulation of the B-cell receptor activates the JAK2/STAT3 signaling pathway in chronic lymphocytic leukemia cells. Blood 123(24):3797–3802

Rozovski U et al (2015) Aberrant LPL expression, driven by STAT3, mediates free fatty acid metabolism in CLL cells. Mol Cancer Res 13(5):944–953

Ruby MA et al (2010) VLDL hydrolysis by LPL activates PPAR-α through generation of unbound fatty acids. J Lipid Res 51:2275

Santos C et al (2012) Lipid metabolism in cancer. FEBS J 279:2610

Shapiro GI et al (2005) Phase I trial of ARQ 501, an Activated Checkpoint Therapy (ACT) agent, in patients with advanced solid tumors. J Clin Oncol 23(16_suppl):3042

Shapovalov Y et al (2011) Mitochondrial dysfunction in cancer cells due to aberrant mitochondrial replication. J Biol Chem 286:22331

Simonnet H (2002) Low mitochondrial respiratory chain content correlates with tumor aggressiveness in renal cell carcinoma. Carcinogenesis 23:759

Spaner DE et al (2013) PPAR-alpha is a therapeutic target for chronic lymphocytic leukemia. Leukemia 27:1090

Stuart SD et al (2014) A strategically designed small molecule attacks alpha-ketoglutarate dehydrogenase in tumor cells through a redox process. Cancer Metab 2:4

Tili E et al (2012) The down-regulation of miR-125b in chronic lymphocytic leukemias leads to metabolic adaptation of cells to a transformed state. Blood 120:2631

Till KJ et al (2015) Expression of functional sphingosine-1 phosphate receptor-1 is reduced by B cell receptor signaling and increased by inhibition of PI3 kinase δ but not SYK or BTK in chronic lymphocytic leukemia cells. In: J Immunol, vol 194, p 2439

Vogelstein B et al (2004) Cancer genes and the pathways they control. Nat Med 10:789

Warburg O (1956) On the origin of cancer cells. Science 123:309
Wise DR et al (2008) Myc regulates a transcriptional program that stimulates mitochondrial glutaminolysis and leads to glutamine addiction. In: Proc Natl Acad Sci U S A, vol 105, p 18782
Yang M et al (2016) Serine and one-carbon metabolism in cancer. Nat Rev Cancer 16:650
Yang L et al (2017) Glutaminolysis: a hallmark of cancer metabolism. Annu Rev Biomed Eng 19:163
Yu M et al (2017) The prognostic value of GLUT1 in cancers: a systematic review and meta-analysis. Oncotarget 8(26):43356–43367
Zhan T et al (2011) Silybin and dehydrosilybin decrease glucose uptake by inhibiting GLUT proteins. J Cell Biochem 112:849
Zhou Q et al (2011) A phase I dose-escalation, safety and pharmacokinetic study of the 2-methoxyestradiol analog ENMD-1198 administered orally to patients with advanced cancer. Investig New Drugs 29:340

Reprogramming of Cancer Cell Metabolism: Warburg and Reverse Warburg Hypothesis

2

Samyukta Narayanan, Anirudh Santhoshkumar, Srijit Ray, and Sitaram Harihar

Abstract

Every cell requires energy which they obtain from oxidative phosphorylation to perform major metabolic functions. This energy requirement is dependent on their metabolic rate, and it is expected that higher the metabolic rate, higher is the amount of energy expended. However, cancer cells have a unique metabolic behavior where they require only a minimal amount of energy, exhibiting a condition called the Warburg effect to survive and proliferate. They undergo glycolysis despite the availability of adequate oxygen (aerobic glycolysis) and obtain less energy as compared to normal cells from this process. This finding has helped many researchers to look for an alternative in treating cancer which is one of the leading causes of death today. This chapter will elucidate on the role of Warburg effect in modulating cancer cell metabolism and describe recent findings on this unique pathway employed by cancer cells. The chapter will also shed light on an alternative model called the reverse Warburg effect that provides an environment rich in energy for tumor growth and discuss the potential of using this pathway for therapeutically targeting cancer cells.

Keywords

Cancer · Metastasis · Metabolism · Glycolysis · Warburg effect · Microenvironment · Oxidative phosphorylation

S. Narayanan · A. Santhoshkumar · S. Ray · S. Harihar (✉)
Department of Genetic Engineering, School of Bioengineering, SRM Institute of Science and Technology, Kattankulathur, Tamil Nadu, India

D. Kumar (ed.), *Cancer Cell Metabolism: A Potential Target for Cancer Therapy*,
https://doi.org/10.1007/978-981-15-1991-8_2

2.1 Introduction

Cancer cells have always been unique; metabolic adaptations have allowed them to evade their targeting by the immune system and helped them to proliferate and survive. Significant research has been done to understand how a cancer cell alters its metabolic behavior and uses it to its own advantage. One such change involves the rewiring of glucose uptake and aerobic glycolysis, where fermentation of glucose to lactate occurs even in the presence of oxygen, popularly termed as the "Warburg effect" (Vander Heiden 2012). Aerobic glycolysis has been shown to be associated with carcinogenesis, alterations in lipid and protein metabolism along with activation and deactivation of oncogenes and tumor suppressor genes, respectively (Fadaka et al. 2017). The dependence of most cancers on aerobic glycolysis for their metabolic requirements is puzzling since it is less efficient and meets only a limited amount of energy requirements when compared to oxidative phosphorylation. Interestingly, this adaptation is also observed in fast multiplying cells, indicating a possible link with faster proliferation rates. Therefore, this dependence on aerobic glycolysis of cancer cells is a key property that can be employed for detection and targeting of cancer cells; however, for this to happen, a complete understanding of the process is essential (Liberti and Locasale 2016; Vazquez et al. 2010).

The Warburg effect was first hypothesized by Otto Heinrich Warburg when his group initially showed that starving cancer cells of glucose and oxygen resulted in cell death (Warburg et al. 1927). Later, working with *Saccharomyces cerevisiae,* Crabtree found a preference for glycolysis over oxidative phosphorylation in ethanol production even in the presence of high amounts of oxygen and glucose, an effect later termed as the "Crabtree effect." This supported the observations made by Warburg leading to the proposition that the preference of cancer cells to glycolysis over oxidative phosphorylation may possibly be due to improper functioning of the mitochondria and that it could also be the base for cancer development (Liberti and Locasale 2016).

Interestingly, increased levels of glycolytic metabolites are not limited to only cancer cells but are also seen in rapidly growing cells, such as the embryonal cells. The gene expression profile of cancer cells undergoing aerobic glycolysis was identical to that of embryonal cells, indicating a common role in promoting cellular proliferation. Embryonal cells employ this mechanism for increased angiogenesis and growth. Furthermore, when the embryonal cells stop proliferating and start differentiating, the genes responsible are switched off with right cues. However, in cancer cells these genes are always on by default contributing to malignancy (Abdel-Haleem et al. 2017).

2.2 Carbohydrate Metabolism in Normal Cells

To understand reprogramming of cancer cell metabolism, an understanding of the normal differentiated cell metabolism is essential. Differentiated cells take up monosaccharides obtained from breaking down of complex carbohydrates for energy production. On digestion, the monosaccharides are released from the gut to the blood stream where they support the cellular metabolic requirements. The glucose levels are mainly regulated by the pancreatic hormones, insulin and glucagon, with more insulin being secreted on increase in blood glucose levels. Glucose gets converted to glycogen in muscles and liver by glycogenesis, and in case of low glucose levels in the blood, the glycogen is broken down to glucose through glycogenolysis by the hormone glucagon. Glucose is the main energy source of a cell; once it enters the cell, it is further broken down to energy-rich molecules like adenosine triphosphate (ATP), nicotinamide adenine dinucleotide (NADH), and flavin adenine dinucleotide (FADH2) by glycolysis, citric acid cycle, and oxidative phosphorylation (Fadaka et al. 2017).

Glycolysis is the major pathway used for energy production in all cells for catabolism of glucose and is employed for energy production and intermediate generation for other pathways. In glycolysis, one glucose molecule is broken down to two pyruvate molecules producing two ATP and two NADH at the expense of one ATP, the pyruvate in presence of oxygen is converted to acetyl-CoA by pyruvate dehydrogenase enzyme, and this acetyl-CoA enters into the citric acid cycle yielding two ATP, six NADH, and two FADH2 molecules (Fadaka et al. 2017). Based on the enzyme used around 32–38 ATP molecules are produced for one glucose molecule.

2.3 Carbohydrate Metabolism in Cancer Cells

Cancer cells have rewired their carbohydrate metabolism to suit their needs, where they rely on glycolysis for energy production and where pyruvate is converted to lactate even in the presence of oxygen, therefore giving the name aerobic glycolysis. Normal differentiated cells convert pyruvate to acetyl-CoA and continue with citric acid cycle and oxidative phosphorylation and produce more ATP molecules whereas only two ATP molecules are produced in aerobic glycolysis and therefore the process is very inefficient. The cancer cells, to overcome this deficiency, convert glucose to lactate at a rate of 10–100 times faster than a normal cell, resulting in the fulfillment of most of their energy needs over a period. Tumor cells also meet their energy needs by employing creatine kinase, an enzyme present in high levels in exercising muscle for increased ATP production (Liberti and Locasale 2016) (Fig. 2.1). It is still left to argue about the benefits that cancer cells derive off Warburg effect or aerobic glycolysis.

Research accumulated over a period has shown that cancer cells rely on aerobic glycolysis for multiple reasons, one being this assures a cancer cell of a constant supply of ATP even in situations where the oxygen supply is limited or where the cells outgrow their oxygen supply (Yoshida 2015). The metabolic intermediates of glycolysis provide raw materials for the cancer cells to proliferate and grow (Adekola et al. 2012). The decreased pH in their microenvironment as a result of the release of lactate will help in enhancing the cancer cells to “break open” the extracellular matrix leading to increased invasiveness and malignancy. The reduced pH also suppresses the immune effectors such as the tumor-infiltrating lymphocytes, making the environment conducive to supporting cancer growth (Jiang 2017; Liberti and Locasale 2016; Gatenby and Gillies 2004).

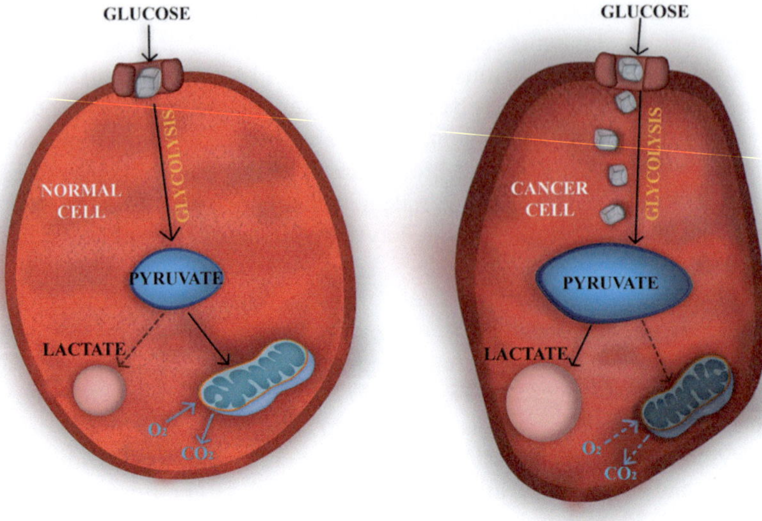

Fig. 2.1 The figure illustrates the difference between a normal cell and a cancer cell in metabolizing glucose. Cancer cells convert the glycolytic end-product pyruvate to lactate (solid arrow) without entering OXPHOS. The lactate generated is secreted to the microenvironment where it acidifies the environment. To make up the energy deficiency, cancer cells take in much more glucose compared to a normal cell. A cancer cell also adapts itself for growing in hypoxic environments due to its reduced dependency on OXPHOS

The Warburg effect has also been shown to impact cell signaling factors and functions in cancer cells. It alters the redox potential of mitochondria regulating the generation of reactive oxygen species (ROS) without affecting cellular proliferation (Fu et al. 2017; Liberti and Locasale 2016; Wu et al. 2013). Warburg effect is also linked with chromatin modulation; acetyl-CoA, a substrate for carrying out histone acetylation is usually controlled by glucose flux. This regulates the expression of genes since histone acetylation would result in increased amounts of euchromatin and ease of access of DNA to transcription factors to transcribe the genes necessary for glucose metabolism. ATP-citrate lyase converts citrate to acetyl-CoA, inhibiting or downregulating its activity results in reduction of histone acetylation, and diverting the cancer cells from normal glucose metabolism to aerobic glycolysis (Liberti and Locasale 2016).

The mechanism by which cancer cells shift their metabolic pathway toward activation of aerobic glycolysis was shown to vary depending on the type of cancer. Under reduced levels of available oxygen, hypoxia-inducible factor 1 (HIF-1) was shown to act as a master regulator of transcription of other genes (Semenza 2010). HIF-1 upregulates the expression of GLUT-1 and GLUT-3 glucose transporters that facilitate cellular glucose uptake (Adekola et al. 2012). HIF-1 overexpression leads cancer cells to become independent of oxygen requirements and depend on aerobic glycolysis for their energy needs (Papandreou et al. 2006). HIF-1 expression also promotes resistance to apoptosis, and upregulates vesicular endothelial growth factor (VEGF) expression leading to increased angiogenesis that leads to cancer malignancy (Lu et al. 2002). Furthermore, mitochondrial gene mutations increase ROS amounts leading to upregulation of HIF-1 levels (Fu et al. 2017; Yu et al. 2017). HIF-1 directly targets and inactivates the enzyme pyruvate dehydrogenase kinase 1 (PDK1) leading to the inactivation of the mitochondrial pyruvate dehydrogenase (PDH) enzyme complex which is required for conversion of pyruvate to acetyl-CoA (Kim et al. 2006). Therefore, this leads to the accumulation of pyruvate and lactate and further inhibition of mitochondrial function. This has been shown to further activate oncogenes such as protein kinase B (PKB/AKT), RAS and MYC leading to increased aerobic glycolysis (Dang 2010; Kim and Dang 2006; Tran et al. 2016; Elstrom et al. 2004; Li et al. 2005; Plas and Thompson 2005). HIF-1 expression also leads to the upregulation of hexokinase 2 (HK2), an enzyme responsible for the conversion of glucose to glucose-6-phosphate. Increased levels of hexokinase are seen in many cancer types, where it has been shown to directly promote tumor initiation and maintenance (Courtnay et al. 2015; Mathupala et al. 2009; Wang et al. 2016).

The loss of p53 or mutant p53, a common feature of cancer cells, was shown to play an important role in shifting of their metabolic behavior to aerobic glycolysis (Kato et al. 2018). Mutated p53 was shown to promote GLUT 1 translocation to plasma membrane, helping drive the Warburg effect (Zawacka-Pankau et al. 2011; Zhang et al. 2013). It was also found to promote actin polymerization by regulating the levels of actin-binding proteins ROCK/RhoA, thereby resulting in high vesicle trafficking rates, essential for translocation of glucose transporters (Zhang et al. 2013). Active p53 is an essential factor for reducing glycolysis rates by increasing the amount of fructose 2,6-bisphosphate in normal cells, something that is lacking in cancer cells (Tran et al. 2016). This results in a greater glycolytic flux, reduced oxidation of pyruvate and reduction in ATP molecules normally generated by oxidative phosphorylation. Active p53 is also helpful in inhibiting mammalian target of rapamycin (mTOR) signaling which is important for cellular proliferation (Kondoh 2012; Matoba et al. 2006). Mutant p53 therefore, promotes cell proliferation in cancer cells by activating the mTOR signaling pathway (Zawacka-Pankau et al. 2011).

The mechanism for maintaining a continuous glycolytic process is active in cancer cells. This involves the upregulation of glycolytic enzymes like phosphofructokinase-1 (PFK-1) in order to maintain a constant glucose flux (Yu et al. 2017). Phosphorylation and inactivation of PDK1 leads to a further reduction in acetyl-CoA levels and promotes glycolysis (Kim and Dang 2005). Furthermore, pyruvate kinase, the enzyme that catalyzes the last step of the glycolytic pathway—conversion of phosphoenolpyruvate (PEP) to pyruvate—exists in two isozymes, PKM1 and PKM2. PKM1 is expressed in normal cells, whereas PKM2 is mainly expressed in rapidly growing cells such as cancer cells (Yang and Lu 2013). PKM2 further exists in its less-efficient dimeric form in cancer cells resulting in diminished enzymatic activity and accumulation of glycolytic intermediates leading to their employment in the synthesis of amino acids and nucleic acids critical for cancer cell proliferation (Kato et al. 2018; Hitosugi et al. 2009). PKM2 increases the expression of c-Myc, an oncogene promoting uncontrolled cellular proliferation (Danhier et al. 2017; Sawayama et al. 2014).

Apart from upregulating glycolytic enzymes, cancer cells also downregulate the expression of several mitochondrial enzymes that are important for oxidative phosphorylation (Gottlieb and Tomlinson 2005). Mitochondrial biogenesis is controlled by the master regulator gene, peroxisome proliferator-activated receptor gamma coactivator 1-alpha (PGC1α), which is downregulated in cancers leading to their switch to glycolytic metabolism (Vyas et al. 2016; Yang and Lu 2013). Mitochondrial gene point mutations causing dysfunction are also known to promote disturbances in cellular bioenergetics and serve as a trigger for tumor cell growth by releasing ROS or small molecule metabolites released by mitochondria (Gonzalez et al. 2014; Hsu et al. 2016; Samudio et al. 2009; Tran et al. 2016).

2.4 Reverse Warburg Effect

The Warburg theory of cancer as puzzling and intriguing effect observed in the tumor cells has also led to the postulation of other hypotheses that counter the initial Warburg effect. One such hypothesis which has been studied upon in the past decade is the reverse Warburg model also known as the "two-component coupling model." The name suggests an interaction between the tumor cells and the nearby stromal cells and possibly energy transfer between the two components. The concept suggests a significant role of the tumor microenvironment in promoting the Warburg effect. The tumor cells induce aerobic glycolysis in the surrounding stromal cells, which in turn promote the growth and proliferation of tumor cells by secreting certain pro-tumorigenic factors (Bonuccelli et al. 2010). The stromal cells, mainly the cancer-associated fibroblasts (CAF), were shown to be manipulated by tumor cell factors to undergo myofibroblastic differentiation and produce energy-rich metabolites like pyruvate which is then used by the tumors for their metabolic activity. The tumor cells can then carry out oxidative phosphorylation (OXPHOS) using these metabolites and enter the citric acid cycle to fulfil their high energy requirements facilitating excessive proliferation and angiogenesis (Pavlides et al. 2009). This suggests a more efficient process of harnessing energy such as ATP molecules and different catabolites like pyruvate, ketone bodies and lactate are transferred to the cancer cells via monocarboxylate transporter molecules (MCT). There is a high level of regulation maintained in the release as well as the transporting of these catabolites (Shan et al. 2018; Wilde et al. 2017).

The reverse Warburg effect has been hypothesized as a mechanism through which metastatic tumor cells modify the microenvironment at ectopic sites leading to the formation of macro metastasis (Wilde et al. 2017). Disseminated tumor cells (DTCs) on reaching the ectopic sites aim to establish secondary tumors; however, very few are successful. Establishing metastasis will require DTCs to regain their tumor initiating abilities in a foreign and sometimes hostile environment. The DTCs do that by adjusting and successfully altering the microenvironment at the distant sites. Various pathways including glycolysis, OXPHOS, fatty acid, and amino acid metabolism have been implicated in cancer metastasis (Hsu and Sabatini 2008).

Several anti-metastatic genes, specifically metastasis suppressor gene family, have been shown to prevent tumor cells from altering the microenvironment or take advantage of the altered microenvironment (Horak et al. 2008; Potter et al. 2016). One of them is KISS1 that has been shown to play an important role in altering cell metabolism by decreasing aerobic glycolysis and increasing OXPHOS and increases mitochondrial biogenesis (Liu et al. 2014; Manley et al. 2017). This results in the reduction of microenvironment acidification, reduced uptake of glucose and lactate secretion, all contributing in their own way to reverse the Warburg effect. KISS1 was also shown to prevent the degradation of PGC1α and stabilize its protein levels leading to increased mitochondrial biogenesis. KISS1 also inhibited HK-II enzyme activity leading to increased apoptosis. Therefore, by preventing microenvironment manipulation, a family of genes was shown to prevent the establishment of metastasis underscoring the importance of the tumor microenvironment and cellular metabolism in the metastatic process.

Different cancer cell types exhibit considerable variation in their metabolic behavior. In breast cancer cells, the Warburg effect is mainly observed in the triple-negative breast cancer cells whereas the reverse Warburg effect has been mainly observed in the luminal phenotype of breast cancer. Several modifications and deviations have been observed to the initial Warburg effect based on many pharmacological applications and a plethora of questions still need to be answered for gaining a complete understanding of the process (Gonzalez et al. 2014).

The autophagy paradox—where a process known commonly as destructive to the cell has been recently shown to promote cancer cell growth and proliferation—is also explained to some extent via the reverse Warburg model. Autophagy is a lysosome-dependent protein degradation process that ultimately leads to the cell's death. In the case of tumor formation, this process seems to have an ambiguous effect. During the early stages of carcinogenesis, it acts as a suppressing mechanism that inhibits growth and inflammation and even provides genetic stability. But in certain conditions, autophagy may act as a survival mechanism for the cancer cells, protecting them from other kinds of cell stress they encounter. The cancer cells induce the Warburg effect onto cancer-associated stromal cells and induce this autophagy process. Inhibition of autophagy makes the cancer cells vulnerable to therapeutic action and chemotherapy and in certain aspects, it mediates the therapeutic effect of anticancer drugs. This paradoxical nature of autophagy as a cell-fate decision component makes the studies on the reverse Warburg effect much more important especially when the modulation of this process will increase the efficacy of the existing anticancer therapeutic drugs (Gonzalez et al. 2014; Wu et al. 2012).

2.5 Diagnostic Significance and Therapeutic Approach

The property of glucose hunger has been employed in positron emission tomography (PET) scans of solid tumors where 18F fluorodeoxyglucose, a non-metabolizable derivative of glucose, is used and is preferentially taken up by tumor cells and rapidly growing cells. As 18F fluorodeoxyglucose cannot be metabolized, it accumulates within cells that rapidly take it up showing the concentrated glucose regions as bright points on the PET scan (Miles and Williams 2008). This will be helpful in identifying localized tumors within the body, in identifying key metabolites, and in developing personalized therapy (Shanmugam et al. 2009).

In order to widen the scope of therapy and medicine, many glycolytic inhibitors and mitochondrial activating factors have been developed as potential anticancer drugs. STF-31, a GLUT-1 inhibitor was shown to inhibit the uptake of glucose in cancer cells, inhibiting the aerobic glycolytic process (Adekola et al. 2012; Barron et al. 2016; Legg et al. 2010). Novel approaches to target the activity of hexokinase enzymes have been developed to disrupt the tumor cell metabolism (Mathupala et al. 2009).

AMP-activated protein kinase (AMPK) is a critical player in maintaining a balance between metabolites in cells. AMPK is normally activated under ATP minimal conditions, where it activates cellular pathways for ATP production. AMPK expression was shown to be downregulated in multiple tumor cell types leading to an upregulation of HIF-1 and switching of tumor cells to aerobic glycolysis. Induction of AMPK expression in tumor cells can serve to help shift tumor cells from aerobic glycolysis to OXPHOS (Faubert et al. 2013). Atg 7, a factor that induces autophagy, in HeLa cells, is seen to be blocking the interaction between fibroblast growth factor (FGF-1) and PKM2 to inhibit phosphorylation of PKM2 at Tyr-105. Inhibiting Atg 7 is seen to be responsible for enhancing the Warburg effect on cells (Feng et al. 2018). Curcumin, a major component of turmeric, was shown to decrease HIF-1α protein levels in many types of cancer such as lung cancer and breast cancer (Semenza 2003). It acts by inhibiting the mTOR signaling pathway leading to the reduction of cancer cell proliferation (Courtnay et al. 2015). It also represses the transcription of HIF-1α under low oxygen conditions leading to downregulation of HIF-1 target expression levels (Finley et al. 2011; Siddiqui et al. 2018).

2.6 Conclusion and Perspective

Since cancer cells utilize a unique metabolic pathway differentiating them from normal cells, this pathway could present an opportunity to specifically target cancer cells. An approach could be starving cancer cells of their metabolic requirements, which means not providing a steady supply of glycolytic substrates and intermediates. The starving strategy will be more pronounced in cancer cells compared to normal cells since they are significantly more dependent on aerobic glycolysis compared to their counterparts. This approach can serve as a supplement to chemotherapy or even as an alternative since clinical chemotherapeutic approaches by itself have resulted in multiple and sometimes severe side effects in patients. In order to bring this to the clinic, it requires a complete understanding of the key genes and metabolites regulating the modified metabolism of cancer cells and targeting their activity. The reverse Warburg effect, if found to be more universal, can help understand the metastatic process in detail. Cancers that metastasize in one individual may not do the same in another; this is due to the inherent differences in genetic makeup, diet, and exposure to the environment. Therefore, a personalized treatment approach is required in tackling cancer and continued understanding of the Warburg/reverse Warburg effects will prove to be a boon in the field of cancer therapeutics. Furthermore, though the Warburg effect widens the horizon of cancer study, it needs to be underscored that it is not a regular and consistent feature in all types of cancer. Studies have indicated surprisingly high levels and degrees of mitochondrial activity in cancer cells (Potter et al. 2016). These observations suggest that approaches for therapeutically targeting cancer cell metabolism may not be a definitive solution for all cancer types and a more holistic approach will be more beneficial. To sum up, Warburg effect may or may not be the permanent answer, but for a concept discovered close to a hundred years ago, we have come a long way in our understanding of the importance of metabolism in cancer.

Acknowledgments The authors would like to thank Keerthika J. Jayachandran for helping them with the graphic design of Fig. 2.1.

Financial support: S.H. laboratory is supported by selective excellence initiative grant from the SRM Institute of Science and Technology.

References

Abdel-Haleem AM, Lewis NE, Jamshidi N, Mineta K, Gao X, Gojobori T (2017) The emerging facets of non-cancerous Warburg effect. Front Endocrinol 8:1–7. https://doi.org/10.3389/fendo.2017.00279

Adekola K, Rosen ST, Shanmugam M (2012) Glucose transporters in cancer metabolism. Curr Opin Oncol 24:650–654. https://doi.org/10.1097/CCO.0b013e328356da72

Barron CC, Bilan PJ, Tsakiridis T, Tsiani E (2016) Facilitative glucose transporters: implications for cancer detection, prognosis and treatment. Metabolism 65:124–139. https://doi.org/10.1016/j.metabol.2015.10.007

Bonuccelli G, Whitaker-Menezes D, Castello-Cros R, Pavlides S, Pestell RG, Fatatis A, Witkiewicz AK, Vander Heiden MG, Migneco G, Chiavarina B, Frank PG, Capozza F, Flomenberg N, Martinez-Outschoorn UE, Sotgia F, Lisanti MP (2010) The reverse Warburg effect: glycolysis inhibitors prevent the tumor promoting effects of caveolin-1 deficient cancer associated fibroblasts. Cell Cycle 9:1960–1971. https://doi.org/10.4161/cc.9.10.11601

Courtnay R, Ngo DC, Malik N, Ververis K, Tortorella SM, Karagiannis TC (2015) Cancer metabolism and the Warburg effect: the role of HIF-1 and PI3K. Mol Biol Rep 42:841–851. https://doi.org/10.1007/s11033-015-3858-x

Dang CV (2010) Rethinking the Warburg effect with Myc micromanaging glutamine metabolism. Cancer Res 70:859–863. https://doi.org/10.1158/0008-5472.CAN-09-3556

Danhier P, Ba P, Payen VL, Grasso D, Ippolito L, Sonveaux P, Porporato PE (2017) Cancer metabolism in space and time: beyond the Warburg effect. Biochim Biophys Acta 1858:556–572. https://doi.org/10.1016/j.bbabio.2017.02.001

Elstrom RL, Bauer DE, Buzzai M, Karnauskas R, Harris MH, Plas DR, Zhuang H, Cinalli RM, Alavi A, Rudin CM, Thompson CB (2004) Akt stimulates aerobic glycolysis in cancer cells. Cancer Res 64:3892–3899. https://doi.org/10.1158/0008-5472.CAN-03-2904

Fadaka A, Ajiboye B, Ojo O, Adewale O, Olayide I, Emuowhochere R (2017) Biology of glucose metabolization in cancer cells. J Oncol Sci 3:45–51. https://doi.org/10.1016/j.jons.2017.06.002

Faubert B, Boily G, Izreig S, Griss T, Samborska B, Dong Z, Dupuy F, Chambers C, Fuerth BJ, Viollet B, Mamer OA, Avizonis D, Deberardinis RJ, Siegel PM, Jones RG (2013) AMPK is a negative regulator of the Warburg effect and suppresses tumor growth in vivo. Cell Metab 17:113–124. https://doi.org/10.1016/j.cmet.2012.12.001

Feng Y, Liu J, Guo W, Guan Y, Xu H, Guo Q, Song X, Yi F, Liu T, Zhang W, Dong X, Cao LL, O'Rourke BP, Cao LL (2018) Atg7 inhibits Warburg effect by suppressing PKM2 phosphorylation resulting reduced epithelial-mesenchymal transition. Int J Biol Sci 14:755–783. https://doi.org/10.7150/ijbs.26077

Finley LWS, Carracedo A, Lee J, Souza A, Egia A, Zhang J, Teruya-Feldstein J, Moreira PI, Cardoso SM, Clish CB, Pandolfi PP, Haigis MC (2011) SIRT3 opposes reprogramming of cancer cell metabolism through HIF1\$α\$ destabilization. Cancer Cell 19:416–428. https://doi.org/10.1016/j.ccr.2011.02.014

Fu Y, Liu S, Yin S, Niu W, Xiong W, Tan M, Li G, Zhou M (2017) The reverse Warburg effect is likely to be an Achilles' heel of cancer that can be exploited for cancer therapy. Oncotarget 8:57813–57825. https://doi.org/10.18632/oncotarget.18175

Gatenby RA, Gillies RJ (2004) Why do cancers have high aerobic glycolysis? Nat Rev Cancer 4:891–899. https://doi.org/10.1038/nrc1478

Gonzalez CD, Alvarez S, Ropolo A, Rosenzvit C, Gonzalez Bagnes MF, Vaccaro MI (2014) Autophagy, Warburg, and Warburg reverse effects in human cancer. Biomed Res Int 2014:1–10. https://doi.org/10.1155/2014/926729

Gottlieb E, Tomlinson IPM (2005) Mitochondrial tumour suppressors: a genetic and biochemical update. Nat Rev Cancer 5:857–866. https://doi.org/10.1038/nrc1737

Hitosugi T, Kang S, Heiden MGV, Chung T-w, Elf S, Lythgoe K, Dong S, Lonial S, Wang X, Chen GZ, Xie J, Gu T-l, Polakiewicz RD, Roesel JL, Boggon TJ, Khuri FR, Gilliland DG, Cantley LC, Kaufman J, Chen J (2009) Tyrosine phosphorylation inhibits PKM2 to promote the Warburg effect and tumor growth. Sci Signal 2:ra73

Horak CE, Lee JH, Marshall JC, Shreeve SM, Steeg PS (2008) The role of metastasis suppressor genes in metastatic dormancy. APMIS 116:586. https://doi.org/10.1111/j.1600-0463.2008.01027.x

Hsu PP, Sabatini DM (2008) Cancer cell metabolism: Warburg and beyond. Cell 134:703. https://doi.org/10.1016/j.cell.2008.08.021

Hsu CC, Tseng LM, Lee HC (2016) Role of mitochondrial dysfunction in cancer progression. Exp Biol Med 241:1281–1295. https://doi.org/10.1177/1535370216641787

Jiang B (2017) Aerobic glycolysis and high level of lactate in cancer metabolism and microenvironment. Genes Dis 4:25–27. https://doi.org/10.1016/j.gendis.2017.02.003

Kato Y, Maeda T, Suzuki A (2018) Cancer metabolism : new insights into classic characteristics. Jpn Dent Sci Rev 54:8–21. https://doi.org/10.1016/j.jdsr.2017.08.003

Kim J-W, Dang CV (2005) Multifaceted roles of glycolytic enzymes. Trends Biochem Sci 30:142–150. https://doi.org/10.1016/j.tibs.2005.01.005

Kim J-w, Dang CV (2006) Cancer's molecular sweet tooth and the Warburg effect. Cancer Res 66:8927–8931. https://doi.org/10.1158/0008-5472.CAN-06-1501

Kim JW, Tchernyshyov I, Semenza GL, Dang CV (2006) HIF-1-mediated expression of pyruvate dehydrogenase kinase: a metabolic switch required for cellular adaptation to hypoxia. Cell Metab 3:177–185. https://doi.org/10.1016/j.cmet.2006.02.002

Kondoh H (2012) Glycolytic enzymes can modulate cellular life span. Cancer Res 65:177–186

Legg PD, Chaplin JF, Williamson RE (2010) Genetic diversity in burley and flue-cured Tobacco1. Crop Sci 17:943. https://doi.org/10.2135/cropsci1977.0011183x001700060032x

Li F, Wang Y, Zeller KI, Potter JJ, Wonsey DR, O'Donnell KA, Kim J-w, Yustein JT, Lee LA, Dang CV (2005) Myc stimulates nuclearly encoded mitochondrial genes and mitochondrial biogenesis. Mol Cell Biol 25:6225–6234. https://doi.org/10.1128/mcb.25.14.6225-6234.2005

Liberti MV, Locasale JW (2016) The Warburg effect : how does it benefit cancer cells ? Trends Biochem Sci 41:211–218. https://doi.org/10.1016/j.tibs.2015.12.001

Liu W, Beck BH, Vaidya KS, Nash KT, Feeley KP, Ballinger SW, Pounds KM, Denning WL, Diers AR, Landar A, Dhar A, Iwakuma T, Welch DR (2014) Metastasis suppressor KISS1Seemsto reverse the Warburg effect by enhancing mitochondrial biogenesis. Cancer Res 74:954. https://doi.org/10.1158/0008-5472.CAN-13-1183

Lu H, Forbes RA, Verma A (2002) Hypoxia-inducible factor 1 activation by aerobic glycolysis implicates the Warburg effect in carcinogenesis. J Biol Chem 277:23111–23115. https://doi.org/10.1074/jbc.M202487200

Manley SJ, Liu W, Welch DR (2017) The KISS1 metastasis suppressor appears to reverse the Warburg effect by shifting from glycolysis to mitochondrial beta-oxidation. J Mol Med 95:951. https://doi.org/10.1007/s00109-017-1552-2

Mathupala SP, Ko YH, Pedersen PL (2009) Hexokinase-2 bound to mitochondria: cancer's stygian link to the "Warburg effect" and a pivotal target for effective therapy. Semin Cancer Biol 19:17–24. https://doi.org/10.1016/j.semcancer.2008.11.006

Matoba S, Kang JG, Patino WD, Wragg A, Boehm M, Gavrilova O, Hurley PJ, Bunz F, Hwang PM (2006) P53 regulates mitochondrial respiration. Science 312:1650–1653. https://doi.org/10.1126/science.1126863

Miles KA, Williams RE (2008) Warburg revisited : imaging tumour blood flow and. Metabolism 8:81–86. https://doi.org/10.1102/1470-7330.2008.0011

Papandreou I, Cairns RA, Fontana L, Lim AL, Denko NC (2006) HIF-1 mediates adaptation to hypoxia by actively downregulating mitochondrial oxygen consumption. Cell Metab 3:187–197. https://doi.org/10.1016/j.cmet.2006.01.012

Pavlides S, Whitaker-Menezes D, Castello-Cros R, Flomenberg N, Witkiewicz AK, Frank PG, Casimiro MC, Wang C, Fortina P, Addya S, Pestell RG, Martinez-Outschoorn UE, Sotgia F, Lisanti MP (2009) The reverse Warburg effect: aerobic glycolysis in cancer associated fibroblasts and the tumor stroma. Cell Cycle 8:3984–4001. https://doi.org/10.4161/cc.8.23.10238

Plas DR, Thompson CB (2005) Akt-dependent transformation: there is more to growth than just surviving. Oncogene 24:7435–7442. https://doi.org/10.1038/sj.onc.1209097

Potter M, Newport E, Morten KJ (2016) The Warburg effect: 80 years on. Biochem Soc Trans 44:1499–1505. https://doi.org/10.1042/bst20160094

Samudio I, Fiegl M, Andreeff M (2009) Mitochondrial uncoupling and the Warburg effect: molecular basis for the reprogramming of cancer cell metabolism. Cancer Res 69:2163–2166. https://doi.org/10.1158/0008-5472.CAN-08-3722

Sawayama H, Ishimoto T, Sugihara H, Miyanari N, Miyamoto Y, Baba Y, Yoshida N, Baba H (2014) Clinical impact of the Warburg effect in gastrointestinal cancer (Review). Int J Oncol 45:1345–1354. https://doi.org/10.3892/ijo.2014.2563

Semenza GL (2003) Targeting HIF-1 for cancer therapy. Nat Rev Cancer 3:721–732. https://doi.org/10.1038/nrc1187

Semenza GL (2010) HIF-1: upstream and downstream of cancer metabolism. Curr Opin Genet Dev 20:51–56. https://doi.org/10.1016/j.gde.2009.10.009

Shan M, Dai D, Vudem A, Varner JD, Stroock AD (2018) Multi-scale computational study of the Warburg effect, reverse Warburg effect and glutamine addiction in solid tumors. PLoS Comput Biol 14:1–30. https://doi.org/10.1371/journal.pcbi.1006584

Shanmugam M, McBrayer SK, Rosen ST (2009) Targeting the Warburg effect in hematological malignancies: from PET to therapy. Curr Opin Oncol 21:531–536. https://doi.org/10.1097/CCO.0b013e32832f57ec

Siddiqui FA, Prakasam G, Chattopadhyay S, Rehman AU, Padder RA, Ansari MA, Irshad R, Mangalhara K, Bamezai RNK, Husain M, Ali SM, Iqbal MA (2018) Curcumin decreases Warburg effect in cancer cells by down-regulating pyruvate kinase M2 via mTOR-HIF1$α$ inhibition. Sci Rep 8:2–10. https://doi.org/10.1038/s41598-018-25524-3

Tran Q, Lee H, Park J, Kim S-h, Park J (2016) Targeting cancer metabolism – revisiting the Warburg effects. Toxicol Res 32:177–193. https://doi.org/10.5487/TR.2016.32.3.177

Vander Heiden MG (2012) Understanding the Warburg effect: the metabolic requirements of cell proliferation. Science 324:1029. https://doi.org/10.1126/science.1160809

Vazquez A, Liu J, Zhou Y, Oltvai ZN (2010) Catabolic efficiency of aerobic glycolysis: the Warburg effect revisited. BMC Syst Biol 4:58

Vyas S, Zaganjor E, Haigis MC (2016) Mitochondria and cancer. Cell 166:555–566. https://doi.org/10.1016/j.cell.2016.07.002

Wang L, Wang J, Xiong H, Wu F, Lan T, Zhang Y, Guo X, Wang H, Saleem M, Jiang C, Lu J, Deng Y (2016) Co-targeting hexokinase 2-mediated Warburg effect and ULK1-dependent autophagy suppresses tumor growth of PTEN- and TP53-deficiency-driven castration-resistant prostate cancer. EBioMedicine 7:50–61. https://doi.org/10.1016/j.ebiom.2016.03.022

Warburg O, Wind F, Negelein E (1927) The metabolism of tumors in the body. J Gen Physiol 8(6):519–530

Wilde L, Roche M, Domingo-Vidal M, Tanson K, Philp N, Curry J, Martinez-Outschoorn U (2017) Metabolic coupling and the reverse Warburg effect in cancer: implications for novel biomarker and anticancer agent development. Semin Oncol 44:198–203. https://doi.org/10.1053/j.seminoncol.2017.10.004

Wu WKK, Coffelt SB, Cho CH, Wang XJ, Lee CW, Chan FKL, Yu J, Sung JJY (2012) The autophagic paradox in cancer therapy. Oncogene 31:939–953. https://doi.org/10.1038/onc.2011.295

Wu C-A, Chao Y, Shiah S-G, Lin W-W (2013) Nutrient deprivation induces the Warburg effect through ROS/AMPK-dependent activation of pyruvate dehydrogenase kinase. Biochim Biophys Acta 1833:1147–1156. https://doi.org/10.1016/j.bbamcr.2013.01.025

Yang W, Lu Z (2013) Nuclear PKM2 regulates the Warburg effect. Cell Cycle 12:3154–3158. https://doi.org/10.4161/cc.26182

Yoshida GJ (2015) Metabolic reprogramming: the emerging concept and associated therapeutic strategies. J Exp Clin Cancer Res 34:1–10. https://doi.org/10.1186/s13046-015-0221-y

Yu L, Chen X, Sun X, Wang L, Chen S (2017) The glycolytic switch in tumors: how many players are involved? J Cancer 8:3430–3440. https://doi.org/10.7150/jca.21125

Zawacka-Pankau J, Grinkevich VV, Hünten S, Nikulenkov F, Gluch A, Li H, Enge M, Kel A, Selivanova G (2011) Inhibition of glycolytic enzymes mediated by pharmacologically activated p53. J Biol Chem 286:41600–41615. https://doi.org/10.1074/jbc.m111.240812

Zhang C, Liu J, Liang Y, Wu R, Zhao Y, Hong X, Lin M, Yu H, Liu L, Levine AJ, Hu W, Feng Z (2013) Tumour-associated mutant p53 drives the Warburg effect. Nat Commun 4:2935. https://doi.org/10.1038/ncomms3935

Molecular Aspects of Cancer Cell Metabolism: Altered Glycolysis and Lipid Metabolism

3

Sandesh Kumar Patel, Deepanshu Verma, and Neha Garg

Abstract

Cancer cells have high proliferation rate and therefore require continuous energy source. Metabolic alteration in pathways like glycolysis and lipid metabolism gives a better chance of survival for cancer cells. Cancer cells produce lactic acid from glucose in the presence of oxygen and suppress tricarboxylic acid (TCA) cycle. This phenomenon is known as the Warburg effect. Cancer cells have the ability to perform de novo synthesis of lipids. These alterations in metabolism of cancer cells provide them multimodal advantages and differentiate them from normal cells. These altered metabolisms can be used for tracking and isolating the cancer cells from normal cell population and further can be targeted for cancer-specific treatment. In this chapter, we have highlighted the cancer cell advantages over normal cell in two specific pathways: Glycolysis and Lipid metabolism. These two strategic pathways are utilized by cancer cells for their survival and progression.

Keywords

Altered metabolism · Glycolysis · Lipogenesis · Warburg effect · Cancer cells

S. K. Patel · D. Verma
School of Basic Sciences and BioX Center, Indian Institute of Technology Mandi, Mandi, Himachal Pradesh, India

N. Garg (✉)
School of Basic Sciences and BioX Center, Indian Institute of Technology Mandi, Mandi, Himachal Pradesh, India

Department of Medicinal Chemistry, Faculty of Ayurveda, Institute of Medical Sciences, BHU, Varanasi, Uttar Pradesh, India
e-mail: neha@iitmandi.ac.in; nehagarg@bhu.ac.in

D. Kumar (ed.), *Cancer Cell Metabolism: A Potential Target for Cancer Therapy*,
https://doi.org/10.1007/978-981-15-1991-8_3

3.1 Introduction

Cell performs sequential reactions in order to provide energy and other essential substrates that help them in maintenance and development. The reactions that cell carries out are known as metabolic pathways, which include glycolysis, tricarboxylic acid (TCA) cycle, pentose phosphate pathway, electron transport chain (ETC), oxidative phosphorylation, lipid biosynthesis, etc. The flux of these pathways depends on requirement of the cell. Modified flux rates due to hypoxia are observed in cancerous cells, which help in their better survival.

Glycolysis, a type of catabolic process, is the initial step in energy production. Its intermediates are required for anabolic precursor synthesis, hence making it the root of all activities in the cell. The final product of the glycolysis, i.e., Pyruvate is sent to tricarboxylic acid (TCA) cycle in which the high energy (38 ATP) and precursor metabolites, CO_2 and H_2O are formed as the final products. Oxygen inhibits the glucose flux (Racker 1974) and favors oxidative phosphorylation. In cancer cells, production of lactic acid occurs from glucose in the presence of oxygen, and this process is known as aerobic oxidation or Warburg effect (Warburg 1956).

Lipid metabolism consists of synthesis and degradation of lipids. Lipids are essential for energy production during fasting conditions, membrane lipid biosynthesis, and other associated functions during the growth of cells. Cancer cells, anywhere in the body, tend to synthesize lipids through de novo mechanism, whereas in normal conditions, de novo synthesis is limited to hepatic cells (Medes et al. 1953; Lee et al. 1995). Due to the rapid growth of tumor cells, fatty acids in the microenvironment can signal the activation of its de novo synthesis (Swinnen et al. 2006). These metabolic alterations in cancer cells enable them to sustain in the low nutrient conditions of the systemic circulations and help them in maintaining the high proliferative rate (Swinnen et al. 2000; Turyn and Schlichtholz 2003).

3.2 Altered Glycolysis

In a cancer cell microenvironment, the rapid growth of the cells outgrows the diffusion limit of blood supply, thereby forming hypoxia conditions. To stabilize it, hypoxia-inducible factors (HIF) initiate several transcriptional programs that help in switching to glycolysis, lower the mitochondrial metabolism, and shunt the respiration to aerobic fermentation. HIF also promote angiogenesis for formation of new blood vessels by inducing factors like vascular endothelial growth factor (VEGF). The fast-growing blood vessels are unsystematic and poorly formed, which limit the oxygen and nutrient supply. This irregular supply of oxygen forces the cell to follow the aerobic fermentation, i.e., altered glycolysis pathway, producing lactate as the by-product.

Studies have shown that the major outcome of the Warburg effect such as increased glycolysis, decreased oxidative phosphorylation, and increased lactate production is the result of oncogene activation. Renin–angiotensin system (RAS) oncogene promotes glycolysis when it is mutated (Dang and Semenza 1999; Ramanathan et al. 2005). Akt kinase (an effector of insulin signaling) on mutation increases the glucose uptake in the cells (Manning and Cantley 2007). Mutation in the p53 gene has a major role in survival and metabolic activity of cancer cells. It prevents the expression of SCO2 (Cytochrome C Oxidase Assembly Protein 2) gene and interferes with mitochondrial respiration chain (Muller and Vousden 2013).

In cancer, glycolysis plays a vital role in the survival of cancer cells. The rate of glycolysis acceleration in cancer cells can be inferred by upregulation of enzymes related to the pathway (e.g., phosphofructokinase 2, glyceraldehyde-3-phosphate dehydrogenase, Hexokinase 2, pyruvate kinase, and glucose transporter 1) (Fig. 3.1) (Furuta et al. 2010; Katabi et al. 1999; Cancers et al. 2002; Danial et al. 2003; Koukourakis et al. 2003, 2005; Isidoro et al. 2004). The Warburg effect compels cells to produce lactic acid after pyruvate synthesis, thus suppressing other catabolic pathways for energy production in the presence of oxygen. Cancer cells tend to follow the fermentation pathway even if the energy produced from fermentation is less than TCA cycle. Glycolysis alone cannot fulfill the requirement of anabolic metabolism, as TCA cycle provides the major precursor for the anabolic metabolism (Butterworth 2005). To compensate the absence of the TCA cycle, cancer cells adapt other metabolic pathways such as pyruvate carboxylation (Fan et al. 2009) and glutaminolysis. According to Warburg, cancer cells have nonfunctional mitochondria which limit them to glycolysis; however, recent studies show that tumor cells have functional mitochondria and enhanced glycolysis has a positive effect on cancer cells (Fantin et al. 2006).

3.3 Altered Lipid Metabolism

Lipid metabolism consists of synthesis and degradation of lipid molecules. Lipid molecules act as the stored energy source in the cell. In the deficiency of oxygen, these stored lipids are utilized as the source of energy through the process of lipolysis. Liver cells convert the lipids to keto bodies. Beyond that, lipid metabolism also provides membrane lipids that are required during cell proliferation or cell regulation (Fig. 3.2). Through previous studies, it has been established that lipid metabolism also plays a crucial role in cancer proliferation (Menendez and Lupu 2007). Cell overcomes the demand of the fatty acids through dietary food or de novo synthesis. The upregulated and continuous de novo lipogenesis fulfills the need of lipid membrane building blocks, backup energy supply for cell proliferation, signaling of lipid molecules, and posttranslational protein modification (Kuhajda et al. 1994; Swinnen et al. 2000; Menendez and Lupu 2007; Piyathilake et al. 2000).

Lipogenesis serves as the crucial step for cancer cell survival, as inhibiting the Fatty acid synthase (FASN) and Acetyl-CoA Carboxylase (ACC) through RNA silencing forces cell to undergo apoptosis (Chajès et al. 2006). Various studies have reported that lipogenesis is controlled through oncogene signaling pathway mainly during the transcriptional, translational, and posttranslational modification processes. Expression of major enzymes like FASN and ACC depends on the oncogene signaling. Growth factor-associated signaling pathways including phosphatidylinositol 3-kinase (PI3K) and mitogen-activated protein kinase (MAPK) control the expression of FASN (Yang et al. 2002; Mashima et al. 2009). One of the examples is prostate adenocarcinoma, wherein the gene copy number of FASN is significantly increased leading to high FASN expression (Shah et al. 2006).

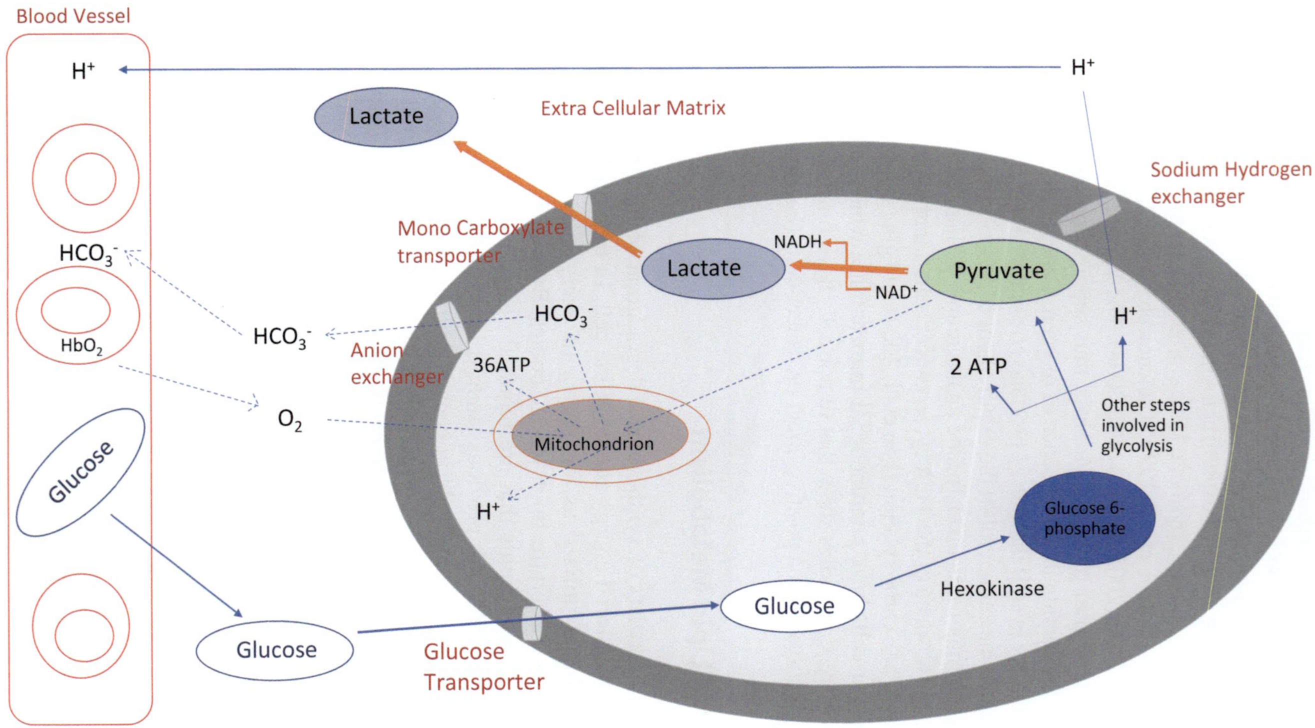

Fig. 3.1 Glucose metabolism in the cell. In normal cells after glycolysis, pyruvate is transported to mitochondria for oxidative phosphorylation which further generates 36 molecules of ATP. Cancer cells perform aerobic fermentation (Warburg effect) leading to pyruvate formation and further lactate production, giving only 2 moles of NADH (shown in bold lines). The oxidative phosphorylation step in cancer cells is downregulated or blocked (shown in dotted lines) (Gatenby and Gillies 2004)

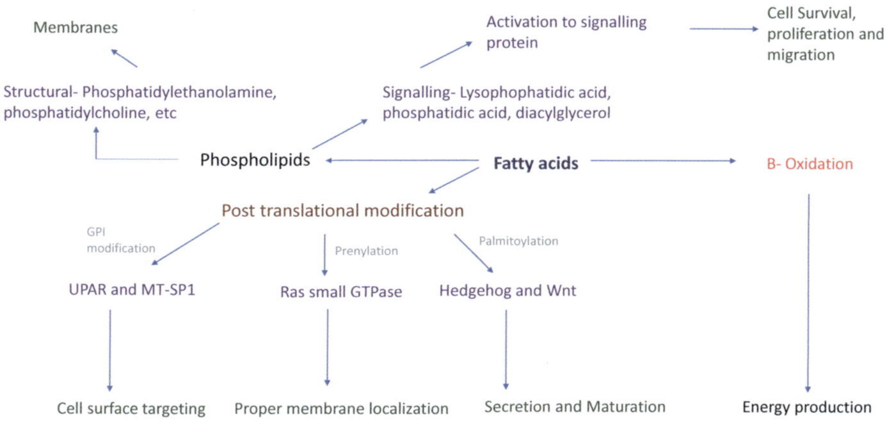

Fig. 3.2 Lipid metabolism plays an important role in the survival of cells. It helps in energy production, proliferation, migration, membrane synthesis, cell surface targeting, membrane localization, secretion, and maturation. The figure was modified from Zhang and Du (2012)

3.4 Link Between Glucose Pathway and Lipid Metabolism in Cancer Cells (De Novo Synthesis)

NADPH and acetyl-CoA generated by glycolysis support the de novo biosynthesis of lipids, which in turn is regulated by tumor suppressor and oncoproteins. Acetyl-CoA is derived from pyruvate using pyruvate dehydrogenase (PDH) in the inner mebrane of mitochondria. Oxaloacetic acide (OAA) present in mitochondria condenses with acetyl-CoA forming Citrate. From TCA cycle, some amount of citrate is pumped out of mitochondria to cytoplasm and by ATP citrate lyase (ACL) is catalyzed to cytosolic acetyl-CoA, which serves as the precursor for fatty acid biosynthesis (Bauer et al. 2005). Akt/Protein kinase B (PKB) directly regulates ACL by phosphorylation, and controls the level of acetyl-CoA in cytoplasm (Berwick et al. 2002).

In fatty acid biosynthesis, large amount of energy is consumed in the form of NADPH. To fulfill this huge energy demand of NADPH, cell uses several pathways in which pentose phosphate (PPP) pathway is predominant (Levine and Puzio-Kuter 2010). Other than PPP pathway, some other pathways are also involved in NADPH generation. Citrate from TCA cycle is exported to cytoplasm and through two independent pathways generates NADPH. In one reaction, isocitrate dehydrogenase 1 (IDH 1) catalyzes citrate to α-ketoglutarate and yields NADPH (Cairns et al. 2011). In another reaction for NADPH production from cytosolic citrate, OAA derived from citrate is catalyzed to malate, which is further converted to pyruvate by malic enzyme harvesting NADPH. Malate from TCA cycle can be exported to cytosol and directly utilized for NADPH production. Malic enzyme is considered to be a lipogenic enzyme as its activity correlates with de novo fatty acid synthesis (Sanz et al. 1997) and in cancer cells it is found to be highly expressed (Fig. 3.3) (Loeber et al. 1994).

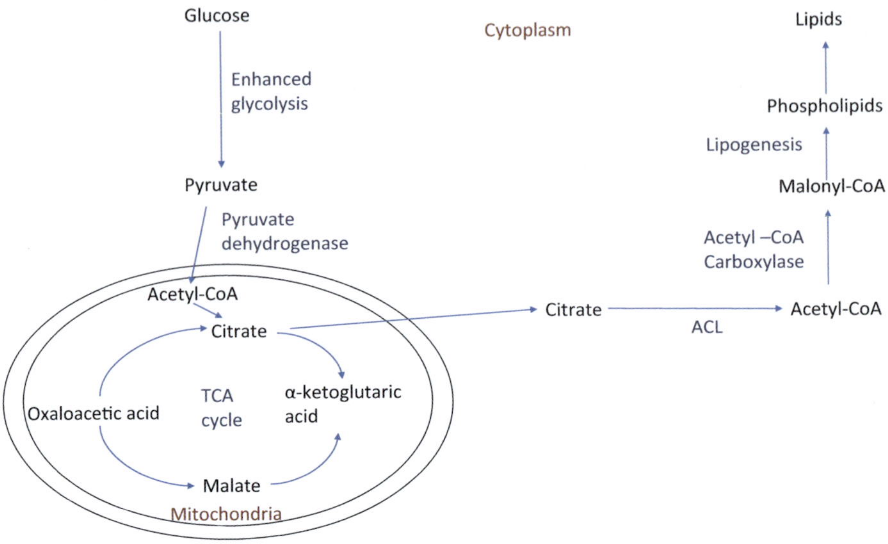

Fig. 3.3 Pictorial representation of the link between the glucose pathway and lipid biosynthesis pathway in cancer cells

3.5 Advantages to Cancer Cells

3.5.1 Glycolysis Pathway

Though glycolysis has low energy production, it provides several benefits to cancer cells. The higher rate of glycolysis compensates ATP requirement of cancer cells (Guppy et al. 1993). Glycolysis intermediates work as the precursor for the other anabolic pathways such as pentose phosphate pathway (PPP) to produce phospholipids, cholesterol, nucleic acids, porphyrins, and NADPH. The carbon that reaches the TCA cycle is extruded as citrate (truncated TCA), which provides a precursor for fatty acids and lipids (DeBerardinis et al. 2007). The association of hexokinase II with mitochondria promotes its integrity and prevents the release of cytochrome c (Gottlob et al. 2001) and another effector of cell death, i.e., pro-apoptotic Bax (Zhao et al. 2007), pro-apoptotic BAD (Danial et al. 2003), and pro-survival Mcl-1 (Rathmell et al. 2003). The high glycolysis rate assures the tumor survival as well as rapid growth. The early production of lactic acid and its release in the surrounding help cancer cells to protect from the attack of immune cells, and the low pH induces an adverse effect on the surrounding healthy cells, helping the cancer cells for invasion and metastasis (Gatenby and Gillies 2004).

3.5.2 Lipid Metabolism

Lipid metabolism provides cells with membrane building blocks and signaling lipid molecules. In cancer cells, endogenously synthesized fatty acids esterified to phospholipids generate pivotal structural lipids that help in intracellular trafficking, migration, polarization, and detergent-resistant microdomain needed for signal transduction (Menendez and Lupu 2007; Swinnen et al. 2006). Lipid molecules such as lysophosphatidic acid (LPA), phosphatidic acid (PA), and diacylglycerol (DAG) have a significant role in signal transduction (Swinnen et al. 2006; Kuhajda et al. 1994). These induce other signaling proteins or bind to G protein-coupled receptor (GPCR) on cell surface. Posttranslational protein modification with lipids, such as covalent modification of Wnt and Hedgehog, plays an important role in maturation and secretion of proteins (Willert et al. 2003; Mann and Beachy 2004). In the glucose-limiting condition, fatty acids through β-oxidation provide energy for the cells, and in cancer cells, it has been reported that fatty acid oxidation is alone capable for cell survival and protection of the cells from induced death. One of the examples is the survival of Akt-overexpressing glioblastoma cells after glucose withdrawal (Buzzai et al. 2005). In some other cancer cells (e.g., prostate cancer), fatty acid oxidation plays a dominant bioenergetic pathway (Liu 2006).

3.6 Differentiating Cancer Cells with the Altered Metabolic Pathways

The altered metabolic pathways can differentiate cancer cells from normal cells. Cancer cells can be determined using the FdG PET (18fluorodeoxyglucose positron emission tomography) technique (Weber et al. 1999). FdG is an analog of glucose which gives fluorescence when is excited. Specificity and sensitivity for this technique are about 90% in most of the cancer cells (Czernin 2002).

3.7 Targeting Cancer Cells Through Altered Metabolism

The altered metabolism in cancer cells plays a pivotal role in overexpressing various proteins and oncogenes, which can be distinct from normal cells. Targeting these altered metabolic proteins/genes can help in the treatment of cancer. 2-Deoxy-D-glucose (2DG) is a synthetic analog of glucose that cannot be metabolized. 2DG competes with glucose for uptake by GLUT1 receptor. Cancer cells have high uptake rate and therefore accumulation of 2DG will be higher in these cells. Coupling 2DG with chemotherapeutic drugs such as propanolol, metformin, and docetaxel inhibits the progression of cancer as well as starves the cancer cells. This particular mechanism has been postulated in prostate cancer and breast cancer (O'Neill et al. 2019; Brohée et al. 2018). Lonidamine, 1-(2,4-dichlorobenzyl)-1-H-indazole-3-carboxylic acid acts as hexokinase inhibitor and shows selectivity for the mitochondrial bound form of this enzyme (Nista et al. 1985). Overexpressed GAPDH (glyceraldehyde-3-phosphate dehydrogenase) in cancer cells makes it as a potential target. In the cell-free system, enzymatically dysfunctional mutant GAPDH inhibits wild-type GAPDH. When this is followed by metabolic stress, it results in the decreased uptake of glucose, hence decreasing cancer growth both in vivo and in vitro (Kunjithapatham and Ganapathy-Kanniappan 2018). The switching of flux from aerobic glycolysis to glucose oxidation occurs by inhibiting pyruvate dehydrogenase kinase (PDK) with dichloroacetate (DCA). This results in the decrease of mitochondrial hyperpolarization, making tumor cells sensitive to apoptosis (Bonnet et al. 2007).

Targeting fatty acid synthesis pathways using pharmacological means can yield selective cytotoxicity in cancer cells which is verified both in vitro and in vivo (Thupari et al. 2001; Barger and Plas 2010). FASN is overexpressed in cancer and therefore some FASN inhibitors were generated such as orlistat, C93, C247, C75, GSK837149A, and Cerulenin (Flavin et al. 2011). These drugs have a proven role in in vitro conditions and genetically induced mouse model/xenograft (Li et al. 2001; Vazquez-Martin et al. 2007a, b). Inhibiting ACL (ATP citrate lyase) by small interfering RNAs (siRNAs) or by chemical inhibitor SB 204990 limits survival of tumor cells in vitro and reduces tumor growth in vivo (Hatzivassiliou et al. 2005; Migita et al. 2008). By using RNAi, ACC-α (acetyl-CoA carboxylase) expression was knocked down. This resulted in inhibition of cell proliferation and induction of caspase-mediated apoptosis in highly lipogenic LNCaP prostate cancer (Brusselmans et al. 2005). 6-Amino-nicotinamide inhibits G6PDH and shows anti-tumorigenic effects in glioblastoma, leukemia, and lung cancer cells (Budihardjo et al. 1998).

3.8 Conclusion

Metabolic alteration in cancer cells helps to sustain and proliferate in harsh conditions by providing sustained source of energy and biomolecules. These altered metabolisms provide cells with better competitive ability over normal cells and help in defense against host immune system. Cancer cells fulfill their energy demands through upregulating glycolysis and lipid metabolism pathways. Intermediates are further utilized in anabolic processes to provide NADPH and precursors for other metabolic pathways like pentose phosphate pathway. Altered metabolisms can be targeted for locating cancer cells in tissue mass and generating cancer-specific treatment. Further research works are underway to target intermediates of altered metabolic pathway and achieve cancer-specific treatments.

References

Barger JF, Plas DR (2010) Balancing biosynthesis and bioenergetics: metabolic programs in oncogenesis. Endocr Relat Cancer 17(4):R287–R304. https://doi.org/10.1677/ERC-10-0106

Bauer DE et al (2005) ATP citrate lyase is an important component of cell growth and transformation. Oncogene 24(41):6314–6322. https://doi.org/10.1038/sj.onc.1208773

Berwick DC et al (2002) The identification of ATP-citrate Lyase as a protein kinase B (Akt) substrate in primary adipocytes. J Biol Chem 277:33895. https://doi.org/10.1074/jbc.M204681200

Bonnet S et al (2007) A mitochondria-K+ channel axis is suppressed in cancer and its normalization promotes apoptosis and inhibits cancer growth. Cancer Cell 11(1):37–51. https://doi.org/10.1016/J.CCR.2006.10.020.

Brohée L et al (2018) Propranolol sensitizes prostate cancer cells to glucose metabolism inhibition and prevents cancer progression. Sci Rep 8(1):7050. https://doi.org/10.1038/s41598-018-25340-9.

Brusselmans K et al (2005) RNA interference-mediated silencing of the *Acetyl-CoA-Carboxylase-α* gene induces growth inhibition and apoptosis of prostate cancer cells. Cancer Res 65(15):6719–6725. https://doi.org/10.1158/0008-5472.CAN-05-0571

Budihardjo II et al (1998) 6-Aminonicotinamide sensitizes human tumor cell lines to cisplatin. Clin Cancer Res 4(1):117–130. Available from: http://www.ncbi.nlm.nih.gov/pubmed/9516960. Accessed 27 Dec 2018

Butterworth PJ (2005) Lehninger: principles of biochemistry. In: Nelson DL, Cox MC (eds) , 4th edn. W. H. Freeman & Co., New York, 1119pp (plus 17pp glossary). ISBN: 0-7167-4339-6 (2004). Cell biochemistry and function. Wiley-Blackwell, 23(4), pp. 293–294. https://doi.org/10.1002/cbf.1216

Buzzai M et al (2005) The glucose dependence of Akt-transformed cells can be reversed by pharmacologic activation of fatty acid β-oxidation. Oncogene 24(26):4165–4173. https://doi.org/10.1038/sj.onc.1208622

Cairns RA, Harris IS, Mak TW (2011) Regulation of cancer cell metabolism. Nat Rev Cancer 11:85–95. https://doi.org/10.1038/nrc2981

Cancers H et al (2002) High expression of inducible 6-phosphofructo-2-kinase/fructose-2,6-bisphosphatase (iPFK-2; PFKFB3) in human cancers. Cancer Res 62:5881–5887

Chajès V et al (2006) Acetyl-CoA carboxylase α is essential to breast cancer cell survival. Cancer Res 63(13):3799–3804. https://doi.org/10.1158/0008-5472.can-05-1489.

Czernin J (2002) Clinical applications of FDG-PET in oncology. Acta Med Austriaca 29:162. https://doi.org/10.1046/j.1563-2571.2002.02042.x

Dang CV, Semenza GL (1999) 1-s2.0-S0968000498013449-main. Available from: https://pdfs.semanticscholar.org/1fd6/65d8b97ac2f055a0daa875d398bdd3bb748c.pdf. Accessed 07 Dec 2018.

Danial NN et al (2003) BAD and glucokinase reside in a mitochondrial complex that integrates glycolysis and apoptosis. Nature 424(6951):952–956. https://doi.org/10.1038/nature01825

DeBerardinis RJ et al (2007) Beyond aerobic glycolysis: transformed cells can engage in glutamine metabolism that exceeds the requirement for protein and nucleotide synthesis. Proc Natl Acad Sci U S A 104(49):19345–19350. https://doi.org/10.1073/pnas.0709747104

Fan TWM et al (2009) Altered regulation of metabolic pathways in human lung cancer discerned by 13C stable isotope-resolved metabolomics (SIRM). Mol Cancer 8:1–19. https://doi.org/10.1186/1476-4598-8-41.

Fantin VR, St-Pierre J, Leder P (2006) Attenuation of LDH-A expression uncovers a link between glycolysis, mitochondrial physiology, and tumor maintenance. Cancer Cell 9(6):425–434. https://doi.org/10.1016/J.CCR.2006.04.023.

Flavin R, Zadra G, Loda M (2011) Metabolic alterations and targeted therapies in prostate cancer. J Pathol 223(2):283–294. https://doi.org/10.1002/path.2809.

Furuta E et al (2010) Metabolic genes in cancer: their roles in tumor progression and clinical implications. Biochim Biophys Acta 1805(2):141–152. https://doi.org/10.1016/j.bbcan.2010.01.005

Gatenby RA, Gillies RJ (2004) Why do cancers have high aerobic glycolysis? Nat Rev Cancer 4(11):891–899. https://doi.org/10.1038/nrc1478

Gottlob K et al (2001) Inhibition of early apoptotic events by Akt/PKB is dependent on the first committed step of glycolysis and mitochondrial hexokinase. Genes Dev 15(11):1406–1418. https://doi.org/10.1101/gad.889901

Guppy M, Greiner E, Brand K (1993) The role of the Crabtree effect and an endogenous fuel in the energy metabolism of resting and proliferating thymocytes. Eur J Biochem. Available from: https://febs.onlinelibrary.wiley.com/doi/pdf/10.1111/j.1432-1033.1993.tb17637.x. Accessed 07 Dec 2018 212:95

Hatzivassiliou G et al (2005) ATP citrate lyase inhibition can suppress tumor cell growth. Cancer Cell 8(4):311–321. https://doi.org/10.1016/j.ccr.2005.09.008

Isidoro A et al (2004) Alteration of the bioenergetic phenotype of mitochondria is a hallmark of breast, gastric, lung and oesophageal cancer. Biochem J 378(1):17–20. https://doi.org/10.1042/bj20031541

Katabi MM et al (1999) Hexokinase type II: a novel tumor-specific promoter for gene-targeted therapy differentially expressed and regulated in human cancer cells. Hum Gene Ther 10:155–164. https://doi.org/10.1089/10430349950018959

Koukourakis MI, Giatromanolaki A, Sivridis E (2003) Lactate dehydrogenase isoenzymes 1 and 5: differential expression by neoplastic and stromal cells in non-small cell lung cancer and other epithelial malignant tumors. Tumor Biol 24(4):199–202. https://doi.org/10.1159/000074430

Koukourakis MI et al (2005) Pyruvate dehydrogenase and pyruvate dehydrogenase kinase expression in non small cell lung cancer and tumor-associated stroma. Neoplasia 7(1):1–6. https://doi.org/10.1593/neo.04373

Kuhajda FP et al (1994) Fatty acid synthesis: a potential selective target for antineoplastic therapy. Proc Natl Acad Sci U S A 91(14):6379–6383. Available from: https://www.pnas.org/content/pnas/91/14/6379.full.pdf. Accessed 07 Dec 2018

Kunjithapatham R, Ganapathy-Kanniappan S (2018) GAPDH with NAD+-binding site mutation competitively inhibits the wild-type and affects glucose metabolism in cancer. Biochim Biophys Acta Gen Subj 1862(12):2555–2563. https://doi.org/10.1016/j.bbagen.2018.08.001

Lee WNP et al (1995) Isotopomer study of lipogenesis in human hepatoma cells in culture: contribution of carbon and hydrogen atoms from glucose. Anal Biochem 226(1):100–112. https://doi.org/10.1006/ABIO.1995.1197

Levine AJ, Puzio-Kuter AM (2010) The control of the metabolic switch in cancers by oncogenes and tumor suppressor genes. Science 330(6009):1340–1344. Available from: http://science.sciencemag.org/. Accessed 03 July 2019

Li JN et al (2001) Pharmacological inhibition of fatty acid synthase activity produces both cytostatic and cytotoxic effects modulated by p53. Cancer Res 61(4):1493–1499. Available from: http://www.ncbi.nlm.nih.gov/pubmed/11245456. Accessed 27 Dec 2018

Liu Y (2006) Fatty acid oxidation is a dominant bioenergetic pathway in prostate cancer. Prostate Cancer Prostatic Dis 9(3):230–234. https://doi.org/10.1038/sj.pcan.4500879

Loeber G et al (1994) Characterization of cytosolic malic enzyme in human tumor cells. FEBS Lett 344(2–3):181–186. https://doi.org/10.1016/0014-5793(94)00386-6

Mann RK, Beachy PA (2004) Novel lipid modifications of secreted protein signals. Annu Rev Biochem 73(1):891–923. https://doi.org/10.1146/annurev.biochem.73.011303.073933

Manning BD, Cantley LC (2007) AKT/PKB signaling: navigating downstream. Cell 129(7):1261–1274. https://doi.org/10.1016/J.CELL.2007.06.009

Mashima T, Seimiya H, Tsuruo T (2009) De novo fatty-acid synthesis and related pathways as molecular targets for cancer therapy. Br J Cancer 100(9):1369–1372. https://doi.org/10.1038/sj.bjc.6605007.

Medes G, Thomas A, Weinhouse S (1953) Metabolism of neoplastia tissue. IV. A study of lipid synthesis in neoplastia tissue slices in vitro. Cancer Res 13(1):27–29. Available from: http://cancerres.aacrjournals.org/content/canres/13/1/27.full.pdf. Accessed 07 Dec 2018

Menendez JA, Lupu R (2007) Fatty acid synthase and the lipogenic phenotype in cancer pathogenesis. Nat Rev Cancer 7:763–777. https://doi.org/10.1038/nrc2222

Migita T et al (2008) ATP citrate lyase: activation and therapeutic implications in non-small cell lung cancer. Cancer Res 68(20):8547–8554. https://doi.org/10.1158/0008-5472.CAN-08-1235

Muller PAJ, Vousden KH (2013) p53 mutations in cancer. Nat Cell Biol 15(1):2–8. https://doi.org/10.1038/ncb2641

Nista A et al (1985) Effect of lonidamine on the aerobic glycolysis of normal and phytohemagglutinin-stimulated human peripheral blood lymphocytes. Exp Mol Pathol 42(2):194–205. https://doi.org/10.1016/0014-4800(85)90027-9

O'Neill S et al (2019) 2-Deoxy-D-glucose inhibits aggressive triple-negative breast cancer cells by targeting glycolysis and the cancer stem cell phenotype. Sci Rep 9(1):3788. https://doi.org/10.1038/s41598-019-39789-9

Piyathilake CJ et al (2000) The expression of fatty acid synthase (FASE) is an early event in the development and progression of squamous cell carcinoma of the lung. Hum Pathol 31(9):1068–1073. https://doi.org/10.1053/hupa.2000.9842

Racker E (1974) History of the Pasteur effect and its pathobiology. Mol Cell Biochem 5(1–2):17–23. https://doi.org/10.1007/BF01874168

Ramanathan A, Wang C, Schreiber SL (2005) Perturbational profiling of a cell-line model of tumorigenesis by using metabolic measurements. Proc Natl Acad Sci U S A 102(17):5992–5997. Available from: https://doi.org/10.1073pnas.0502267102. Accessed 07 Dec 2018

Rathmell JC et al (2003) Akt-directed glucose metabolism can prevent Bax conformation change and promote growth factor-independent survival. Mol Cell Biol 23(20):7315–7328. https://doi.org/10.1128/MCB.23.20.7315-7328.2003

Sanz N et al (1997) Malic enzyme and glucose 6-phosphate dehydrogenase gene expression increases in rat liver cirrhogenesis. Br J Cancer 75(4):487–492. Available from: https://www.ncbi.nlm.nih.gov/pmc/articles/PMC2063320/pdf/brjcancer00181-0025.pdf. Accessed 03 July 2019

Shah U et al (2006) Fatty acid synthase gene overexpression and copy number gain in prostate adenocarcinoma. Hum Pathol 37(4):401–409. https://doi.org/10.1016/j.humpath.2005.11.022

Swinnen JV et al (2000) Selective activation of the fatty acid synthesis pathway in human prostate cancer. Int J Cancer 88(2):176–179. https://doi.org/10.1002/1097-0215(20001015)88:2<176::AID-IJC5>3.0.CO;2-3

Swinnen JV, Brusselmans K, Verhoeven G (2006) Increased lipogenesis in cancer cells: new players, novel targets. Curr Opin Clin Nutr Metab Care 9(4):358–365. https://doi.org/10.1097/01.mco.0000232894.28674.30

Thupari JN, Pinn ML, Kuhajda FP (2001) Fatty acid synthase inhibition in human breast cancer cells leads to malonyl-CoA-induced inhibition of fatty acid oxidation and cytotoxicity. Biochem Biophys Res Commun 285(2):217–223. https://doi.org/10.1006/bbrc.2001.5146

Turyn J, Schlichtholz B (2003) Increased activity of glycerol 3-phosphate dehydrogenase and other lipogenic enzymes in human bladder cancer. Horm Metab Res 35:565. https://doi.org/10.1055/s-2003-43500

Vazquez-Martin A et al (2007a) Inhibition of Fatty Acid Synthase (FASN) synergistically enhances the efficacy of 5-fluorouracil in breast carcinoma cells. Oncol Rep 18(4):973–980. Available from: http://www.ncbi.nlm.nih.gov/pubmed/17786362. Accessed 27 Dec 2018

Vazquez-Martin A et al (2007b) Pharmacological blockade of fatty acid synthase (FASN) reverses acquired autoresistance to trastuzumab (Herceptin by transcriptionally inhibiting "HER2 super-expression" occurring in high-dose trastuzumab-conditioned SKBR3/Tzb100 breast cancer cells). Int J Oncol 31(4):769–776. Available from: http://www.ncbi.nlm.nih.gov/pubmed/17786307. Accessed 27 Dec 2018

Warburg O (1956) On the origin of cancer cells. Science 123(3191):309–314. Available from: https://www.jstor.org/stable/pdf/1750066.pdf?casa_token=5qFi60CIl5AAAAAA:sGLocysgOcLbvtPk1K7nH2OTqEy-AAxQSh1eSandEn1ZF7-CnV0odV-vmpcbZtQNti16w9qJYzFmMbOP2y-EhEZTLWDXLuoKW8D3lYpUSHENhEc_59xoDzg. Accessed 10 Dec 2018

Weber WA, Avril N, Schwaiger M (1999) Aktuelles forum relevance of positron emission tomography (PET) in oncology. Strahlenther Onkol. Available from: https://link.springer.com/content/pdf/10.1007/s000660050022.pdf. Accessed 07 Dec 2018

Willert K et al (2003) Wnt proteins are lipid-modified and can act as stem cell growth factors. Nature 423(6938):448–452. https://doi.org/10.1038/nature01611

Yang Y-A et al (2002) Activation of fatty acid synthesis during neoplastic transformation: role of mitogen-activated protein kinase and phosphatidylinositol 3-kinase. Exp Cell Res 279(1):80–90. https://doi.org/10.1006/EXCR.2002.5600

Zhang F, Du G (2012) Dysregulated lipid metabolism in cancer. World J Biol Chem 3(8):167. https://doi.org/10.4331/wjbc.v3.i8.167

Zhao Y et al (2007) Glycogen synthase kinase 3 and 3 mediate a glucose-sensitive antiapoptotic signaling pathway to stabilize Mcl-1. Mol Cell Biol 27(12):4328–4339. https://doi.org/10.1128/MCB.00153-07

Understanding the Metabolic Cross Talk Between Cancer Cells and Cancer-Associated Fibroblasts

4

Anthony Michael Alvarado, Levi Kent Arnold, and Sufi Mary Thomas

Abstract

The tumor microenvironment (TME) is a heterogeneous, complex, and dynamic setting in which both invading tumor and local stromal cells reside, coevolve, and form a metabolic symbiosis that dictates downstream steps of cancer development and progression. Besides tumor cells, cancer-associated fibroblasts (CAFs) are the predominant cell type found in the majority of solid tumor microenvironment. It is recognized that cancer cells induce a metabolic phenotype in CAFs that is conducive to cancer progression. In addition, CAFs produce nutrients and metabolites, which are utilized by the tumor for energy production, proliferation, invasion, and migration. However, the precise mechanisms whereby CAFs contribute to the process remain uncertain. CAFs are believed to contribute to tumor metabolism through the production of high energy intermediates to fuel glycolytic, oxidative, amino acid, and fatty acid metabolism of cancer cells. This chapter consolidates recent findings regarding

A. M. Alvarado
Department of Neurosurgery, University of Kansas Medical Center, Kansas City, KS, USA
e-mail: aalvarado3@kumc.edu

L. K. Arnold
Department of Otolaryngology, University of Kansas Medical Center, Kansas City, KS, USA

Department of Cancer Biology, University of Kansas Medical Center, Kansas City, KS, USA
e-mail: larnold6@kumc.edu

S. M. Thomas (✉)
Department of Otolaryngology, University of Kansas Medical Center, Kansas City, KS, USA

Department of Cancer Biology, University of Kansas Medical Center, Kansas City, KS, USA

Department of Anatomy and Cellular Biology, University of Kansas Medical Center, Kansas City, KS, USA
e-mail: sthomas7@kumc.edu

D. Kumar (ed.), *Cancer Cell Metabolism: A Potential Target for Cancer Therapy*,
https://doi.org/10.1007/978-981-15-1991-8_4

the metabolic cross talk occurring between CAFs and cancer cells within the tumor microenvironment.

Keywords
Cancer-associated fibroblasts · Tumor microenvironment · Metabolism · Metabolites · Cancer therapy

4.1 Introduction

Tumorigenesis is classically considered a process driven by dysregulated and uninhibited growth and proliferation driven by cancer cells. However, tumors are multicellular tissues that comprise not only tumor cells but also resident cells in the local stroma. Stromal cells that compose the tumor microenvironment (TME) include fibroblasts, heme and lymph endothelial cells, pericytes, neuronal cells, adipocytes, microbiota, and inflammatory immune cells (Weber and Kuo 2012). Thus, the TME is a heterogeneous population of cells, constituting the stromal network engaged in complex interactions with cancer cells (Alkasalias et al. 2018). The crucial role of the TME in tumor progression has been demonstrated in the literature and has prompted further evaluation of the underlying interactions between cancer cells and stromal cells (Weber and Kuo 2012; Huang et al. 2014). However, the mechanisms facilitating these interactions are not fully understood.

Fibroblasts contribute a significant portion to the cell composition of most solid tumors. They are influenced by external stimuli from the microenvironment or nearby neoplastic cells through secreted growth factors and cytokines and adopt a reactive phenotype termed cancer-associated fibroblasts (CAFs). It is increasingly recognized that various cancers exploit resident and infiltrating nontumoral cells for their own benefit with CAFs being commonly implicated in cancer progression (Zhang et al. 2015; Liao et al. 2018). CAFs are rich within the TME and promote tumorigenicity by many avenues to foster proliferation, migration, and invasion (Pietras and Ostman 2010; Weber and Kuo 2012; Alkasalias et al. 2018).

Cells within the TME are in extensive metabolic cross talk contributing to tumor progression (Giatromanolaki et al. 2012; Kalluri 2016; Fu et al. 2017; Lyssiotis and Kimmelman 2017; Alkasalias et al. 2018). Studies reveal metabolic coupling that occurs between fibroblast and cancer cells. This has been documented in many malignancies, including breast, prostate, head and neck, and lymphomas (Witkiewicz et al. 2012; Pan et al. 2015; Mikkilineni et al. 2017; Kumar et al. 2018). Existing literature highlights a pro-tumorigenic role for CAFs via secretion of growth factors, cytokines, chemokines, and extracellular matrix degradation (Pan et al. 2015).

Present literature has focused on how CAFs induce ECM remodeling and secrete cytokines and growth factors to promote tumor growth, invasion, and metastasis. However, current investigations aim to appraise the metabolic cross talk existing between cancer cells and CAFs (Weber and Kuo 2012; Zhang et al. 2015). Despite literature suggesting CAFs fuel tumor growth and establish metabolic cross talk with cancer cells, the precise mechanisms by which this occurs is not fully understood. In this chapter the evolution of CAFs and the metabolic mechanisms by which they cross talk with cancer cells will be discussed as this may offer insights into the regulation of tumor progression of future therapeutic targets in oncologic treatment (LeBleu and Kalluri 2018).

4.2 Normal Fibroblast Function and CAF Origin

Fibroblasts reside in the connective tissue and are involved in synthesizing components of the extracellular matrix including collagen, orchestrating wound healing, and influencing local cell types through secretion of various cytokines and growth factors (Micke and Ostman 2005). Ordinarily they retain a quiescent phenotype, yet, in the setting of chronic inflammation, such as carcinoma, they can be stimulated to a tumor-promoting state (Beacham and Cukierman 2005). CAFs have properties distinct from normal fibroblasts and aggressively promote tumorigenesis as has been described in various cancers, including head and neck, breast, and prostate cancer (Orimo et al. 2005; Kumar et al. 2018; Liao et al. 2018).

The origin of CAFs is largely unknown with studies reporting various cell types implicated as predecessors including normal fibroblasts, pericytes, smooth muscle cells, fibrocytes, or mesenchymal stem cells (MSCs) (Fig. 4.1) (Huang et al. 2014; Kalluri 2016; Alkasalias et al. 2018; Santi et al. 2018). Multipotent MSCs

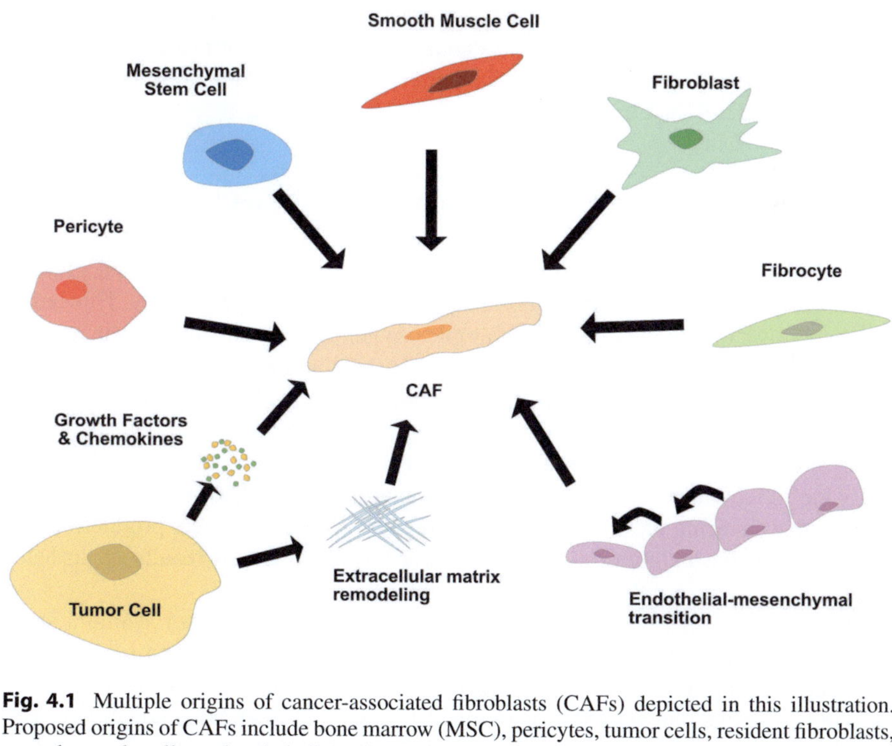

Fig. 4.1 Multiple origins of cancer-associated fibroblasts (CAFs) depicted in this illustration. Proposed origins of CAFs include bone marrow (MSC), pericytes, tumor cells, resident fibroblasts, smooth muscle cells, and endothelial cells via EndMT. *HSC* hematopoietic stem cell, *MSC* mesenchymal stem cell, *EndMT* endothelial-mesenchymal transition

participate in tissue repair and maintenance under normal homeostasis and serve comparable roles in malignancy. MSCs migrate to developing tumors with great affinity and are influenced by numerous factors including monocyte chemotactic protein-1 (MCP-1), stromal cell-derived factor (SDF-1), interleukin-6 (IL-6), and basic fibroblast growth factor (bFGF) (Cuiffo and Karnoub 2012). In several cancers, including breast and pancreatic carcinoma, CAFs comprise up to 80% of the tumor biomass because of widespread desmoplasia generating mechanical forces that contribute to tumor progression (Gonzalez et al. 2016). In melanoma and pancreatic cancer, endothelial cells are subjected to endothelial-mesenchymal transition (EMT) mediated by autocrine and paracrine TGF-β signaling that transitions them to CAF precursors (Zeisberg et al. 2007). This elucidates that CAFs represent a cellular state as opposed to a specific cell type.

Irrespective of origin, previous studies have shown that transformation growth factor beta (TGF-β) is implicated in the transformation and activation processes of CAFs (Wen et al. 2015; Liao et al. 2018). TGF-β expression has been shown to positively correlate with CAF formation and provide a protective role against apoptosis in breast cancer. More so, TGF-β-induced autophagy can promote tumor growth and CAF production (Liu et al. 2016). Additionally, epigenetic alternations, changes in expression of noncoding RNAs, and aberrant activation of signal axis are often observed in CAF formation (Liao et al. 2018). Compared to normal fibroblast, CAFs demonstrate downregulation of IDH3α allowing accumulation of HIF-1α, which promotes glycolysis through increasing glucose uptake, and upregulation of glycolytic enzymes under normal oxygen conditions (Zhang et al. 2015). Thus, uncovering how CAFs contribute to cancer metabolism or reprogramming may serve as a chemotherapeutic target in cancer treatment (Gonzalez et al. 2016; Alkasalias et al. 2018; Liao et al. 2018).

4.3 The "Warburg and Reverse Warburg Effect"

In the 1920s, Otto Warburg proposed that cancer cells exhibit enhanced glucose metabolism compared to normal tissue despite abundant oxygen supply. This led to the postulation that in the presence of ample oxygen, tumor cells prefer glucose and produce more lactate compared to normal cells (Warburg et al. 1927). This process recognized as the "Warburg effect" is the fundamental and metabolic characteristic of cancer and is associated with metabolic reprogramming of cancer cells (Fig. 4.2) (Xing et al. 2015; Avagliano et al. 2018). Why certain cancer cells prefer this relatively inefficient process for energy production remains largely unknown. Literature suggest that favoring elevated glucose metabolism results in lactate production and secretion into the neighboring tumor–stroma interface, which results in an acid-mediated invasion into the microenvironment.

However, this theory only partially explains tumor metabolism. Tumors are a heterogeneous mixture of cells, both stromal and cancerous, populating the TME with certain cells preserving a glycolytic phenotype while others predominately utilizing oxidative phosphorylation (Xing et al. 2015). CAFs further add complexity

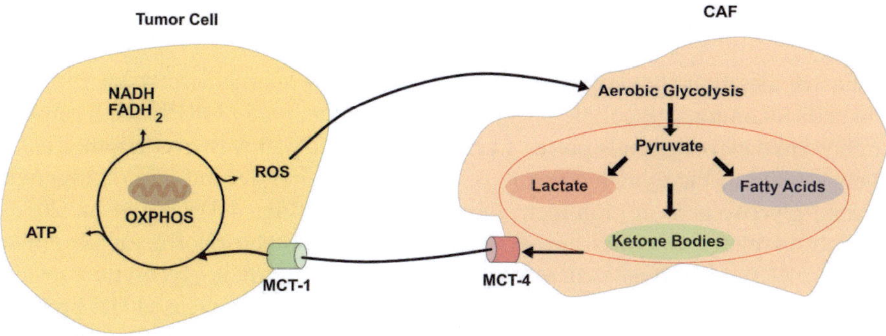

Fig. 4.2 The reverse Warburg effect. Cancer cells produce reactive oxygen species (ROS) which induce oxidative stress in neighboring fibroblasts, triggering aerobic glycolysis and production of high energy metabolites, that are in turn transported to adjacent cancer cells to fuel anabolic activities

by producing metabolic intermediates that are taken up by cancer cells to meet metabolic demands, maintain ATP production, and provide alternative carbon sources to fuel tumor metabolism (Weber and Kuo 2012; Xing et al. 2015; Gentric et al. 2017; Wu et al. 2017).

The "reverse Warburg effect" describes a two-cell, cancer metabolism model in which cancer cells and CAFs are metabolically coupled. In a murine model, nude mice co-injected with human breast cancer cells and murine stromal fibroblasts (wild-type versus Cav-1 deficient) demonstrated Cav-1 deficient stromal fibroblasts promoted tumor growth with upregulation of glycolytic enzymes (Pavlides et al. 2009; Bonuccelli et al. 2010b; Fu et al. 2017). However, others have found opposing results regarding CAFs metabolism. Stromal CAFs studied in breast cancer were shown to recycle tumor-derived lactate that was either utilized for their own energetic necessities or converted to pyruvate, which was secreted and metabolized through glycolysis by tumor cells (Patel et al. 2017). Ultimately, it can be inferred that tumor metabolism is a dynamic process whereby tumor cells must retain a metabolic flexibility with metabolism favoring current tumor metabolic needs and metabolites produced by the microenvironment.

The metabolic coupling of CAFs and cancer cells allows tumors to respond to variations in nutrient availability to maximize cellular proliferation and invasion (Wilde et al. 2017; Gouirand et al. 2018). These effects are further amplified by the coupling of monocarboxylate transporters (MCTs). MCTs assist in lactate shuttling to maintain intracellular pH and serve as a nutrient exchange in the TME. Various isotypes exist in both normal and tumorigenic tissue and assist with release and uptake of lactate to fuel metabolism. This CAF-cancer cell model exemplifies the complexity of the TME, illustrating that cells with different metabolic phenotypes coexist and act together to foster tumor growth (Martinez-Outschoorn et al. 2012a, b; Martinez-Outschoorn et al. 2014).

4.4 CAFs and Glucose Utilization

Extensive metabolic heterogeneity exists in the tumor microenvironment with certain cells retaining a glycolytic phenotype while others prefer OXPHOS. It remains largely unknown why cells prefer a certain metabolic pathway over another but is likely related to the dynamic nature of the tumor niche. Several reports highlight aerobic glycolysis as a prominent feature of CAFs (Fig. 4.3) (Wu et al. 2017). Glycolysis-related enzymes hexokinase-2 (HK2) and 6-phosphofructokinase liver type (PFKL) are upregulated in CAFs, thus sustaining their glycolytic capacity (Zhang et al. 2015; Avagliano et al. 2018). In other studies, increased HK2 protein levels were observed during CAFs differentiation induced by TGF-β1. Glycolytic enzymes lactate dehydrogenase (LDH) and the M2 isoform of pyruvate kinase (PKM2) are upregulated in breast cancer CAFs (Wu et al. 2017). Downregulation of α subunit of the isocitrate dehydrogenase 3 complex (IDH3α) prompted metabolic switch from oxidative phosphorylation to glycolysis in CAFs with overexpression of IDH3α preventing CAF formation. Additionally, reduced IDH3α expression reduced the ratio of α-ketoglutarate (α-KG) to succinate and fumarate, resulting in stabilization of HIF-1α, which in turn promoted glycolysis in CAFs. Accumulation of HIF-1α promoted glycolysis by increasing glucose intake, upregulating expression of glycolytic enzymes, and inhibiting oxidative phosphorylation under normoxic conditions (Zhang et al. 2015). These observations suggest that a complex metabolic symbiosis coexists between cancer cells and CAFs.

CAFs have been identified to secrete exosomes into the microenvironment further fueling tumor metabolism. Exosomes are nanometer-sized vesicles that carry multiple biological components, such as proteins, nucleic acids and lipids. Exosomes

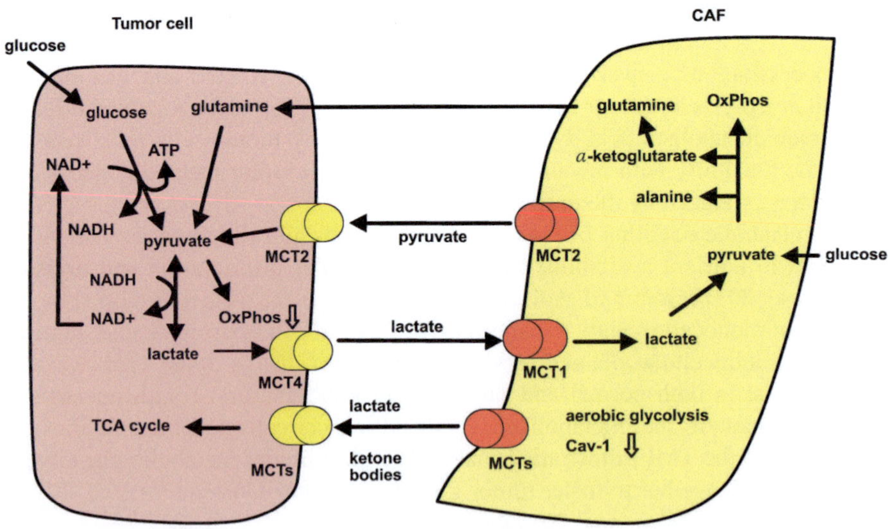

Fig. 4.3 Model of cancer-associated fibroblast (CAF) and tumor cell metabolic cooperation in the tumor microenvironment, demonstrating exchange of metabolic substrates for growth and survival

isolated from prostate cancer patient-derived CAFs inhibited mitochondrial oxidative phosphorylation and increased glycolysis and glutamine-dependent reductive carboxylation in cancer cells. Using 13C-labeled isotope it was shown that CAF-derived exosomes contained metabolites, including amino acids, lipids, and components of the TCA cycle (Zhao et al. 2016). Reciprocally, bladder carcinoma-secreted exosomes triggered differentiation of fibroblasts to CAFs by exosome-mediated TGFβ transfer and SMAD pathway activation. This further elucidates to the complexity of the tumor-stromal interactions and how CAFs are regulated and influence tumor metabolism (Ringuette Goulet et al. 2018).

Reciprocal signaling involving basic fibroblast growth factor (bFGF) and hepatocyte growth factor (HGF) has been implicated between CAF and HNSCC. CAF-secreted HGF induced glycolysis in head and neck squamous cell carcinoma (HNSCC) cells and in return HNSCC-secreted bFGF promoted OXPHOS in CAFs illustrating this complex interaction (Kumar et al. 2018). In colorectal cancer (CRC), stromal-derived HGF from the microenvironment protected CRC cells from glucose starvation-induced apoptosis promoting resistance to angiogenesis inhibitors and anti-glycolytic agents (Mira et al. 2017). Prostate cancer cells contacting CAFs were reprogrammed toward aerobic metabolism with decrease in GLUT1 expression and increased lactate uptake via MCT1. Interaction of CAFs and prostate cancer cells demonstrated that following the activation of CAFs there was a shift toward glycolytic metabolism through a HIF-1 and oxidative stress-dependent extrusion of lactate via MCT4. Lactate served as a metabolic by-product that was shuttled back to prostate cancer cells via MCT1, which was used for TCA, fueling cancer cell proliferation (Fiaschi et al. 2012; Giatromanolaki et al. 2012). Activated fibroblast exhibited increased glucose transporter GLUT1 expression and lactate production which was extruded via monocarboxylate transporter-4 (MCT4). MCT4 is the main extruder of lactate from cells to prevent intracellular accumulation and high expression of HIF-1 could potentially modulate MCT4 expression in pancreatic ductal adenocarcinoma (PDAC) (Wu et al. 2017). In PDAC, CAFs utilized glucose predominately for glycolytic intermediates, whereas glutamine was used for the TCA cycle. Compared to PDAC cell lines, CAFs were resistant to glucose withdrawal but sensitive to glutamine depletion demonstrating the altered and rerouted metabolism of CAFs (Knudsen et al. 2016). In contrast, MDA-MB-231 breast cancer cells demonstrated significantly greater glycolytic capacity than CAFs when extracellular acidification rate (ECAR) was measured via the Seahorse XF96 Analyzer. More so, CAFs secreted several lactate-oxidative metabolites (LOMs) that provided energetic value to tumor cells. These findings further implicate the complex metabolic relationship between CAFs and tumor cells and the dynamic metabolism that exists to fuel tumorigenesis based on current needs (Patel et al. 2017).

Transporters potentially act as biomarkers to identify patients with high-risk cancer. Lactate acidifies the microenvironment and activates matrix metalloproteinase-9 (MMP-9) facilitating developing chemotherapy resistance (Fiaschi et al. 2012). Thus, the reliance of CAFs on aerobic glycolysis with lactate and pyruvate uptake by cancer cells could promote anabolic activities. Two immortalized fibroblast populations, CL3 and CL4, favor different metabolic pathways for energy production and their metabolic interaction with breast cancer cells. CL4 fibroblasts, which favor aerobic glycolysis, were co-injected with human breast cancer cells in a xenograft model and showed drastically enhanced tumor growth compared to CL3 fibroblast, which favored oxidative metabolism at baseline. Thus, CL4 fibroblast acts as a model for mimicking the "glycolytic phenotype" of CAFs (Migneco et al. 2010). Additionally, CL3 and CL4 fibroblasts failed to form tumors when injected alone without epithelial cancer cells, signifying the metabolic coupling that occurs between tumor cells and CAFs. These insights into the utilization of glucose and lactate in neoplastic cells and CAFs may be challenging in the future treatment of numerous tumors.

4.5 CAFs and Metabolic Coupling of Oxidative Metabolism

CAFs undergo aerobic glycolysis and extrude lactate via monocarboxylate transporter-4 (MCT4) to supply nutrients to adjacent cancer cells, thereby driving mitochondrial biogenesis and oxidative metabolism. This metabolic cross talk involves transport of energy-rich substrates from the CAFs to anabolic cancer cells in a reverse Warburg manner (Fig. 4.2). Analysis of co-cultured MCF7 breast cancer cells and normal fibroblasts demonstrated the existence of a stromal-epithelial lactate shuttle, whereby breast cancer cells induced MCT4 expression in CAFs while MCT1 regulation was observed in cancer cells; whereas in monoculture, neither cell type expressed MCT4 (Whitaker-Menezes et al. 2011). Further, MCT4 immunostaining of human breast cancer tissue microarrays demonstrated high stromal MCT4 levels, which were associated with loss of stromal caveolin-1 (Cav-1) (Witkiewicz et al. 2012).

MCT1 has also been found to be overexpressed in lung cancer cell lines, colorectal carcinomas, and invasive cervical carcinoma (Pavlides et al. 2012). This suggests that cancer cells utilize lactate potentially to serve as fuel for the TCA cycle and oxidative phosphorylation, supporting a reverse Warburg effect. In pancreatic ductal adenocarcinoma (PDAC), cultured CAFs derived from tumor exhibited elevated basal levels of HIF1α that was both necessary and sufficient to regulate MCT4 expression (Knudsen et al. 2016). Analysis of cultured CAFs demonstrated that most cells expressed high levels of MCT4 protein and RNA relative to PDAC tumor cell lines. It was also demonstrated that CAFs harboring high MCT4 levels also harbored high levels of HIF1α (Knudsen et al. 2016).

The microenvironment of Classical Hodgkin Lymphoma (cHL) is composed predominately of noncancerous cells, such as tumor-associated macrophages (TAMs) and lymphocytes, which have been shown to promote tumor growth via cross talk with cancer cells. Comparison of relapsed versus remission cHL patients demonstrated that aggressive cHL displays high mitochondrial metabolism in cancer cells and high glycolysis in TAMs compared to reactive lymph nodes (Mikkilineni et al. 2017), further supporting the complexity of the TME and metabolic cross talk. In HNSCC, extensive cross talk exists within the TME and different metabolic compartments (oxidative vs. glycolytic). Assessment of the metabolic state of cancer cells using biomarkers reported OXPHOS is a common feature to both normal stem cells and proliferating cancer cells (TOMM20+/COXC+) with MCT4 expression highly specific for CAFs. These findings support the concept that oxidative stress is a key hallmark of human tumors that drives high-energy metabolism in adjacent proliferating mitochondrial-rich cancer cells via the paracrine transfer of mitochondrial fuels (L-lactate and ketone bodies) (Curry et al. 2013).

4.6 Amino Acid Metabolism and CAFs

Glutamine is essential for proliferating cancer cell mitochondria and is utilized to replenish the TCA cycle with oxaloacetic acid. It serves as a nitrogen donor for nucleotide and amino acid synthesis, and for protein translation (Wise and Thompson 2010; Romero et al. 2015; Tsun and Possemato 2015; Wu et al. 2017). Glutamine serves as the amino acid most frequently used by cancer cells, a process termed "glutamine addiction" (Fig. 4.3). Metabolic profiling of breast tumors and tumor-adjacent normal tissue demonstrated 2-hydroxyglutarate (2HG) was over fourfold higher in tumor tissue compared to normal tissue. This was functionally linked to both glutamine metabolism and MYC activation, resulting in a global increase in DNA methylation and poorer clinical outcome (Terunuma et al. 2014). These findings add to prior studies elucidating to a relationship between MYC activation and glutamine utilization in tumor cells (Li and Simon 2013).

Cancer cells are capable of assimilating glutamine from the tumor microenvironment. In a recent study, metabolomic profiling of CAFs revealed an overall catabolic state in which CAFs produce several potent metabolic substrates for tumorigenic use, including glutamine (Pavlides et al. 2012; Wu et al. 2017). The effects of glutamine on metabolism in the breast cancer TME were evaluated with MCF7 breast cancer cells cultured with CAFs. Co-culture results revealed cancer cells showed reduced glutamine synthesis, increased glutamine catabolism, and increased expression of glutamine uptake transporter SLC6A14 (Ko et al. 2011). In pancreatic cancer, CAFs metabolize glutamine to TCA intermediates, which was demonstrated with U13C-glutamine (Knudsen et al. 2016). Analyses of enzymes implicated in glutamine metabolism indicated CAFs expressed high levels of glutamine (GLS1) and glutamate dehydrogenase (GLUD1) responsible for metabolism of glutamine in the TCA cycle. Application of GLS1 and GLUD1 inhibitors BPTES and EGCG, respectively, inhibited the growth of CAFs and further demonstrated the dependency of CAFs on glutamate for oxidative phosphorylation (Knudsen et al. 2016).

Cystine has been implicated to foster drug resistance in chronic lymphocytic leukemia (CLL) cells. Mesenchymal stromal cells consume cystine and convert to cysteine, which is released into the surrounding microenvironment and taken up by CLL cancer cells for glutathione (GSH) production. High GSH expression in CLL tumor cells augments survival and reduced drug cytotoxicity (Zhang et al. 2015). This is in opposition to literature suggesting that loss of p62 in stromal cells impairs GSH production and facilitates tumor growth through secretion of cytokines and growth factors and CAF interaction (Valencia et al. 2014).

The impact of mTOR inhibition in cancer cells has been evaluated, but how it affects metabolic reprogramming in specific cancers is unknown. Studies have demonstrated that compensatory upregulation of glutamine metabolism in mTOR kinase inhibitors promotes resistance. Metabolomic studies in GBM cells revealed that glutaminase (GLS) and glutamate levels were elevated following mTOR kinase inhibitor treatment, which were confirmed in the xenograft model (Tanaka et al. 2015). These results provide insight into the metabolic reprogramming of amino acid metabolism that occurs between cancer cells and CAFs provide building blocks for cancer cell growth and to evade therapeutic treatments.

4.7 Ketone Utilization and CAFs

Ketones are end-products of aerobic glycolysis and intermediate-products generated by fatty acid catabolism. Additionally, ketones are produced from ketogenic amino acids. Catabolic fibroblasts generate ketones serving as mitochondria fuels that promote tumor cell growth and dissemination during starvation (Figs. 4.2 and 4.3). Tumorigenesis is a state of nutrient deprivation due to highly metabolic cancer cells, where ketones are generated from lipid metabolism in poor glucose or lipid rich tissue and serve as fuel (Martinez-Outschoorn et al. 2012a, b; Wu et al. 2017).

CAFs secrete ketone bodies that are consumed by tumor cells for anabolic metabolism and oxidative phosphorylation like lactate. In a co-culture study evaluating human MCF7 breast cancer cells and hTERT-immortalized fibroblasts, it was demonstrated that enzymes required for ketone body production (HMGCS2, HMGCL, and BDH1) were upregulated in CAFs, compared to human breast cancer cells which exhibited higher expression of enzymes associated with ketone re-utilization (ACAT1) and mitochondrial biogenesis (HSP60) (Martinez-Outschoorn et al. 2012a, b). These findings support the "two-compartment tumor metabolism" model and intricate metabolic relationship within the tumor microenvironment. Cav-1 deficiency can escalate autophagy in the stroma and promote ketone body generation (Pavlides et al. 2010).

Compared to lactate, ketones are more powerful fuels for mitochondria, yielding greater energy and decreased oxygen consumption. Hydroxybutyrate increased proliferation almost threefold in cancer cells (Bonuccelli et al. 2010a). It was shown that ketone body production is associated with gene overexpression in CAFs, as opposed to re-utilization (Pavlides et al. 2010; Martinez-Outschoorn et al. 2012a, b). Mitochondrial 3-hydroxy-3-methylglutaryl CoA synthase 2, the rate limiting enzyme in ketogenesis, is overexpressed in CAFs (Martinez-Outschoorn et al. 2012a, b). Conversely, cancer cells upregulate genes associated with ketone re-utilization, which are directed to mitochondria for OXPHOS and TCA cycle intermediates (Martinez-Outschoorn et al. 2012a, b; Martinez-Outschoorn et al. 2014). Understanding the relationship between autophagy and ketogenesis is complex and remains of debate. Ketones potentially act in a paracrine fashion and mimic principles of lactate transportation via MCTs.

4.8 Pentose Phosphate Pathway

The pentose phosphate pathway (PPP) is a fundamental component of cellular metabolism and is crucial for cancer cells. In tumorigenesis, glucose metabolism is altered and affects metabolic pathways requiring glucose utilization such as the PPP. The PPP, also referred to as the hexose monophosphate shunt, converges with glycolysis and is linked by the generation of glucose-6-phosphate (G6P) (Kowalik et al. 2017). The generation of pentose phosphates ensures nucleic acid synthesis and NADPH production, which are favorable for tumorigenesis.

Glucose-6-phosphate dehydrogenase (G6PD) activity has been documented to be upregulated in hepatocellular carcinoma (HCC) (Hacker et al. 1982; Stumpf and Bannasch 1994; Kowalik et al. 2017). Cancer cells must synthesize nitrogenous compounds in the form of nucleotides and NEAAs for continued growth and survival. Glutamine is a precursor nitrogen donor in multiple enzymatic steps of purine synthesis (phosphoribosyl pyrophosphate (PRPP) amidotransferase, phosphoribosylformylglycinamidine (FGAM) synthetase, GMP synthetase). Additionally, it contributes to the enzymatic steps of carbamoyl phosphate synthetase II and CTP synthetase in pyrimidine (Wise and Thompson 2010).

Though there is a paucity of research evaluating CAFs and the pentose phosphate pathway, the rate limiting enzyme glucose-6-phosphate dehydrogenase (G6PD) is a target of various malignancies and can act as a potential therapeutic strategy against cancer.

Ultimately, the metabolic interactions between CAFs and cancer cells and the metabolic reprogramming that has been documented in solid malignancies are complex and remain largely undetermined. Perhaps metabolic programming, beyond aerobic glycolysis, is a more dynamic process whereby tumor-stromal interaction adapts to current cancer cell needs to facilitate growth and progression. To further delineate the complex interactions between CAFs and cancer cells, preclinical imaging techniques may shed insight into the mechanisms and interactions that occur in the TME to promote tumorigenesis. In vivo magnetic resonance imaging (MRI) and near-infrared fluorescence (NIRF) imaging assist in CAF imaging with the use of imaging probes. Further, positron emission tomography (PET) and 13C-MRS can be applied to evaluate glucose uptake (reflecting glucose metabolism) and downstream derived metabolites (Ramamonjisoa and Ackerstaff 2017; Blomme et al. 2018).

4.9 Conclusion

The tumor microenvironment comprises not only cancer cells, but also CAFs and other supporting cells. CAFs play a pivotal role in cancer metabolism by producing high-energy metabolites and releasing them into the TME where they are subsequently taken up by cancer cells and used as an energy source for growth and progression. Metabolic products of CAF metabolism such as lactate, ketone bodies, and amino acids are necessary for cancer cell growth. Therefore, it is widely accepted that CAF-mediated metabolism plays a key role in tumorigenesis and that targeting the metabolic cross talk between CAFs and cancer cells can serve as prospective therapeutic targets. As a result, ongoing research investigations attempt to exploit areas of metabolic vulnerability by targeting glycolysis, lactate metabolism, glutaminolysis, ketone bodies and ketosis, and fatty acid metabolism. How cancer cells metabolically reprogram fibroblast to facilitate tumorigenesis can help in understanding the effects of cancer cells within the tumor microenvironment and how targeting CAFs with chemotherapeutic agents can inhibit tumor progression.

Acknowledgments This work was supported by the NIH grant CA227838 to S.M.T. and The National Cancer Institute Cancer Center Support Grant to the University of Kansas Cancer Center, P30CA168524.

References

Alkasalias T, Moyano-Galceran L, Arsenian-Henriksson M, Lehti K (2018) Fibroblasts in the tumor microenvironment: shield or spear? Int J Mol Sci 19(5). https://doi.org/10.3390/ijms19051532

Avagliano A, Granato G, Ruocco MR, Romano V, Belviso I, Carfora A, Montagnani S, Arcucci A (2018) Metabolic reprogramming of cancer associated fibroblasts: the slavery of stromal fibroblasts. Biomed Res Int 2018:6075403

Beacham DA, Cukierman E (2005) Stromagenesis: the changing face of fibroblastic microenvironments during tumor progression. Semin Cancer Biol 15(5):329–341

Blomme A, Van Simaeys G, Doumont G, Costanza B, Bellier J, Otaka Y, Sherer F, Lovinfosse P, Boutry S, Palacios AP, De Pauw E, Hirano T, Yokobori T, Hustinx R, Bellahcene A, Delvenne P, Detry O, Goldman S, Nishiyama M, Castronovo V, Turtoi A (2018) Murine stroma adopts a human-like metabolic phenotype in the PDX model of colorectal cancer and liver metastases. Oncogene 37(9):1237–1250

Bonuccelli G, Tsirigos A, Whitaker-Menezes D, Pavlides S, Pestell RG, Chiavarina B, Frank PG, Flomenberg N, Howell A, Martinez-Outschoorn UE, Sotgia F, Lisanti MP (2010a) Ketones and lactate "fuel" tumor growth and metastasis: evidence that epithelial cancer cells use oxidative mitochondrial metabolism. Cell Cycle 9(17):3506–3514

Bonuccelli G, Whitaker-Menezes D, Castello-Cros R, Pavlides S, Pestell RG, Fatatis A, Witkiewicz AK, Vander Heiden MG, Migneco G, Chiavarina B, Frank PG, Capozza F, Flomenberg N, Martinez-Outschoorn UE, Sotgia F, Lisanti MP (2010b) The reverse Warburg effect: glycolysis inhibitors prevent the tumor promoting effects of caveolin-1 deficient cancer associated fibroblasts. Cell Cycle 9(10):1960–1971

Cuiffo BG, Karnoub AE (2012) Mesenchymal stem cells in tumor development: emerging roles and concepts. Cell Adhes Migr 6(3):220–230

Curry JM, Tuluc M, Whitaker-Menezes D, Ames JA, Anantharaman A, Butera A, Leiby B, Cognetti DM, Sotgia F, Lisanti MP, Martinez-Outschoorn UE (2013) Cancer metabolism, stemness and tumor recurrence: MCT1 and MCT4 are functional biomarkers of metabolic symbiosis in head and neck cancer. Cell Cycle 12(9):1371–1384

Fiaschi T, Marini A, Giannoni E, Taddei ML, Gandellini P, De Donatis A, Lanciotti M, Serni S, Cirri P, Chiarugi P (2012) Reciprocal metabolic reprogramming through lactate shuttle coordinately influences tumor-stroma interplay. Cancer Res 72(19):5130–5140

Fu Y, Liu S, Yin S, Niu W, Xiong W, Tan M, Li G, Zhou M (2017) The reverse Warburg effect is likely to be an Achilles' heel of cancer that can be exploited for cancer therapy. Oncotarget 8(34):57813–57825

Gentric G, Mieulet V, Mechta-Grigoriou F (2017) Heterogeneity in cancer metabolism: new concepts in an old field. Antioxid Redox Signal 26(9):462–485

Giatromanolaki A, Koukourakis MI, Koutsopoulos A, Mendrinos S, Sivridis E (2012) The metabolic interactions between tumor cells and tumor-associated stroma (TAS) in prostatic cancer. Cancer Biol Ther 13(13):1284–1289

Gonzalez L, Eiro N, Fernandez-Garcia B, Gonzalez LO, Dominguez F, Vizoso FJ (2016) Gene expression profile of normal and cancer-associated fibroblasts according to intratumoral inflammatory cells phenotype from breast cancer tissue. Mol Carcinog 55(11):1489–1502

Gouirand V, Guillaumond F, Vasseur S (2018) Influence of the tumor microenvironment on cancer cells metabolic reprogramming. Front Oncol 8:117

Hacker HJ, Moore MA, Mayer D, Bannasch P (1982) Correlative histochemistry of some enzymes of carbohydrate metabolism in preneoplastic and neoplastic lesions in the rat liver. Carcinogenesis 3(11):1265–1272

Huang L, Xu AM, Liu S, Liu W, Li TJ (2014) Cancer-associated fibroblasts in digestive tumors. World J Gastroenterol 20(47):17804–17818

Kalluri R (2016) The biology and function of fibroblasts in cancer. Nat Rev Cancer 16(9):582–598

Knudsen ES, Balaji U, Freinkman E, McCue P, Witkiewicz AK (2016) Unique metabolic features of pancreatic cancer stroma: relevance to the tumor compartment, prognosis, and invasive potential. Oncotarget 7(48):78396–78411

Ko YH, Lin Z, Flomenberg N, Pestell RG, Howell A, Sotgia F, Lisanti MP, Martinez-Outschoorn UE (2011) Glutamine fuels a vicious cycle of autophagy in the tumor stroma and oxidative mitochondrial metabolism in epithelial cancer cells: implications for preventing chemotherapy resistance. Cancer Biol Ther 12(12):1085–1097

Kowalik MA, Columbano A, Perra A (2017) Emerging role of the pentose phosphate pathway in hepatocellular carcinoma. Front Oncol 7:87

Kumar D, New J, Vishwakarma V, Joshi R, Enders J, Lin F, Dasari S, Gutierrez WR, Leef G, Ponnurangam S, Chavan H, Ganaden L, Thornton MM, Dai H, Tawfik O, Straub J, Shnayder Y, Kakarala K, Tsue TT, Girod DA, Van Houten B, Anant S, Krishnamurthy P, Thomas SM (2018) Cancer-associated fibroblasts drive glycolysis in a targetable signaling loop implicated in head and neck squamous cell carcinoma progression. Cancer Res 78(14):3769–3782

LeBleu VS, Kalluri R (2018) A peek into cancer-associated fibroblasts: origins, functions and translational impact. Dis Model Mech 11(4):dmm029447

Li B, Simon MC (2013) Molecular pathways: targeting MYC-induced metabolic reprogramming and oncogenic stress in cancer. Clin Cancer Res 19(21):5835–5841

Liao Z, Tan ZW, Zhu P, Tan NS (2018) Cancer-associated fibroblasts in tumor microenvironment – accomplices in tumor malignancy. Cell Immunol 343:103729

Liu FL, Mo EP, Yang L, Du J, Wang HS, Zhang H, Kurihara H, Xu J, Cai SH (2016) Autophagy is involved in TGF-beta1-induced protective mechanisms and formation of cancer-associated fibroblasts phenotype in tumor microenvironment. Oncotarget 7(4):4122–4141

Lyssiotis CA, Kimmelman AC (2017) Metabolic interactions in the tumor microenvironment. Trends Cell Biol 27(11):863–875

Martinez-Outschoorn UE, Lin Z, Whitaker-Menezes D, Howell A, Lisanti MP, Sotgia F (2012a) Ketone bodies and two-compartment tumor metabolism: stromal ketone production fuels mitochondrial biogenesis in epithelial cancer cells. Cell Cycle 11(21):3956–3963

Martinez-Outschoorn UE, Lin Z, Whitaker-Menezes D, Howell A, Sotgia F, Lisanti MP (2012b) Ketone body utilization drives tumor growth and metastasis. Cell Cycle 11(21):3964–3971

Martinez-Outschoorn UE, Lisanti MP, Sotgia F (2014) Catabolic cancer-associated fibroblasts transfer energy and biomass to anabolic cancer cells, fueling tumor growth. Semin Cancer Biol 25:47–60

Micke P, Ostman A (2005) Exploring the tumour environment: cancer-associated fibroblasts as targets in cancer therapy. Expert Opin Ther Targets 9(6):1217–1233

Migneco G, Whitaker-Menezes D, Chiavarina B, Castello-Cros R, Pavlides S, Pestell RG, Fatatis A, Flomenberg N, Tsirigos A, Howell A, Martinez-Outschoorn UE, Sotgia F, Lisanti MP (2010) Glycolytic cancer associated fibroblasts promote breast cancer tumor growth, without a measurable increase in angiogenesis: evidence for stromal-epithelial metabolic coupling. Cell Cycle 9(12):2412–2422

Mikkilineni L, Whitaker-Menezes D, Domingo-Vidal M, Sprandio J, Avena P, Cotzia P, Dulau-Florea A, Gong J, Uppal G, Zhan T, Leiby B, Lin Z, Pro B, Sotgia F, Lisanti MP, Martinez-Outschoorn U (2017) Hodgkin lymphoma: a complex metabolic ecosystem with glycolytic reprogramming of the tumor microenvironment. Semin Oncol 44(3):218–225

Mira A, Morello V, Cespedes MV, Perera T, Comoglio PM, Mangues R, Michieli P (2017) Stroma-derived HGF drives metabolic adaptation of colorectal cancer to angiogenesis inhibitors. Oncotarget 8(24):38193–38213

Orimo A, Gupta PB, Sgroi DC, Arenzana-Seisdedos F, Delaunay T, Naeem R, Carey VJ, Richardson AL, Weinberg RA (2005) Stromal fibroblasts present in invasive human breast carcinomas promote tumor growth and angiogenesis through elevated SDF-1/CXCL12 secretion. Cell 121(3):335–348

Pan B, Liao Q, Niu Z, Zhou L, Zhao Y (2015) Cancer-associated fibroblasts in pancreatic adenocarcinoma. Future Oncol 11(18):2603–2610

Patel BB, Ackerstaff E, Serganova IS, Kerrigan JE, Blasberg RG, Koutcher JA, Banerjee D (2017) Tumor stroma interaction is mediated by monocarboxylate metabolism. Exp Cell Res 352(1):20–33

Pavlides S, Tsirigos A, Migneco G, Whitaker-Menezes D, Chiavarina B, Flomenberg N, Frank PG, Casimiro MC, Wang C, Pestell RG, Martinez-Outschoorn UE, Howell A, Sotgia F, Lisanti MP (2010) The autophagic tumor stroma model of cancer: role of oxidative stress and ketone production in fueling tumor cell metabolism. Cell Cycle 9(17):3485–3505

Pavlides S, Vera I, Gandara R, Sneddon S, Pestell RG, Mercier I, Martinez-Outschoorn UE, Whitaker-Menezes D, Howell A, Sotgia F, Lisanti MP (2012) Warburg meets autophagy: cancer-associated fibroblasts accelerate tumor growth and metastasis via oxidative stress, mitophagy, and aerobic glycolysis. Antioxid Redox Signal 16(11):1264–1284

Pavlides S, Whitaker-Menezes D, Castello-Cros R, Flomenberg N, Witkiewicz AK, Frank PG, Casimiro MC, Wang C, Fortina P, Addya S, Pestell RG, Martinez-Outschoorn UE, Sotgia F, Lisanti MP (2009) The reverse Warburg effect: aerobic glycolysis in cancer associated fibroblasts and the tumor stroma. Cell Cycle 8(23):3984–4001

Pietras K, Ostman A (2010) Hallmarks of cancer: interactions with the tumor stroma. Exp Cell Res 316(8):1324–1331

Ramamonjisoa N, Ackerstaff E (2017) Characterization of the tumor microenvironment and tumor-stroma interaction by non-invasive preclinical imaging. Front Oncol 7:3

Ringuette Goulet C, Bernard G, Tremblay S, Chabaud S, Bolduc S, Pouliot F (2018) Exosomes induce fibroblast differentiation into cancer-associated fibroblasts through TGFbeta signaling. Mol Cancer Res 16(7):1196–1204

Romero IL, Mukherjee A, Kenny HA, Litchfield LM, Lengyel E (2015) Molecular pathways: trafficking of metabolic resources in the tumor microenvironment. Clin Cancer Res 21(4):680–686

Santi A, Kugeratski FG, Zanivan S (2018) Cancer associated fibroblasts: the architects of stroma remodeling. Proteomics 18(5–6):e1700167

Stumpf H, Bannasch P (1994) Overexpression of glucose-6-phosphate-dehydrogenase in rat hepatic preneoplasia and neoplasia. Int J Oncol 5(6):1255–1260

Tanaka K, Sasayama T, Irino Y, Takata K, Nagashima H, Satoh N, Kyotani K, Mizowaki T, Imahori T, Ejima Y, Masui K, Gini B, Yang H, Hosoda K, Sasaki R, Mischel PS, Kohmura E (2015) Compensatory glutamine metabolism promotes glioblastoma resistance to mTOR inhibitor treatment. J Clin Invest 125(4):1591–1602

Terunuma A, Putluri N, Mishra P, Mathe EA, Dorsey TH, Yi M, Wallace TA, Issaq HJ, Zhou M, Killian JK, Stevenson HS, Karoly ED, Chan K, Samanta S, Prieto D, Hsu TY, Kurley SJ, Putluri V, Sonavane R, Edelman DC, Wulff J, Starks AM, Yang Y, Kittles RA, Yfantis HG, Lee DH, Ioffe OB, Schiff R, Stephens RM, Meltzer PS, Veenstra TD, Westbrook TF, Sreekumar A, Ambs S (2014) MYC-driven accumulation of 2-hydroxyglutarate is associated with breast cancer prognosis. J Clin Invest 124(1):398–412

Tsun ZY, Possemato R (2015) Amino acid management in cancer. Semin Cell Dev Biol 43:22–32

Valencia T, Kim JY, Abu-Baker S, Moscat-Pardos J, Ahn CS, Reina-Campos M, Duran A, Castilla EA, Metallo CM, Diaz-Meco MT, Moscat J (2014) Metabolic reprogramming of stromal fibro-

blasts through p62-mTORC1 signaling promotes inflammation and tumorigenesis. Cancer Cell 26(1):121–135
Warburg O, Wind F, Negelein E (1927) The metabolism of tumors in the body. J Gen Physiol 8(6):519–530
Weber CE, Kuo PC (2012) The tumor microenvironment. Surg Oncol 21(3):172–177
Wen S, Niu Y, Yeh S, Chang C (2015) BM-MSCs promote prostate cancer progression via the conversion of normal fibroblasts to cancer-associated fibroblasts. Int J Oncol 47(2):719–727
Whitaker-Menezes D, Martinez-Outschoorn UE, Lin Z, Ertel A, Flomenberg N, Witkiewicz AK, Birbe RC, Howell A, Pavlides S, Gandara R, Pestell RG, Sotgia F, Philp NJ, Lisanti MP (2011) Evidence for a stromal-epithelial "lactate shuttle" in human tumors: MCT4 is a marker of oxidative stress in cancer-associated fibroblasts. Cell Cycle 10(11):1772–1783
Wilde L, Roche M, Domingo-Vidal M, Tanson K, Philp N, Curry J, Martinez-Outschoorn U (2017) Metabolic coupling and the reverse Warburg effect in cancer: implications for novel biomarker and anticancer agent development. Semin Oncol 44(3):198–203
Wise DR, Thompson CB (2010) Glutamine addiction: a new therapeutic target in cancer. Trends Biochem Sci 35(8):427–433
Witkiewicz AK, Whitaker-Menezes D, Dasgupta A, Philp NJ, Lin Z, Gandara R, Sneddon S, Martinez-Outschoorn UE, Sotgia F, Lisanti MP (2012) Using the "reverse Warburg effect" to identify high-risk breast cancer patients: stromal MCT4 predicts poor clinical outcome in triple-negative breast cancers. Cell Cycle 11(6):1108–1117
Wu D, Zhuo L, Wang X (2017) Metabolic reprogramming of carcinoma-associated fibroblasts and its impact on metabolic heterogeneity of tumors. Semin Cell Dev Biol 64:125–131
Xing Y, Zhao S, Zhou BP, Mi J (2015) Metabolic reprogramming of the tumour microenvironment. FEBS J 282(20):3892–3898
Zeisberg EM, Potenta S, Xie L, Zeisberg M, Kalluri R (2007) Discovery of endothelial to mesenchymal transition as a source for carcinoma-associated fibroblasts. Cancer Res 67(21):10123–10128
Zhang D, Wang Y, Shi Z, Liu J, Sun P, Hou X, Zhang J, Zhao S, Zhou BP, Mi J (2015) Metabolic reprogramming of cancer-associated fibroblasts by IDH3alpha downregulation. Cell Rep 10(8):1335–1348
Zhao H, Yang L, Baddour J, Achreja A, Bernard V, Moss T, Marini JC, Tudawe T, Seviour EG, San Lucas FA, Alvarez H, Gupta S, Maiti SN, Cooper L, Peehl D, Ram PT, Maitra A, Nagrath D (2016) Tumor microenvironment derived exosomes pleiotropically modulate cancer cell metabolism. Elife 5:e10250

Metabolic Cross Talk Between Cancer Cells and Tumor Microenvironment

5

Satish S. Poojary, Maryam Ghufran, Ananya Choudhary, and Mehreen Aftab

Abstract

An obscure metabolic network controls the activities of the cancer cells and their microenvironment which still continues to be unraveled. Cancer cells modify the biochemistry of the extracellular environment, which bring about multiple consequences on the phenotypes of non-tumor cells residing in the close vicinity of the tumor and also the extracellular matrix. Reciprocally, metabolism and the signaling feedback of cancer cells are affected by the microenvironment. Here we discuss our existing understanding of alterations in metabolism during cancer progression and how metabolic cross talk between cancer cells and their so-called microenvironment is affected during this process.

Keywords

Tumor microenvironment · Metabolic cross talk · Cancer metabolism · Hypoxia

5.1 Introduction

Uncountable processes can be directly impacted by metabolites from signaling to gene expression. They allow ATP production and redistribution of carbons to nucleotide, protein, and fatty acid synthesis to support their physiological functions. The changes in metabolite levels can affect both pathway regulation and gene expression more particularly because of the effects of these metabolites on chromatin modifications, thus influencing the cell state. There appears to be bi-directional cross talk between metabolism and epigenetics wherein multiple epigenetic enzymes act as

S. S. Poojary (✉) · M. Ghufran · A. Choudhary · M. Aftab
Amity Institute of Molecular Medicine & Stem Cell Research (AIMMSCR), Amity University Uttar Pradesh (AUUP), Noida, Uttar Pradesh, India
e-mail: spoojary@amity.edu

D. Kumar (ed.), *Cancer Cell Metabolism: A Potential Target for Cancer Therapy*, https://doi.org/10.1007/978-981-15-1991-8_5

regulators for re-adjusting metabolism according to the nutrient changes. Metabolites availability is influenced by alterations in microbiome which affects signaling, cell proliferation, and chromatin. Both Sirtuins and PARP enzymes get impacted with the changes in metabolites, with age. This influences diverse pathways which include epigenetics and DNA repair (Canto et al. 2013).

5.2 Metabolites Role as Signaling Molecules in Cancer

Signal transduction and gene expression in neighboring cells can be regulated by metabolites exchange within the tumor microenvironment (TME) for example, lactate functions as a signaling molecule directly and it leads to angiogenic response (Romero-Garcia et al. 2016). Nitrogen and Redox balance, bioenergetics, and biosynthesis are also regulated by metabolites exchange. Additionally, lactate can also take part in signaling through binding directly in N-MYC downstream-regulated gene (NDRG3) and activation of a Hypoxia-inducible factor 1a (HIF-1a)-dependent angiogenic program (Fig. 5.1).

The physiological mechanism shown above works in collaboration with canonical H1F-la response to actuate blood vessel formation and is acculturated by tumors (Park et al. 2015).

Lactate signaling molecules in cancer directly affecting several additional growth-promoting signaling pathways have also been reported. Moreover, immune cells can be directly affected by abundant lactate in the tumor microenvironment (TME). Lactate affects various immune cell functions like T cell proliferation, cytokine production, and cytotoxic activity of CD8+ T cells and NK (Romero-Garcia et al. 2016), so it has also got an immunosuppressive role. Lactate has been reportedly functioning as a signaling molecule, even though its role in metabolic pathway reconnect has yet to be fully explained.

Even though high level of lactate is typical to tumor, the way in which lactate enters endothelial cells and encourages angiogenesis thereby creating vascular perfusion to growing tissues has not been completely understood. Lactate increases the level of Gas6, Ang1 and probably VEGF by entering through MCT1 transporter. Lactate occupies the PI3K/Akt pathway passing through ligand-mediated activation

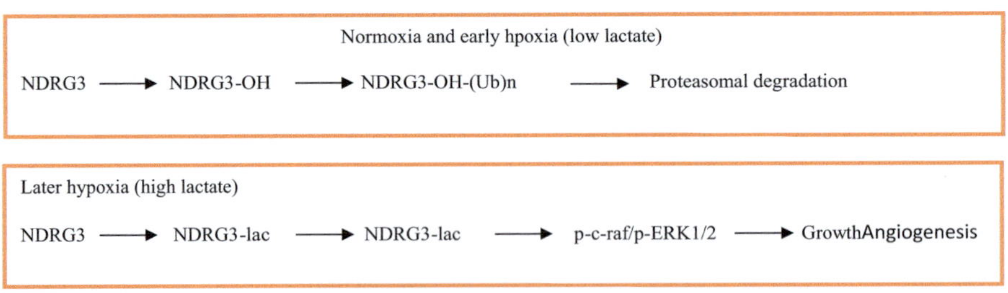

Fig. 5.1 A scheme outlining the regulatory mechanism for prolonged hypoxia responses involving lactate and NDRG3

of three receptor tyrosine kinases (RTKs) Axl, Tie2, and VEGFR-2, which is essential for angiogenesis. These ligands are also produced by other cell types (Ruan and Kazlauskas 2013). Using pharmacological inhibitors, deactivating the ligands of these receptor tyrosine kinases and inhibiting their kinase activity, eliminate cells' ability to respond to lactate. The mechanism by which lactate communicates with endothelial cells previously unacknowledged is a chance to improve our knowledge and understanding of the angiogenic program and to control it (Fig. 5.2).

Growth signaling increases the cellular demand for reduced nitrogen besides increasing the consumption of carbon in biosynthetic pathways. Nitrogen-containing molecules, viz., nucleotides, nonessential amino acids, and polyamines, are synthesized by a proliferating cell. For the biosynthesis of purines and pyrimidine bases, the amide group of glutamine is an essential donor of nitrogen (Tedeschi et al. 2013).

The role of purinergic signaling besides modulating multiple steps in tumor progression also plays a role in a number of physiological and patho-physiological processes (Di Virgilio and Adinolfi 2017). Participation of extracellular nucleotides and nucleosides is there in all the main phases of tumor progression but with opposite effects, which depends on the specific receptor subtype that is activated (Di Virgilio and Adinolfi 2017). To respond and to transduce signaling by adenosine and associated nucleotides (i.e., ATP, ADP, AMP), all the cells involved in the TME express the machinery required for doing so. Generally, nucleotide phosphates are released into the TME either by transport or passively by dying cells. Antitumor properties are exhibited by nucleotide phosphates by facilitating antigen presentation on dendritic cells and cancer cell clearance by T cells (Haskó et al. 2008). Nucleotide hydrolases are overexpressed by tumor infiltrating immune cells in advanced cancers which convert adenosine nucleotides into potently immunosuppressive molecule of adenosine nucleoside. The immunosuppressive T cells are the only immune cells that express the full complement of surface endonucleases (CD39 and CD73) which convert adenine nucleotides into adenosine, and adenosine levels are typically one to two orders of magnitude higher in tumors in comparison to normal tissues (Deaglio et al. 2007). The observations given above indicate

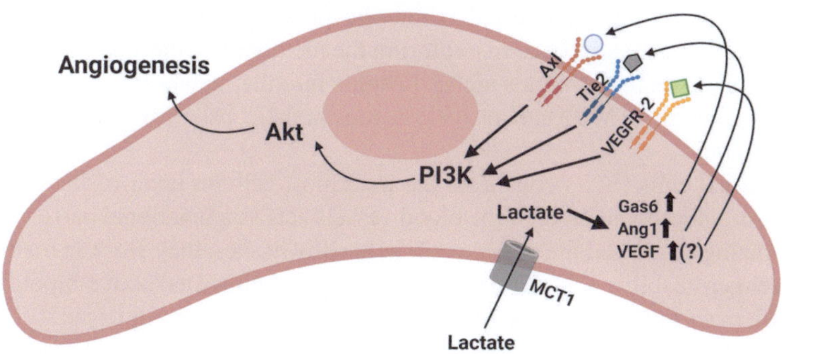

Fig. 5.2 Model for lactate-dependent activation of PI3K/Akt and promotion of angiogenesis (adapted from Ruan and Kazlauskas 2013)

that adenosine nucleotides accumulate in tumor tissue and are converted into adenosine, which suppresses the antitumor immune response.

Accumulation of ATP and adenosine is caused by hypoxia in the tumor core. This promotes CD73, CD39, A2AR, and A2BR expression. Additionally, hypoxia also promotes expression of P2X7R and D73, and this stimulates angiogenesis. Nucleotides and their receptors promote extracellular matrix degradation and tissue invasion (P2X7R and P2Y2R), tumor cell migration, extravasation and metastatic dissemination (P2Y2R, P2X7R, and P2Y12R) (Synnestvedt et al. 2002).

Metabolites are substrates and products of enzymes that are derived from reactions in central carbon metabolism which regulate the epigenome. Thus, the abundance of metabolites regulates gene expression. Cytosolic acetyl-CoA is the key metabolite that builds up when cell metabolizes more glucose than needed for bioenergetic support. Cytosolic acetyl-CoA is the required substrate for enzymes that acetylate histones, other proteins and S-adenosyl methionine (SAM). It provides acetyl and methyl groups that decorate histones and DNA. Histone and DNA methylation is sensitive to alteration in SAM levels which has been demonstrated by a number of recent reports (Shyh-Chang et al. 2013; Towbin et al. 2012). Acetylation has activated gene signatures involved in anabolic glucose metabolism significantly. These changes led to increased glycolytic flux and mitochondrial activity. It is enticing to speculate that these changes lead to increases in the Ac-CoA pools and thus act in a feed-forward manner to potentiate an anabolic metabolic program (Lyssiotis and Kimmelman 2017).

Cancer cells alter the chemical composition of the extracellular milieu, which exerts pleiotropic effects on the phenotypes of normal cells that reside in the vicinity of the tumor, as well as the extracellular matrix. Reciprocally, the microenvironment affects the metabolism and signaling responses of cancer cells themselves.

5.3 Targeting Endothelial Cell Metabolism for Antiangiogenic Therapy

There has been a paradigm shift in the area of cancer metabolism from an atomistic approach of studying the internal metabolic processes that feed the cancer cell towards an integrated approach of exploring the metabolic communications between different cell types in the tumor niche. Insights into the metabolic nexus of a tumor microenvironment (TME) can provide a mechanistic base for future therapeutic investigations.

Endothelial cells (ECs) constitute the innermost cellular layer of the circulatory system. The endothelial layer of the blood vessels acts as a functional barrier between the circulating blood and the vessel wall. In healthy tissues, they work in maintaining the vessel permeability and regulate the exchange of nutrients, active biomolecules, and waste macromolecules between the blood and the underlying tissue.

The "angiogenic switch" marks the onset of "neo-vascularization" of the avascularized hyperplasic tumors. Angiogenesis is a cumulative effect of rapid expansion, migration, and differentiation of endothelial cells (Ausprunk and Folkman 1977).

The metabolic processes utilized by the ECs have recently been acclaimed as major regulating factors in the angiogenic process. In order to realize their high energy demands and biomass production during vessel sprouting and remodeling, ECs switch to an altered metabolism. Normalizing these metabolic perturbations in ECs has propounded the translational potential in inhibiting angiogenesis.

De Bock et al. (2013) computed the flux of metabolic signaling in EC monolayers using radioactive labeled substances and found out that ECs are generally highly glycolytic when compared to other kinds of cells. Although sufficient amounts of dissolved oxygen from blood are regularly available to the ECs, they prefer anaerobic glycolysis over oxidative phosphorylation. This finding was confirmed by silencing phosphofructokinase-2/fructose-2,6-bisphosphatase (PFKFB3)—the key rate-determining enzyme, which led to reduced vessel formation, whereas activation or obstruction of mitochondrial respiration did not affect the vessel sprouting and stalk formation. The dependence of ECs on anaerobic metabolism for energy generation gives them a selective advantage during sprouting into avascular tissues having low oxygen levels, while sparing glucose for other cells or for biomass production (Verdegem et al. 2014). Later, metabolic profiling of endothelial cells isolated from tumors in mice showed that, of all the central metabolism pathways, glycolytic pathway had the highest fraction of upregulated genes including the PFKFB3 gene (Cantelmo et al. 2016). The three-fold higher glycolytic flux in ECs did not link glucose oxidation to ATP generation but assimilated more glucose in RNA and DNA bioproduction, suggesting that tumor endothelial cells relayed more glucose carbons towards biomass synthesis. Haplo-deficiency or inactivation of PFKFB3 in ECs displayed no significant effect on tumor growth. However, invasion, intravasation, and metastasis of tumor cells were reduced in effect improving chemotherapy of primary and metastatic tumors. Glycolysis reduction via inhibition of the PFKFB3 mechanistically lowers VE-cadherin endocytosis in ECs, which strengthens the vascular barrier, whereas upregulation of N-cadherin keeps pericyte quiescent and adhesive. Also lowering glycolysis decreases the expression of cancer cell adhesion molecules in ECs by decreasing NF-κB signaling (Cantelmo et al. 2016).

Another study showed that reduced flux of mitochondrial fatty acid oxidation (FAO) can also result in impaired proliferation in mouse ECs causing vascular sprouting defects. Loss of the rate-limiting enzyme, carnitine palmitoyltransferase 1 (CPT1a) reduces FAO flux and limits cell multiplication in human umbilical vein endothelial cells (HUVEC) (Schoors et al. 2015). Likewise, Schoors demonstrated that silencing of the long-chain acyl-CoA dehydrogenase (ACADVL) turned down proliferation in arterial ECs. CPT1a knock-down (KD) did not impair EC proliferation by disturbing the redox balance of the cells or by altering ROS measure to toxic levels. But, since fatty acids are carbon reserves for the Krebs cycle intermediates, CPT1a KD compromised de novo deoxyribonucleotide biosynthesis by reducing aspartate and dNTP pools in ECs. Interestingly, addition of acetate restored the levels of aspartate and dNTPs and rescued the sprouting defects suggesting its role in biomass production. Furthermore, the utilization of fatty acids for DNA synthesis is selectively high in ECs than any other primary cells except fibroblasts. Pharmacological agents inhibiting CPT1 or lowering FAO can be strategically used for blocking angiogenesis without compromising the metabolism of other normal cells (Fig. 5.3).

However, unlike the previous study, where PFKFB3 affected both endothelial growth and motility, FAO selectively regulates EC turnover and shows no effect on migration. These findings altogether suggest that distinct endothelial metabolic signals operate distinct functions in sprouting vessels.

The long-standing notion that angiogenesis is governed by genetic pro-angiogenic signals only is being challenged by recent evidences to consider the role of metabolic pathways in endothelial cells. Tumor vessels exhibit an abnormal phenotype in having a leaky interface, facilitating the metastatic spread of cancer cells. Till date, targeting of angiogenic factors or their cognate receptor molecules has been the center of interest for all antiangiogenic strategies. Lowering hyperglycolysis in tumor ECs has been shown to be beneficial in preclinical tumor models. Further investigations concerning how ECs alter their other metabolic pathways influencing vessel formation may set the stage for the development of novel anti-angiogenic therapies in tackling pathological and particularly tumor angiogenesis.

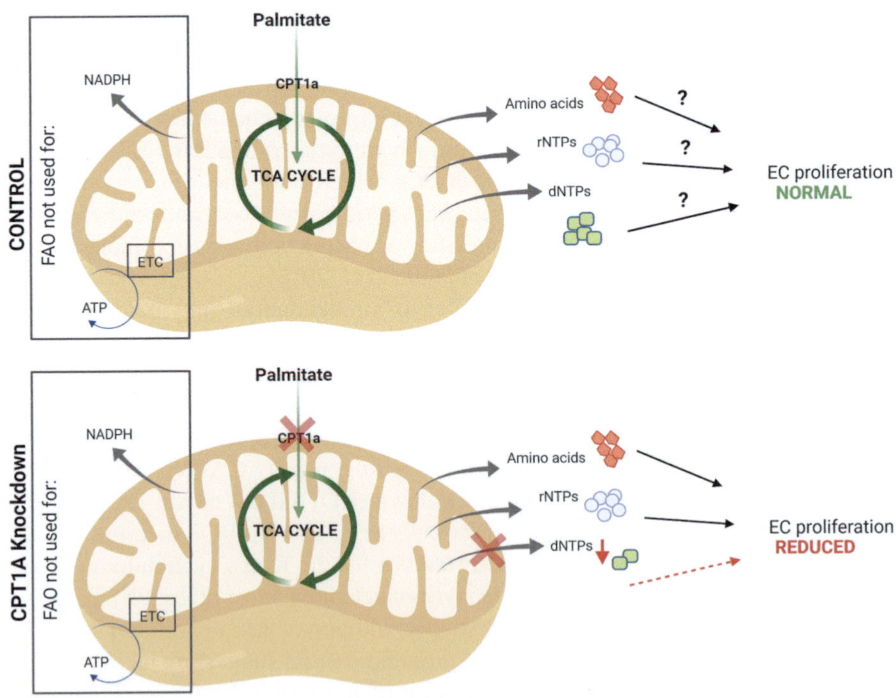

Fig. 5.3 Fatty acid-derived carbons utilized for the generation of amino acids and dNTP and rNTP precursors (adapted from Schoors et al. 2015)

5.4 Role of Extracellular Vesicles in Metabolic Cross Talk and TME

Metabolism within a cell is highly regulated and is considered a vital part of the cell "regulome." It facilitates the cellular participation in systemic and pathway-driven regulatory processes. Metabolic transitions within cell systems mediate cellular adaptations and can have multiple regulatory consequences (Grüning et al. 2010). Relative to normal cells, the cancer cell metabolism is dysregulated, and these alterations support the acquisition and maintenance of malignancy (De Berardinis and Chandel 2016).

The tumor microenvironment (TME) is a complex extracellular environment conducive to tumor growth. It is a key factor in multiple stages of disease progression such as localized resistance, immune-escape and distant metastasis (Milane et al. 2015). Tumors consistently modify their microenvironment and resultantly establish an aberrant ecosystem. Understanding the nature of tumor–stromal cell interactions and their co-evolution is vital to determine what drives cancer (Marusyk and Polyak 2010). Numerous in vitro and xenograft study models have shown increased proliferation, invasiveness, tumorigenicity, and metastatic potential of immortalized epithelial or cancer cells as a result of tumor–stromal interactions (Poltavets et al. 2018).

Beyond the cellular components, TME consists of parallel noncellular elements such as extracellular matrix (ECM), composed of structural proteins. ECM regulates TME via intercepting extracellular signals from the microenvironment to maintain cancer stem cell (CSC) "stemness" or induce heterogeneous tumor differentiations. ECM also regulates CSC behaviors by modulating intercellular signaling and immune surveillance (Shain et al. 2015). MicroRNAs (miRs) and exosomes are also being considered as critical components of the tumor microenvironment and regulators of the TME (Schiavoni et al. 2013).

Exosomes facilitate transfer of bioactive molecules between cancer and stromal cells in TME. This intercellular cross talk alters several biological functions in recipient cells. Multiple hallmarks of cancer have shown to be impacted by this exosome-mediated intercellular communication, including immunomodulation, stromal cell reprogramming, remodeling of the ECM, and onset of drug resistance (Tai et al. 2018). Tumor-released exosomes often transport transforming growth factor beta (TGFβ) from cancers to normal stromal fibroblasts (Webber et al. 2010). In contrast, exosomes derived from cancer-associated fibroblast (CAF) inhibit the mitochondrial oxidative phosphorylation process to regulate cancer (Zhao et al. 2016).

Recent studies have uncovered that exosomes also mediate communication between cancer cells and immune cells and aid the polarization of macrophages (Zhao et al. 2016). Tumor-derived exosomes secrete remodeling enzymes such as MMP2 or MMP9, causing degradation of ECM, leading to cancer invasion and metastasis. Furthermore, acquisition of drug resistance is found to be exosome mediated in some cancers.

Secreted exosomal cargo bears a strong resemblance to the parental cell. Thus real-time detection of modulations within exosomal carriers could provide insightful information about TME. Knowledge thus obtained will be beneficial in better diagnosis, prognosis, and disease monitoring (Zhao et al. 2016). Exosomes are not only key biomarkers but are also emerging as promising micro-carriers used to encapsulate and deliver targeted therapies.

References

Ausprunk DH, Folkman J (1977) Migration and proliferation of endothelial cells in preformed and newly formed blood vessels during tumor angiogenesis. Microvasc Res 14:53

Cantelmo AR, Conradi LC, Brajic A, Goveia J, Kalucka J, Pircher A et al (2016) Inhibition of the glycolytic activator PFKFB3 in endothelium induces tumor vessel normalization, impairs metastasis, and improves chemotherapy. In: Cancer Cell, vol 30, p 968

Canto C, Suave AA, Bai P (2013) Crosstalk between poly(ADP-ribose) polymerase and sirtuin enzymes. Mol Asp Med 34:1168

De Berardinis RJ, Chandel NS (2016) Fundamentals of cancer metabolism. Sci Adv 2(5):e1600200

De Bock K, Georgiadou M, Schoors S, Kuchnio A, Wong BW, Cantelmo AR et al (2013) Role of PFKFB3-driven glycolysis in vessel sprouting. Cell 154(3):651–663

Deaglio S, Dwyer KM, Gao W, Friedman D, Usheva A, Erat A et al (2007) Adenosine generation catalyzed by CD39 and CD73 expressed on regulatory T cells mediates immune suppression. J Exp Med 204:1257

Di Virgilio F, Adinolfi E (2017) Extracellular purines, purinergic receptors and tumor growth. Oncogene 36(3):293–303

Grüning NM, Lehrach H, Ralser M (2010) Regulatory crosstalk of the metabolic network. Trends Biochem Sci 35:220

Haskó G, Linden J, Cronstein B, Pacher P (2008) Adenosine receptors: therapeutic aspects for inflammatory and immune diseases. Nat Rev Drug Discov 7:759

Lyssiotis CA, Kimmelman CA (2017) Metabolic interactions in the tumor microenvironment. Trends Cell Biol 27:863–875

Marusyk A, Polyak K (2010) Tumor heterogeneity: causes and consequences. Biochim Biophys Acta 1805:105

Milane L, Singh A, Mattheolabakis G, Suresh M, Amiji MM (2015) Exosome mediated communication within the tumor microenvironment. J Control Release 219:278

Park KC, Lee DC, Yeom YI (2015) NDRG3-mediated lactate signaling in hypoxia. BMB Rep 48:301

Poltavets V, Kochetkova M, Pitson SM, Samuel MS (2018) The role of the extracellular matrix and its molecular and cellular regulators in cancer cell plasticity. Front Oncol 8:431

Romero-Garcia S, Moreno-Altamirano MMB, Prado-Garcia H, Sánchez-García FJ (2016) Lactate contribution to the tumor microenvironment: mechanisms, effects on immune cells and therapeutic relevance. Front Immunol 7:52

Ruan GX, Kazlauskas A (2013) Lactate engages receptor tyrosine kinases Axl, Tie2, and vascular endothelial growth factor receptor 2 to activate phosphoinositide 3-kinase/AKT and promote angiogenesis. J Biol Chem 288:21161

Schiavoni G, Gabriele L, Mattei F (2013) The tumor microenvironment: a pitch for multiple players. Front Oncol 3:90

Schoors S, Bruning U, Missiaen R, Queiroz KCS, Borgers G, Elia I et al (2015) Fatty acid carbon is essential for dNTP synthesis in endothelial cells. Nature 520(7546):192–197

Shain KH, Dalton WS, Tao J (2015) The tumor microenvironment shapes hallmarks of mature B-cell malignancies. Oncogene 34:4673

Shyh-Chang N, Locasale JW, Lyssiotis CA, Zheng Y, Teo RY, Ratanasirintrawoot S et al (2013) Influence of threonine metabolism on S-adenosylmethionine and histone methylation. Science 339:222

Synnestvedt K, Furuta GT, Comerford KM, Louis N, Karhausen J, Eltzschig HK et al (2002) Ecto-5′-nucleotidase (CD73) regulation by hypoxia-inducible factor-1 mediates permeability changes in intestinal epithelia. J Clin Invest 110:993

Tai YL, Chen KC, Hsieh JT, Shen TL (2018) Exosomes in cancer development and clinical applications. Cancer Sci 109:2364

Tedeschi PM, Markert EK, Gounder M, Lin H, Dvorzhinski D, Dolfi SC et al (2013) Contribution of serine, folate and glycine metabolism to the ATP, NADPH and purine requirements of cancer cells. Cell Death Dis 4:e877

Towbin BD, González-Aguilera C, Sack R, Gaidatzis D, Kalck V, Meister P et al (2012) Step-wise methylation of histone H3K9 positions heterochromatin at the nuclear periphery. Cell 150:934

Verdegem D, Moens S, Stapor P, Carmeliet P (2014) Endothelial cell metabolism: parallels and divergences with cancer cell metabolism. Cancer Metab 2:19

Webber J, Steadman R, Mason MD, Tabi Z, Clayton A (2010) Cancer exosomes trigger fibroblast to myofibroblast differentiation. Cancer Res 70:9621

Zhao H, Yang L, Baddour J, Achreja A, Bernard V, Moss T et al (2016) Tumor microenvironment derived exosomes pleiotropically modulate cancer cell metabolism. Elife 5:e10250

Role of Autophagy in Cancer Cell Metabolism

6

Diego A. Pedroza, Vaishali Chandel, Dhruv Kumar, Prakash Doddapattar, M. S. Biradar, Rajkumar Lakshmanaswamy, Shrikanth S. Gadad, and Ramesh Choudhari

The original version of this chapter was revised with the correction received from the author. The correction to this chapter can be found at https://doi.org/10.1007/978-981-15-1991-8_12

D. A. Pedroza
Graduate School of Biomedical Sciences, Texas Tech University Health Sciences Center El Paso, El Paso, TX, USA

V. Chandel · D. Kumar
Amity Institute of Molecular Medicine & Stem Cell Research (AIMMSCR), Amity University Uttar Pradesh (AUUP), Noida, Uttar Pradesh, India

P. Doddapattar
Department of Internal Medicine, University of Iowa, Iowa City, IA, USA

M. S. Biradar
Shri B. M. Patil Medical College, Hospital and Research Centre, BLDE (Deemed to be University), Vijayapur, Karnataka, India

R. Lakshmanaswamy
Graduate School of Biomedical Sciences, Texas Tech University Health Sciences Center El Paso, El Paso, TX, USA

Center of Emphasis in Cancer Research, Department of Molecular and Translational Medicine, Paul L. Foster School of Medicine, Texas Tech University Health Sciences Center El Paso, El Paso, TX, USA

S. S. Gadad
Graduate School of Biomedical Sciences, Texas Tech University Health Sciences Center El Paso, El Paso, TX, USA

Center of Emphasis in Cancer Research, Department of Molecular and Translational Medicine, Paul L. Foster School of Medicine, Texas Tech University Health Sciences Center El Paso, El Paso, TX, USA

Cecil H. and Ida Green Center for Reproductive Biology Sciences and Division of Basic Reproductive Biology Research, Department of Obstetrics and Gynecology, University of Texas Southwestern Medical Center, Dallas, TX, USA

D. Kumar (ed.), *Cancer Cell Metabolism: A Potential Target for Cancer Therapy*,
https://doi.org/10.1007/978-981-15-1991-8_6

Abstract

Autophagy is a complex process that plays a central role in maintaining cellular homeostasis by breaking down macromolecules and utilizing the metabolites as energy. This allows cells to maintain efficient ATP levels and promote cell survival by recycling macromolecules or dysfunctional organelles. Macromolecule degradation takes place in the lysosome and is identified as macroautophagy, microautophagy, or chaperone-mediated autophagy. Autophagy is also activated in response to cellular nutrient starvation as low glucose levels will cause cells to break down amino acids, such as glutamine. Glutaminolysis is able to support the tricarboxylic acid (TCA) cycle and when cells undergo severe starvation they can produce adequate ATP and NADPH levels. The underlying mechanism of autophagy is regulated by specific genes, primarily known as autophagy-related genes (ATGs). Although autophagy is critical for normal cell maintenance, cancer cells utilize autophagy to eliminate the demanding metabolic stress that is put on the cells allowing them to continue to grow and divide. Cancers with elevated autophagy activity are able to regulate important proliferative signaling pathways, including the PI3K/AKT/mTOR. Mutations in tumor suppressor genes, *KRAS*, *Tp53*, *BRCA2*, and *PTEN* have demonstrated the ability to activate autophagy, allowing for further uncontrolled growth of cancers. Autophagy has dual effects; normal cells can utilize it to promote autophagic cell death under stressful conditions, while cancer cells use it to induce chemo-resistance, promote cellular growth and division even under stressful metabolic conditions. Patients that present with elevated genes associated with autophagy could benefit from pharmacological inhibition of autophagy and targeted therapies to those genes. Here, we complied the role of autophagy regulation in cancer and cancer cell metabolism.

Keywords

Autophagy · Metabolism · Tumor microenvironment · Chemotherapy

6.1 Introduction

6.1.1 Autophagy and Cancer

Autophagy is an integral part of cellular homeostasis; it is a catabolic process that regulates metabolism by breaking down and degrading organelles and macromolecules such as proteins (Germic et al. 2019). Cells maintain certain levels of energy and get rid of toxins to remain in optimum conditions; autophagy mechanism keeps

R. Choudhari (✉)
Center of Emphasis in Cancer Research, Department of Molecular and Translational Medicine, Paul L. Foster School of Medicine, Texas Tech University Health Sciences Center El Paso, El Paso, TX, USA

Shri B. M. Patil Medical College, Hospital and Research Centre, BLDE (Deemed to be University), Vijayapur, India these optimum conditions under control. When macromolecules are broken down, cells not only clear unwanted molecules but also functionally restore intermediate metabolites, which can be utilized as a resourceful material for the cells (Germic et al. 2019). The molecular mechanism of autophagy is under the control of specific set of genes, termed autophagy-related genes (*ATG*) (Thumm et al. 1994). Within these, *BECN1/BECLIN1* (the mammalian homolog of yeast Vps30/Atg6) and *MAP1LC3B/LC3B* (microtubule-associated protein 1 light chain 3 beta) a homolog of yeast *ATG8,* are the most studied ATG genes (Racanelli et al. 2018). Intracellular degradation is carried out by the lysosome, whereby cytosolic organelles and proteins can be taken to the lysosome by autophagy. Dysfunctional mitochondrial accumulation, endoplasmic reticulum, and other cytosolic proteins result in autophagy defect (Pandareesh et al. 2018). Three classes of autophagy have been described, macroautophagy, microautophagy, and chaperone-mediated autophagy (Fig. 6.1)

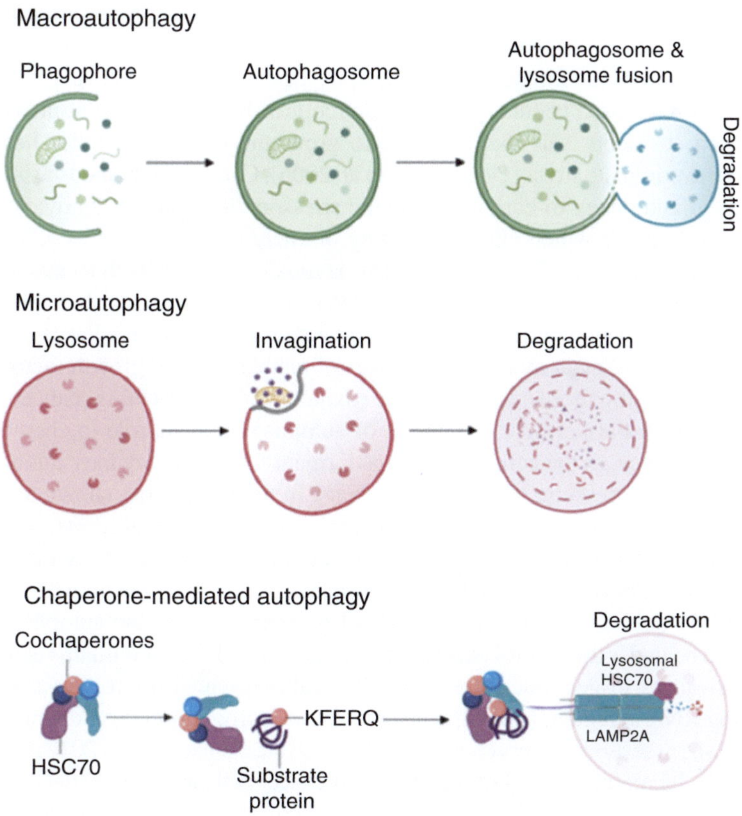

Fig. 6.1 *Macroautophagy* utilizes a phagophore to form an autophagosome that fuses with the lysosome, thereby degrading the internal material in the autolysosome. *Microautophagy* targets small pieces located in the cytoplasm engulfing them by lysosomal or endosomal membrane vacuoles consisting of multivesicular bodies by inward invagination (Sahu et al. 2011). *Chaperone-mediated autophagy* co-chaperones and cytosolic chaperones HSC70 first recognize proteins with a (Lys-Phe-Glu-Arg-Gln) KFERQ-like pentapeptide sequence, once recognized by the lysosome-associated membrane protein 2A (LAMP2A) receptor they are transferred to the lysosomal lumen (Mizushima and Komatsu 2011; Cuervo and Wong 2014)

(Mizushima and Komatsu 2011). The three autophagy forms mainly differ by the way the cargo is delivered to the lysosome. Cellular stress has a major role to play in autophagy stimulation, whether there is a lack of oxygen, energy, growth factors, or amino acids. However, in a nutrient-rich environment, mTOR complex 1 (mTORC1) is able to inactivate the ULK1 (Atg1 homolog) complex, leading to the activation of the PI3K-III complex which can act on phagophore formation to promote autophagosome and autophagolysosome degradation (Mizushima and Komatsu 2011).

Although autophagy is the main recycling system for the cell, it also performs a broad spectrum of functions including energy metabolism and ATP maintenance, cell survival in response to energy depletion, deprivation of nutrients, or growth factor depletion, and getting rid of damaged or dysfunctional organelles (Youle and Narendra 2011), to assure protein turnover and maintain organelle quality control, ensuring mitochondrial homeostasis and controlling pathways associated with cell death such as apoptosis (Galluzzi et al. 2008). Autophagy also plays a critical and important role in the regulation of adaptive immune response by the regulation of antigen presentation and lymphocyte development, inflection of cytokine signaling, and introduction of the innate immune system (Racanelli et al. 2018).

In cancer, increased cellular proliferation requires high metabolic turnover due to the induced stress on cells that continue to grow and divide and relies heavily on autophagy to eliminate stress (Degenhardt et al. 2006). Cancer cell homeostasis requires activation of autophagy to combat metabolic stressors like nutrient deprivation, cytotoxicity like hypoxia which allows recycling of energy sources such as ATP that are vital to sustain survival (Yang et al. 2011a). Hypoxic tumor cells that remain distant from blood vessels can induce autophagy and in turn activate Hypoxia-Inducible Factor 1-alpha (*HIF-1α*) which plays a role in cellular responses to systemic levels of oxygen. Activation of *HIF-1α* can modulate the levels of platelet-derived growth factor, vascular endothelial growth factor, and nitric oxide synthase enabling cancer growth (Semenza 2010). Furthermore, activation of autophagy plays a role in chemo and/or radiation resistance, as the cells remain in a dormant form and may later initiate tumor formation and progression. Inhibiting autophagy in tumor cells has shown to enhance the potential of cancer targeting drugs on these tumors (Lu et al. 2008; Yang et al. 2011a). Studies have demonstrated that human cancer cell lines carrying *HRAS* or *KRAS* mutations have abnormally increased levels of autophagy even when nutrients are plentiful (Guo et al. 2011). Low levels of glucose may activate autophagy which itself could be under the control of AMP-activated protein kinase (Williams et al. 2009). Recent advances in genomic information have also revealed the role of coding and noncoding RNA in regulating autophagy, metabolic reprogramming, and other biological processes in several cancers (Sun et al. 2015, 2018a; Camacho et al. 2018; Choudhari et al. 2019). Increased activity of autophagy in cancer cells most likely degrades intracellular energy reserves such as proteins and glycogen to bypass starvation from the lack of glucose and amino acids (Lin et al. 2019). Additionally, cancer cells with high autophagy activity regulated by the PI3K/AKT/mTOR pathway increase the cell survival even under acidic conditions from glycolysis (Wojtkowiak et al. 2012). Autophagy is also a pathway that is involved in identifying and eliminating intracellular pathogens (Colombo 2007), and engulfing apoptotic cells (Qu et al. 2007). However, the effect of these events on cancer is controversial. Autophagy possesses a complex function in

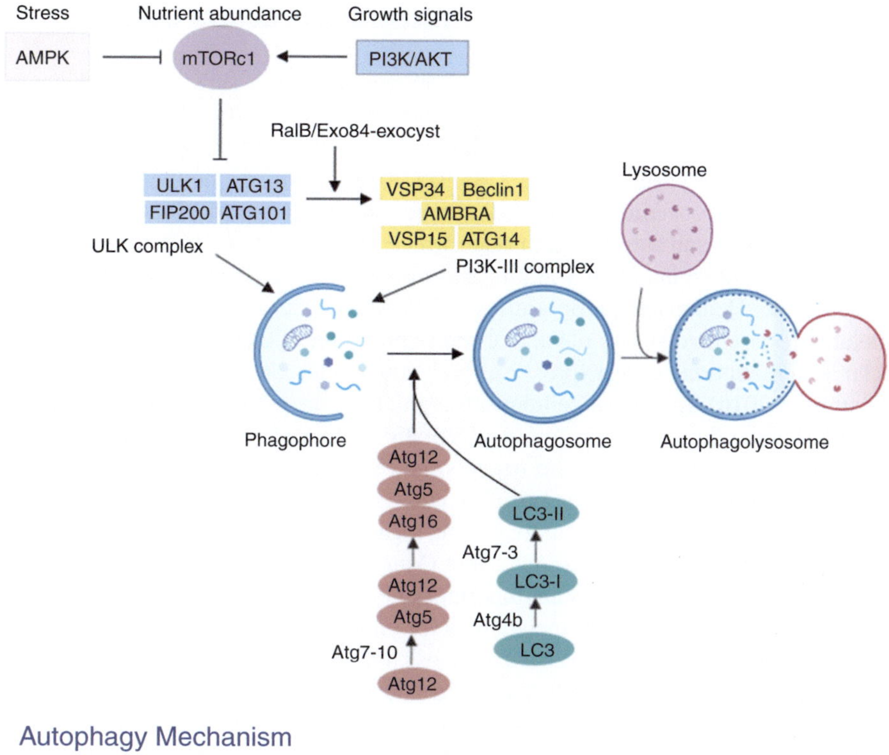

Fig. 6.2 Once autophagy is started, a kinase complex consisting of *UKL1*, *ATG13*, *RB1CC1/FIP200*, and *ATG101* is translocated into the endoplasmic reticulum. Upon activation, the autophagy-specific phosphoinositide 3-kinase (PI3K) signaling complex, comprised of class III phosphatidylinositol-3-phosphate (PtdIns3P), a second messenger, (PIK3C3/VPS34, PIK3R4/VPS15, Beclin 1, ATG14/barkor, and Ambra1), is regulated by the UKL1 complex in the endoplasmic reticulum, promoted by RalB and an Exo84-containing exocyst complex. Starvation also leads to the recruitment of Beclin1 to the PI3-kinase complex; enabling Bcl-2 and Beclin 1 to form an endoplasmic reticulum-associated complex. However, under a nutrient-rich environment and upon phosphorylation of Bcl-2, JNK1 is released. Production of PtdIns3P recruits double FYVE-containing protein 1 (DFCP1) and leads to formation of the omegasome, an endoplasmic reticulum-specific subcompartment where autophagosome biogenesis takes place (Axe et al. 2008; Mizushima and Komatsu 2011; Eskelinen 2019)

human malignancies, which depends on drugs used, tumor subtypes and stages, tumor suppressor genes, and driving oncogenes (White 2012). Autophagy plays a role in tumor suppression, as well as cancer cell survival, especially in response to chemotherapy (Kimmelman and White 2017). In addition, autophagy is implicated in various diseases including infection, liver diseases, inflammation, cancer, neurodegenerative disorders, cardiovascular, and aging (Levine and Kroemer 2008; Choi et al. 2013). Autophagy activation can lead to programmed cell death through *ATG7* and *Beclin 1*, induced by caspase-8 inhibition (Yu et al. 2004). It seems that the autophagy mechanism can be paradoxical in nature as it can become active and be utilized as a protective mechanism to induce chemo-resistance, or under too much stress; however, autophagy may promote autophagic cellular death (Fig. 6.2) (Li et al. 2017).

6.1.2 Autophagy and Metabolic Alteration in Cancer Cells

Recently, studies on cancer and cell metabolism have further substantiated that cancer requires altered metabolism for the cancer cells to survive and proliferate. Metabolic stress in cancer cells and tumor microenvironment occurs due to the lack of nutrients and oxygen (Lozy and Karantza 2012). To overcome the stress, during tumorigenesis, oncogenic mutations direct the cancer cell to reprogram itself for cellular metabolism and autophagy, through which required nutrients are acquired from the environment to maintain viability and tumor biomass (Pavlova and Thompson 2016; Vander Heiden and DeBerardinis 2017). Altered extracellular and intracellular metabolites are involved in metabolic reprogramming of cancer cell, effecting cellular differentiation, gene expression, and tumor microenvironment (Pavlova and Thompson 2016). In normal cellular differentiation, the cells metabolize glucose to carbon dioxide through oxidation of glycolytic pyruvate in the TCA cycle. NADH produced by glucose metabolism triggers the oxidative phosphorylation to amplify the ATP, with minimal production of lactate. However, cancer cells contradict the normal cell process to produce more lactate, regardless of oxygen availability, termed as "aerobic glycolysis" or Warburg effect (Vander Heiden et al. 2009). In addition, mitochondrial metabolism has an important role in ATP generation, redox signaling, and biosynthesis of important metabolites for tumor growth (Weinberg and Chandel 2015; Kimmelman and White 2017). Glucose and glutamine are the two main nutrients that play a critical role in biosynthesis and survival of cells. Evidence suggests that the autophagy regulates aerobic regulation, linked to proliferation and growth of cancer cells. In breast cancer, RNA interference or genetic knockout of autophagy regulator genes such as *ATG5, and ATG3* in *HRAS* and *KRAS* mutant cells significantly reduce glycolysis and attenuate the proliferation and Ras-mediated anchorage-independent growth (Lock et al. 2011). In *KRAS* mutated pancreatic ductal adenocarcinoma (PDAC) mice, *ATG7* and *ATG5* deficient mice acquired low grade premalignant pancreatic lesions but failed to develop high-grade PDAC (Rosenfeldt et al. 2013). However, *KRAS* oncogenic mice lacking *p53,* maintain low levels of autophagy, combined loss of *p53* and *ATG7* significantly increases glycolytic and pentose phosphate pathway to promote PDAC (Rosenfeldt et al. 2013). 6-Phosphofructo-2-kinase/fructose-2,6-bisphosphatases (PFKFBs), an important regulator of the glycolytic enzyme phosphofructokinase-1 (PFK-1), are upregulated in breast, ovarian, glioma, pancreatic, lymphoma, colon, and thyroid cancer cell lines (Atsumi et al. 2002). In colon adenocarcinoma cells, inhibition of PFKFB3 by siRNA or PFKFB3 inhibitor 3-(3-pyridinyl)-1-(4-pyridinyl)-2-propen-1-one (3PO) increases autophagy and decreases glucose uptake (Klarer et al. 2014). Hexokinase-II (HK-II), another key enzyme in glycolysis, induces autophagy and overcomes the metabolic stress (Zhang et al. 2014). In glucose deprivation, HK-II binds to mTOR and limits its activity to suppress autophagy and induce cell death under glucose starvation (Roberts et al. 2014). Pyruvate kinase M2 (PKM2) effects the glucose metabolism in cancer; activated PKM2 inhibited the growth of xenograft tumors, suggesting that high pyruvate suppresses cancer growth (Anastasiou et al. 2012). Chaperone-mediated autophagy effects the pyruvate kinase, degrades PKM2 and enhances the glycolytic intermediate and favors the tumor progression (Lv et al. 2011). However, in contrast, a recent study reported that aberrant expression of PKM2 promotes the tumorigenesis in various cancers, including lung, breast, liver, esophagus, and gastric (Wang et al. 2017a). Knockdown of PKM2 inhibited the PI3K/AKT signaling pathway, activated autophagy, and regressed the tumor growth in gastric cancer (Wang et al. 2017a). Gene mutation and amplification in upstream receptor tyrosine kinases (RTKs) governs the autophagic metabolism and glucose uptake in cancer cells. Oncogenic signaling pathways such as PI3K/AKT, RAS, and c-Myc upregulate the glucose transporter GLUT1 to increase glucose consumption in cells (Murakami et al. 1992; Osthus et al. 2000). Glutamine, another important enzyme in glycolysis, acts as a nitrogen source for biosynthesis of nucleotide, glucosamine-6-phosphate, and nonessential amino acids. In cancers, like glucose, glutamine also acts as a glycolytic intermediate and supports the Warburg effect. Reports suggest that glutamine is upregulated in cancers and promotes tumorigenesis (Mannava et al. 2008). The transcription factor c-Myc, upregulated in proliferative cells, induces glutamine transporters SN2 and ASCT2 and regulates the phosphoribosyl pyrophosphate synthetase (PRPS2), carbamoyl phosphate synthetase, and glutamine-utilizing enzyme glutaminase (GLS1), promotes the glutamine uptake, and converts it into glutamate; later, accumulated glutamate in the cells enters TCA cycle (Eberhardy and Farnham 2001; Wise et al. 2008). Further, TCA cycle generates NADPH to maintain redox pathway through glutaminolysis in pancreatic cancer, establishing the fact that reprogramming of glutamine is driven by oncogenic *KRAS* by suppressing the important metabolic enzymes (Son et al. 2013). In glioblastoma, inhibiting mTOR induces the expression of glutaminase and confers drug resistance (Tanaka et al. 2015). Therefore, glutamine expressed through autophagy is crucial for the survival and cancer growth. Taken together, it is evident that cancer cell alters the metabolic changes to support their survival and proliferation during tumorigenesis.

6.1.3 Roles of Autophagy in Cancers

6.1.3.1 Breast Cancer

Breast cancer is the most frequently diagnosed cancer in women and is the second leading cause of cancer-related deaths with approximately one in eight US women being diagnosed with breast cancer in her lifetime (Siegel et al. 2019). Breast cancers are identified by the clinical histopathological identification of the estrogen receptor (ER), progesterone receptor (PR), and human epidermal growth factor receptor 2 (HER2) or lack thereof. Overall, 70–80% of all breast cancers present as hormone receptor positive (ER, PR-positive), 10–15% are classified as HER2 overexpressing, and 10–15% are identified as triple-negative breast cancers (TNBC) (ER, PR, and HER2-negative) (Konecny et al. 2003). Breast cancer treatment relies on the presence of ER, and these breast cancers are treated with ER-targeted therapy including Tamoxifen, Fulvestrant, or in the case of postmenopausal women Anastrozole. HER2-overexpressing patients are administered, Herceptin and TNBC patients rely on chemotherapy and/or radiation. Unfortunately, clinical and epidemiological data show high resistance to endocrine therapy, such as tamoxifen (Chang 2012). Because autophagy has been demonstrated to play a pivotal role in cancer survival, it has since become a therapeutic target as it is able to sensitize cancer cells to anticancer drugs (True and Matthias 2012). TNBCs are able to utilize autophagy to maintain high proliferative status by inducing cancer-associated fibroblasts (CAFs) which play a major role in cancer progression (Han et al. 2018). Protein conversion levels of Beclin1 and LC3-II/I in CAFs are greater than in normal fibroblasts (NFs) (Wang et al. 2017b). A cancer/testis antigen, TFDP3, belonging to the transcription factor DP (TFDP) family, overexpressed in MDA-MB-231 TNBC cells, has the capability to induce autophagy by altering the expression of autophagy marker light chain 3 (LC3) and elevating the autophagosomes during chemotherapy (Ding et al. 2018). Because of this, chemotherapeutic injury to cytoplasmic organelles or damage to the DNA can be repaired by autophagy; thus, autophagy and TFDP3 work in tandem to promote chemotherapy resistance (Ding et al. 2018). Tamoxifen active metabolites have the capability to activate autophagy, increasing the survival of ER-positive breast cancer cells (Samaddar et al. 2008). Tamoxifen resistant cells demonstrate high autophagosome turnover compared to tamoxifen responsive cells (Cook et al. 2012; Nagelkerke et al. 2014). Interestingly, silencing autophagy involved genes, *ATG5*, *ATG7*, or *BECN/BECLIN1*, recovers tamoxifen sensitivity in the breast cancer cells (Qadir et al. 2008). A cancer progression-related gene, metastasis-associated 1 (MTA1), has been shown to be overexpressed in breast cancer cells. Pathophysiological invasive and metastatic characteristics are also associated with acquired tamoxifen resistance in ER-positive breast cancer cells by activating the AMPK pathway upon induction of autophagy (Lee et al. 2018).

6.1.3.2 Ovarian Cancer

Over 22,500 new cases of ovarian cancers are expected to be diagnosed in the United States in 2019, and 13,980 women are expected to die from the disease in the same year (Siegel et al. 2019). Although ovarian cancer accounts for 2.5% of all female malignancies, approximately 5% of female cancer-related deaths occur because of late stage diagnosis leading to low survival rates (Torre et al. 2018). Women diagnosed with advanced ovarian cancers generally undergo optimal cytoreductive surgery and platinum-based chemotherapy (Kim et al. 2017). Approximately 80% of patients diagnosed with non-advanced ovarian cancers respond to first-line chemotherapy; unfortunately over 70% of patients diagnosed with advance stage develop drug resistance and cancer recurs within 5 years. (Heintz et al. 2006; Monk and Coleman 2009). Clinical trials of targeted therapies such as pazopanib, cediranib, tyrosine kinase inhibitors (TKI), and olaparib, a poly(ADP-ribose) polymerase (PARP) inhibitor, are being conducted for recurrent ovarian cancers (Kim et al. 2017). Because autophagy plays a role in apoptosis and proliferation in ovarian cancers, the signaling mechanisms associated with apoptosis and proliferation tie in with ovarian cancer development by autophagy regulation (Zhan et al. 2016). Autophagy activation has been demonstrated to restrict ovarian cancer development by inhibiting the Ras/MAP kinase and PI3K/AKT/mTOR signaling pathways (Bai et al. 2015). However, danusertib, an aurora kinase inhibitor (AKI), and monepantel, an amino-acetonitrile derivative (AAD), induce autophagy and apoptosis in ovarian cancer cells by the disruption of the PI3K/AKT/mTOR/p70S6K signaling pathway (Bahrami et al. 2014; Zi et al. 2015). Also, activation of the p38 MAPK and JNK pathway by neferine, a bisbenzylisoquinoline alkaloid, induces autophagy in ovarian cancer cells (Xu et al. 2016). The tumor suppressors p53 and phosphatase and tensin homolog (PTEN) play a major role in cancer development. In over 96% of high-grade ovarian cancers, p53 has been shown to be mutated, promoting tumor metastasis (Ren et al. 2016). PTEN is an upstream suppressor of the PI3K pathway and mutated PTEN is also highly common in ovarian cancers (Zhang et al. 2016). PTEN activates autophagy by regulating the PI3K/AKT/mTOR pathway upon the dephosphorylation of Phosphatidylinositol (3,4,5)-triphosphate (PIP3) (Arico et al. 2001). Targeting autophagy has become a major focus, for example, in ovarian cancers, PDZ-binding kinase (PBK) has been shown to be highly upregulated in high-grade serous ovarian carcinoma (HGSOC) tissues and ovarian cancer cells (Ma et al. 2019a, b). PBK is associated with cell proliferation, DNA damage response, migration, and invasion (Ayllon and O'Connor 2007; Joel et al. 2015; Hinzman et al. 2018). PBK has been shown to promote autophagy through the ERK/mTOR pathway and attenuated ovarian cancer cell sensitivity to cisplatin (Ma et al. 2019a, b). Therefore, targeting PBK could lead to an indirect targeting of autophagy and autophagy-related pathways, possibly becoming a therapy for women with ovarian carcinomas.

6.1.3.3 Brain Cancer

An estimated 23,820 new cases of brain and primary central nervous system tumors will be diagnosed in 2019 in the Unites States and 17,760 people are expected to die from this disease (Siegel et al. 2019). The most common and deadly brain tumors are gliomas, with glioblastoma (GBM) accounting for 54% of all gliomas, the most aggressive form of brain cancer (Kohler et al. 2011). GBM patients have a 5-year survival rate of less than 5% (Van Meir et al. 2010). Even after diagnosis, surgery, radiation, and chemotherapies, the average life expectancy is only 14 months (Van Meir et al. 2010). GBMs can be classified into four molecular subtypes—proneural, classical, mesenchymal, and neural—dependent on the frequency of associated mutations to *p53*, *NF1*, *PTEN*, *PDGFRA*, *and EGFR* (Verhaak et al. 2010). Mutations observed in brain tumors such as *PTEN*, *p53*, *EGFR*, *AKT*, and *NF1* also play a role in autophagy regulation (Kaza et al. 2012). Amplification of EGFR, and deletion of NF-1 and PTEN remain as the most frequent mutations observed in gliomas (Verhaak et al. 2010). These mutations are responsible for the survival and chemo-resistance of gliomas, as the signaling mechanisms interact with the PI3K/AKT/mTOR pathway (Cheng et al. 2009). The chemotherapeutic agent temozolomide (TMZ) is one of the options given to patients with GBMs following surgical resection; however, combination of TMZ and radiation has shown to significantly improve patient survival (Cheng et al. 2009). The interesting factor is that both radiation and TMZ induce autophagy in glioma cells (Kaza et al. 2012). This TMZ-induced autophagy has the capability to promote the survival of glioblastoma cells

(Amaravadi et al. 2016). Further, suppressing the autophagy related 4C cysteine peptidase *(ATG4C)*, a gene involved in TMZ-induced autophagy, increased the sensitivity of glioblastoma cells to TMZ (Wen et al. 2019). Aside from those therapies, the combination of autophagy inhibitors and metabolism inhibitors could have synergistic effects due to lower oxidative phosphorylation and high-energy consumption of cancer cells. The role of autophagy in gliomas is not well understood; therefore, targeting autophagy in brain cancer has not seen much success. However, ongoing research on cell signaling and metabolism mechanisms can lead to better understanding of autophagy in brain cancers.

6.1.3.4 Lymphoma Cancer

Lymphoma is a cancer of the immune system which develops due to gene mutations in the lymphocytes (white blood cells). Lymphomas are categorized into two different groups: (1) Hodgkin's lymphoma (LH) and (2) non-Hodgkin's lymphoma (NHL). Among both, NHL is the most common lymphoma. Diffused large B cell lymphoma (DLBCL) alone accounts for 30–40% of B-NHL. Based on the gene expression, DLBCL is further divided into (a) the activated B cell like (ABC) DLBCL, (b) the germinal center B cell like (GCB) DLBCL, and (c) primary mediastinal B cell lymphoma (PMBCL). The CHOP chemotherapy combination (cyclophosphamide, doxorubicin, vincristine, and prednisone) has been the back bone of front-line chemotherapy for most NHLs, with addition of anti-CD 20 monoclonal rituximab antibody R-CHOP to treat diffused B cell lymphoma; however, treatment has shown no promise in patients, with every third patient reported to relapse with ~90% fatality (Amin et al. 2017). Unfortunately, patients with leukemia or lymphoma still have an unsatisfactory prognosis. Accumulating evidence suggests that autophagy is essential for normal hemostasis and leukemia or lymphoma developments. Recent report suggests that *CUL4B* regulate autophagy by activating JNK phosphorylation in B cell lymphoma suggesting that inhibiting autophagy may lead to cancer growth (Li et al. 2019). Double hit B cell lymphomas with translocation involving *MYC* and *BCL-2* or *BCL-6* included in WHO classified as high-grade B cell (Friedberg 2017). Interestingly, BCL-2 directly binds to *BECN1* and inhibits autophagy, correlating to patients with decreased *BCL-2* which carries an increased *BECN1* expression and has a good prognosis (Nicotra et al. 2010; Huang et al. 2011). Moreover, heterozygous $Becn1^{+/-}$ mice has a high incidences of lymphomas, liver, and lung cancers (Qu et al. 2003), and constitutive repression of autophagy in *BCL-6* induced DLBCL, contributes to lymphomagenesis (Bertolo et al. 2013). Nevertheless, the autophagy switches to adaptive strategy by clearing the damaged cell components and survives bioenergetic stress (Kiffin et al. 2004), and it can also play a role in cell death (Mizushima et al. 2008). Inhibition of autophagy either with chloroquine or ATG5 short hairpin RNA (shRNA) activated p53 and induced tumor cell death in B cell lymphoma (Amaravadi et al. 2007). Energy balance of the cell is controlled by AMPK, usually downregulated in most cancers due to the upregulation of mammalian target of rapamycin (mTOR), and promotes T-cell and B-cell lymphoma (Shi et al. 2012). The mTOR pathway under stress conditions regulates autophagy especially to anticancer drugs, AMPK activator, metformin arrests T and B cell lymphoma growth by inhibiting mTOR signaling without activating AKT (Shi et al. 2012). ALCL T-cell NHL is predominantly driven by *NPM-ALK* oncogene and is a constitutively active tyrosine kinase, described in mouse models for NPM-ALK tumorigenesis (Chiarle et al. 2008; Choudhari et al. 2016). Crizotinib is the most advanced ALK tyrosine kinase inhibitor often used to treat ALK-related malignancies. However, T cell NHL conferred a drug resistance to crizotinib (Gambacorti Passerini et al. 2014). The role of autophagy in ALK+ ALCL T cell lymphoma is not been well established; a recent study showed that, upon ALK inactivation and autophagy inhibition through combined treatment with crizotinib and chloroquine has better effect on ALK+ ALCL T cell lymphoma (Mitou et al. 2015). In addition, ALK fusion oncogene activates several signaling pathways including the PI3K/Akt/mTOR and Ras/MEK/ERK (Marzec et al. 2007; McDermott et al. 2008), and play a role in the regulation of autophagy (Cagnol and Chambard 2010; Janku et al. 2011). Therefore, targeting MAP-kinase kinase (MEK) in combination with ALK has shown a potent therapeutic effect in T cell lymphoma (Menotti et al. 2019). Taken together, it is evident that autophagy could be a promising target for lymphoma treatment.

6.1.3.5 Pancreatic Cancer

Pancreatic cancer is a highly fatal cancer, with around 56,770 newly diagnosed cases every year (Siegel et al. 2019). It is the seventh leading cause of death from cancer, accounting for approximately 432,000 deaths worldwide (Bray et al. 2018). Unfortunately, the late diagnosis and failure to the treatment in pancreatic cancer results in a dismal 5-year survival of 6% (Ying et al. 2016). Pancreatic cancer develop high resistance to radiotherapy and chemotherapeutic drugs (Li et al. 2004; Ben-Josef and Lawrence 2008). The altered metabolic and survival pathways in the pancreatic cancers are due to the resistance exerted through different therapeutic approaches. Nearly 85% of pancreatic cancer are PDAC, which harbors mutations in *KRAS*, *CDKN2A*, *INK4A/ARF*, *p53*, *SMAd4*, *BRCA2*, and effective treatment or inhibitors are yet to be developed (Van Cutsem et al. 2004; Hezel et al. 2006; Ryan et al. 2014). The role of autophagy in cancer is referred to as a "double edge sword" because of its characteristic nature to suppress or promote tumorigenesis depending on cellular context or tumor stage (Shintani and Klionsky 2004). Extreme resistance for standard therapy has propelled to think that combination and alternative therapies in treating the aggressive nature of PDAC cancers. Evidence suggests that basal autophagy is elevated in pancreatic cancers and is required for the proliferation both in vivo and in vitro (Yang et al. 2011b). Autophagy inhibition uses either siRNA-mediated silencing or pharmacological inhibition-induced ROS activation by impacting mitochondrial metabolism (Yang et al. 2011b). *FoxO3* controls autophagy-regulated transcription genes such as *Bnip3* and *LC3*, transcription upregulation of *LC3* in mammalian cells during starvation is dependent on *FoxO3*, blocked by *AKT* activation to inhibit autophagy activation during tumorigenesis (Mammucari et al. 2007; He 2009; Perera et al. 2015). Epigenetic changes, histone acetyl transferase (HATs), and histone deacetylase transferase (HDACs) regulate autophagy in pancreatic cancers (Rikiishi 2010). HDACi or inhibition of HATs, hyperacetylates histones to activate autophagy (Shandilya et al. 2009; Arif et al. 2010; Rikiishi 2010). Conditional deletion of *p53* crossed with conditional *Atg5* allele in KRAS-driven pancreatic model showed that deficient autophagy increased Pancreatic Intraepithelial Neoplasia (PanIN) tumor initiation but inhibits PanIN progression to become high-grade PDAC (Yang et al. 2014). Also, in another study, mice lacking *Atg5* or *Atg7* showed that PanIN progression to high-grade PDAC was blocked (Rosenfeldt et al. 2013). In cerulein-induced pancreatitis mouse models, loss of autophagy initiated by deletion of *Atg5* activated lkB kinase (IKK)-related kinase, TBK1, PD-L1, T cell infiltration and neutrophils (Yang et al. 2016). Further, defective autophagy upregulated PD-L1 modulating IFNy signaling pathway and activated the JAK pathway to inhibit KRAS-driven pancreatic cancer (Yang et al. 2016). In contrast to these studies, mice lacking *p53* with oncogenic *KRAS*, autophagy loss could not block tumor progression (Rosenfeldt et al. 2013). Autophagy may be very important in preventing tumorigenesis in healthy and premalignant tissues but can promote cancer progression in already established pancreatic tumors. Therefore, the above findings support autophagy as a double edged sword process. Importantly, it is time to carefully evaluate the use of autophagy inhibitors during premalignant and during late tumor progression.

6.1.3.6 Lung Cancer

Lung cancer is the leading cause of mortality worldwide, with an average of 15% survival for 5 years non-small cell lung cancer (NSCLC) accounts for ~85% of all lung cancers (Ettinger et al. 2013). It is classified into distinct histologic subtypes: squamous cell carcinoma, large cell carcinoma, and adenocarcinomas. NSCLC is further subclassified based on the mutation in *EGFR*, *KRAS*, *BRAF* or gene rearrangement in the *ROS1* or *ALK* loci (Ambrogio et al. 2016). *KRAS* is the most commonly mutated in lung adenocarcinoma, affecting ~30% of patients with overall worst survival (Lohinai et al. 2017). The drugs developed to target the mutant *KRAS* have failed, creating a space for alternative therapeutic approaches. Evidence suggests that the regulation of autophagy is critical in maintaining cellular homeostatic and tumorigenesis. Genetically engineered mouse (GEM) tumor models are the most studied lung cancer model, driven by *KRAS* oncogene. In NSCLC, the *p53* mutation is associated with spontaneous *KRAS* activation and promotes hyperplasia to adenocarcinoma (Johnson et al. 2001). In NSCLC mouse model, autophagy-regulated gene *ATG7* deleted with *KRAS*^{G12D} activation showed dysfunctional mitochondria, activated *p53* to arrest proliferation, further altering the tumor phenotype from adenomas and carcinomas to oncocytomas (benign tumors) (Guo et al. 2013). Furthermore, in *p53* and *ATG7*-deficient tumor-derived cell lines showed starvation survival and formed lipidic cyst instead of tumors, suggesting cancer growth with distinct roles in metabolism for both tumor suppressor and oncogenes (Guo et al. 2013). In *BRAF*^{v600E}-induced lung tumor, deletion of *ATG7* induced oxidative stress and early tumor development, but in later stage of tumorigenesis *ATG7*-deficiency showed defective mitochondria, reduced proliferation and tumor burden resulting in conversion of adenocarcinoma to oncocytomas (Strohecker et al. 2013), suggesting the role of autophagy in tumor progression at different cellular context. *Beclin-1* induces autophagy by the activation of lipid kinase VPS34 and Beclin-1/VPS34/vps15, a core autophagic component (Funderburk et al. 2010). *JNK1* disrupts Bcl-2/Beclin 1 complex by phosphorylating multisite of *Bcl-2* to stimulate starvation-induced autophagy (Wei et al. 2008). Further, Na/K-ATPase inhibitor and cardiac glycoside ouabain induce *JNK1* activation and negatively regulate *Bcl-2* to limit *Bcl-2/Beclin-1* interaction resulting in caspase-independent autophagic cell death in NSCLC cells (Trenti et al. 2014; Felippe Goncalves-de-Albuquerque et al. 2017). *GATA6* enhances autophagy and confers TKI resistant in NSCLC cells (Ma et al. 2019a, b). In TKI-resistant NSCLC, basal level of autophagy is not significantly high compared to the sensitive NSCLC cells and erlotinib treatment enhanced autophagy activity with increased expression of *GATA6*. Further, knockdown of *GATA6* reduced autophagy and cell viability significantly suggesting that targeting *GATA6* and autophagy together along with TKI can be beneficial to overcome drug resistance in NSCLC (Ma et al. 2019a, b). In contrast, another study suggests that knockdown of *ATG5* and *Beclin-1* autophagy induces radiation resistance in NSCLC (Kim et al. 2008). In addition, recent report suggests that silencing of *SIRT1* and *SIRT2* induces apoptosis and differentially regulates the autophagy in cancer cells (Ma et al. 2014). *SIRT1* deacetylates *ATG5*, silencing of *ATG5* induced cellular apoptosis in NSCLC and on the other hand, inhibiting *SIRT1/2* regulates pro-survival autophagy by acetylating *HSPA5* and activated *ATF4* and *DDIT4* to inhibit mTOR signaling pathway in NSCLC (Lee et al. 2008; Mu et al. 2019). Therefore, combination treatment with *SIRT1/2* inhibitors and pharmacological inhibiting autophagy can be an effective therapeutic strategy for cancer therapy. Taken together, these studies suggest that detailed role of autophagy in tumorigenesis still needs to be further investigated. It is evident from the present studies that combination therapy targeting autophagy and specific signaling pathways can provide a viable option in treating resistant lung cancer.

6.1.4 Conclusion

Autophagy is tightly regulated through cellular processes under stressful environment, including damaged organelles, nutrient deprivation, and anticancer therapy. Although autophagy is overall the main recycling system for the cell, it rather has a broad spectrum of functions including: energy metabolism and ATP maintenance, cell survival in response to energy depletion, deprivation of nutrients or growth factors, as well as getting rid of damaged or dysfunctional organelles (Youle and Narendra 2011). In most advanced stage, cancer cell require autophagy to alter the metabolic reprogramming for their development and survival. Despite the role of autophagy is controversial in cancer development, cancer cell needs autophagy to provide metabolite and intermediate precursor and nutrients to promote the cancer cell growth and survival, and on the other hand, autophagy suppresses tumor growth and progression in healthy and premalignant tumors. The multiple roles of autophagy and its complex interplay with cancer metabolism are yet to be elucidated. However, from recent studies, it is clear that autophagy is involved in stress response,

Table 6.1 Expression of Autophagy related genes in cancer metabolism

Gene	Expression	Function	References
Beclin 1	Down	Increased expression of Beclin 1 is negatively associated with advanced, histological grade, and overall increased survival	Shen et al. (2008) and Cai et al. (2014)
ATG5, ATG7	Down	ATG5 and ATG7 inhibit autophagy induction when downregulated in ovarian cancer cells	Correa et al. (2015)
p53	Down	Wild-type tumor suppressor, *p53* sensitizes drug-resistant ovarian cancer cells to chemotherapeutic agents by decreasing autophagy	Kong et al. (2012)
PTEN	Down	Increased drug resistance has been observed when low levels of PTEN are present reducing autophagy activity in cancer	Ying et al. (2015)
p62	Up	Advanced stage, residual tumor presence, and low survival rates correlate with high expression of p62 in ovarian cancers	Iwadate et al. (2014)
FSIP1	Up	Positively regulates the invasion and proliferation of TNBC cells, upon silencing promotes drug resistance by the activation of autophagy	Liu et al. (2018)
IL-12	Up	Promotes autophagy in breast cancer cells by the activation of AMPK and PI3K/AKT	Lin et al. (2017)
Bcl-2	Up	Inhibits autophagy, by targeting Beclin-1 and promoting breast cancer cell growth	Oh et al. (2011)
AMBRA1	Up	Upregulated in breast cancer cells can sensitize cancer cells to epirubicin (EPI), promoting them to undergo autophagy or apoptosis	Sun et al. (2018b)
LC3	Up	Knockdown of LC3 inhibits autophagy, suppresses cell proliferation, colony formation, migration/invasion, and promotes apoptosis in cancer	Yang et al. (2011b) and Hamurcu et al. (2018)
AEG-1	Up	Hypoxia-induced autophagy, chemo-resistance in T cell lymphoma	Yan et al. (2018)
LITAF	Down	BCL-6 target gene regulates autophagy in B cell lymphoma	Bertolo et al. (2013)

metabolism, chemotherapy resistance, metastasis, and apoptosis (Lee et al. 2018). Autophagy has a dual functional or "double edged sword" role in the regulation of cell death and survival in tumor initiation and progression depending on the cellular context of tumor stage (Shintani and Klionsky 2004). Autophagy acts as a tumor suppressor during early tumorigenesis where *Beclin1*, an autophagy responsible gene, controls the early tumor formation; however, heterozygous *Beclin*$^{-/+}$ condition in mouse showed a marked increase in lung, lymphoma, and liver cancer (Kondo et al. 2005). In addition, phosphatidylinositol 3-phosphate kinase (PI3K)–AKT–mTOR signaling pathway induced autophagy and glucose uptake during cancer progression. Furthermore, the mutations in *KRAS*, *CDKN2A*, *INK4A/ARF*, *p53*, *SMAd4*, *BRCA2*, *p53*, *NF1*, *PTEN*, *PDGFRA* genes activate autophagy. HIF-1α has a critical role in cellular responses to systemic levels of oxygen (Table 6.1). Here, autophagy is activated in tumor cells present in the inner mass of the cancer to survive or become dormant under stress condition from low oxygen and low nutrients (Semenza 2010). Activation of autophagy by mutations, stress conditions, and low nutrient promoted the cancer cell to acquire resistance toward chemotherapy and radiotherapy (Ben-Josef and Lawrence 2008; Semenza 2010; Verhaak et al. 2010; Yang et al. 2011a). Multifaceted behavior and complex nature of autophagy in different cancers raises some important questions. How and when do physiological, metabolic or genetic conditions drive autophagy towards cancer cell survival or cell death? How exactly does autophagy play a role in cancer development and progression? If recycling by autophagy provides substrates for metabolism and promotes cancer survival, is this true in all other cancers? Does inhibition or activation of autophagy and intercellular metabolite in cancer help to treat the disease? What is the best inhibition or activation targets in cancer cell metabolism and autophagy pathway to treat the disease? Does combinational drug inhibition of autophagy and metabolic process beneficial or does it have off target effects in cancer treatments? Does autophagy inactivation and uptake of glucose and glutamine in cancer cell confer resistance or adaptive mechanisms? Does the organelle malfunction or metabolic insufficiency contribute to increased oxidative stress in autophagy regulation? Does autophagy act as a biomarker in human cancers and their association with the disease prognosis be correlated? Can manipulation of autophagy, inhibition or induction of autophagy can improve the therapeutic outcome in cancer patients? Understanding the molecular mechanism of how autophagy is involved in metabolic reprogramming including glucose and glutamine regulation in cancer is vital? Addressing these few questions in detail will help to better understand the catabolic process of autophagy in cancer. Thus, exploiting autophagy and metabolic process in cancer can be a potential therapeutic option for treating advanced cancers and other diseases.

Acknowledgments S.S.G. is supported by a first-time faculty recruitment award from the Cancer Prevention and Research Institute of Texas (CPRIT; RR170020).

References

Amaravadi R, Kimmelman AC, White E (2016) Recent insights into the function of autophagy in cancer. Genes Dev 30(17):1913–1930

Amaravadi RK, Yu D, Lum JJ, Bui T, Christophorou MA, Evan GI, Thomas-Tikhonenko A, Thompson CB (2007) Autophagy inhibition enhances therapy-induced apoptosis in a Myc-induced model of lymphoma. J Clin Invest 117(2):326–336

Ambrogio C, Nadal E, Villanueva A, Gomez-Lopez G, Cash TP, Barbacid M, Santamaria D (2016) KRAS-driven lung adenocarcinoma: combined DDR1/Notch inhibition as an effective therapy. ESMO Open 1(5):e000076

Amin AD, Peters TL, Li L, Rajan SS, Choudhari R, Puvvada SD, Schatz JH (2017) Diffuse large B-cell lymphoma: can genomics improve treatment options for a curable cancer? Cold Spring Harb Mol Case Stud 3(3):a001719

Anastasiou D, Yu Y, Israelsen WJ, Jiang JK, Boxer MB, Hong BS, Tempel W, Dimov S, Shen M, Jha A, Yang H, Mattaini KR, Metallo CM, Fiske BP, Courtney KD, Malstrom S, Khan TM,

Kung C, Skoumbourdis AP, Veith H, Southall N, Walsh MJ, Brimacombe KR, Leister W, Lunt SY, Johnson ZR, Yen KE, Kunii K, Davidson SM, Christofk HR, Austin CP, Inglese J, Harris MH, Asara JM, Stephanopoulos G, Salituro FG, Jin S, Dang L, Auld DS, Park HW, Cantley LC, Thomas CJ, Vander Heiden MG (2012) Pyruvate kinase M2 activators promote tetramer formation and suppress tumorigenesis. Nat Chem Biol 8(10):839–847

Arico S, Petiot A, Bauvy C, Dubbelhuis PF, Meijer AJ, Codogno P, Ogier-Denis E (2001) The tumor suppressor PTEN positively regulates macroautophagy by inhibiting the phosphatidylinositol 3-kinase/protein kinase B pathway. J Biol Chem 276(38):35243–35246

Arif M, Vedamurthy BM, Choudhari R, Ostwal YB, Mantelingu K, Kodaganur GS, Kundu TK (2010) Nitric oxide-mediated histone hyperacetylation in oral cancer: target for a water-soluble HAT inhibitor, CTK7A. Chem Biol 17(8):903–913

Atsumi T, Chesney J, Metz C, Leng L, Donnelly S, Makita Z, Mitchell R, Bucala R (2002) High expression of inducible 6-phosphofructo-2-kinase/fructose-2,6-bisphosphatase (iPFK-2; PFKFB3) in human cancers. Cancer Res 62(20):5881–5887

Axe EL, Walker SA, Manifava M, Chandra P, Roderick HL, Habermann A, Griffiths G, Ktistakis NT (2008) Autophagosome formation from membrane compartments enriched in phosphatidylinositol 3-phosphate and dynamically connected to the endoplasmic reticulum. J Cell Biol 182(4):685–701

Ayllon V, O'Connor R (2007) PBK/TOPK promotes tumour cell proliferation through p38 MAPK activity and regulation of the DNA damage response. Oncogene 26(24):3451–3461

Bahrami F, Pourgholami MH, Mekkawy AH, Rufener L, Morris DL (2014) Monepantel induces autophagy in human ovarian cancer cells through disruption of the mTOR/p70S6K signalling pathway. Am J Cancer Res 4(5):558–571

Bai H, Li H, Li W, Gui T, Yang J, Cao D, Shen K (2015) The PI3K/AKT/mTOR pathway is a potential predictor of distinct invasive and migratory capacities in human ovarian cancer cell lines. Oncotarget 6(28):25520–25532

Ben-Josef E, Lawrence TS (2008) Chemoradiotherapy for unresectable pancreatic cancer. Int J Clin Oncol 13(2):121–126

Bertolo C, Roa S, Sagardoy A, Mena-Varas M, Robles EF, Martinez-Ferrandis JI, Sagaert X, Tousseyn T, Orta A, Lossos IS, Amar S, Natkunam Y, Briones J, Melnick A, Malumbres R, Martinez-Climent JA (2013) LITAF, a BCL6 target gene, regulates autophagy in mature B-cell lymphomas. Br J Haematol 162(5):621–630

Bray F, Ferlay J, Soerjomataram I, Siegel RL, Torre LA, Jemal A (2018) Global cancer statistics 2018: GLOBOCAN estimates of incidence and mortality worldwide for 36 cancers in 185 countries. CA Cancer J Clin 68(6):394–424

Cagnol S, Chambard JC (2010) ERK and cell death: mechanisms of ERK-induced cell death—apoptosis, autophagy and senescence. FEBS J 277(1):2–21

Cai M, Hu Z, Liu J, Gao J, Liu C, Liu D, Tan M, Zhang D, Lin B (2014) Beclin 1 expression in ovarian tissues and its effects on ovarian cancer prognosis. Int J Mol Sci 15(4):5292–5303

Camacho CV, Choudhari R, Gadad SS (2018) Long noncoding RNAs and cancer, an overview. Steroids 133:93–95

Chang M (2012) Tamoxifen resistance in breast cancer. Biomol Ther (Seoul) 20(3):256–267

Cheng CK, Fan QW, Weiss WA (2009) PI3K signaling in glioma—animal models and therapeutic challenges. Brain Pathol 19(1):112–120

Chiarle R, Voena C, Ambrogio C, Piva R, Inghirami G (2008) The anaplastic lymphoma kinase in the pathogenesis of cancer. Nat Rev Cancer 8(1):11–23

Choi AM, Ryter SW, Levine B (2013) Autophagy in human health and disease. N Engl J Med 368(7):651–662

Choudhari R, Minero VG, Menotti M, Pulito R, Brakebusch C, Compagno M, Voena C, Ambrogio C, Chiarle R (2016) Redundant and nonredundant roles for Cdc42 and Rac1 in lymphomas developed in NPM-ALK transgenic mice. Blood 127(10):1297–1306

Choudhari R, Sedano MJ, Harrison AL, Subramani R, Lin KY, Ramos EI, Lakshmanaswamy R, Gadad SS (2019) Long noncoding RNAs in cancer: from discovery to therapeutic targets. Adv Clin Chem. https://doi.org/10.1016/bs.acc.2019.08.003

Colombo MI (2007) Autophagy: a pathogen driven process. IUBMB Life 59(4–5):238–242
Cook KL, Shajahan AN, Warri A, Jin L, Hilakivi-Clarke LA, Clarke R (2012) Glucose-regulated protein 78 controls cross-talk between apoptosis and autophagy to determine antiestrogen responsiveness. Cancer Res 72(13):3337–3349
Correa RJ, Valdes YR, Shepherd TG, DiMattia GE (2015) Beclin-1 expression is retained in high-grade serous ovarian cancer yet is not essential for autophagy induction in vitro. J Ovarian Res 8:52
Cuervo AM, Wong E (2014) Chaperone-mediated autophagy: roles in disease and aging. Cell Res 24(1):92–104
Degenhardt K, Mathew R, Beaudoin B, Bray K, Anderson D, Chen G, Mukherjee C, Shi Y, Gelinas C, Fan Y, Nelson DA, Jin S, White E (2006) Autophagy promotes tumor cell survival and restricts necrosis, inflammation, and tumorigenesis. Cancer Cell 10(1):51–64
Ding LY, Chu M, Jiao YS, Hao Q, Xiao P, Li HH, Guo Q, Wang YD (2018) TFDP3 regulates the apoptosis and autophagy in breast cancer cell line MDA-MB-231. PLoS One 13(9):e0203833
Eberhardy SR, Farnham PJ (2001) c-Myc mediates activation of the cad promoter via a post-RNA polymerase II recruitment mechanism. J Biol Chem 276(51):48562–48571
Eskelinen EL (2019) Autophagy: supporting cellular and organismal homeostasis by self-eating. Int J Biochem Cell Biol 111:1–10
Ettinger DS, Akerley W, Borghaei H, Chang AC, Cheney RT, Chirieac LR, D'Amico TA, Demmy TL, Govindan R, Grannis FW Jr, Grant SC, Horn L, Jahan TM, Komaki R, Kong FM, Kris MG, Krug LM, Lackner RP, Lennes IT, Loo BW Jr, Martins R, Otterson GA, Patel JD, Pinder-Schenck MC, Pisters KM, Reckamp K, Riely GJ, Rohren E, Shapiro TA, Swanson SJ, Tauer K, Wood DE, Yang SC, Gregory K, Hughes M, National Comprehensive Cancer (2013) Non-small cell lung cancer, version 2.2013. J Natl Compr Cancer Netw 11(6):645–653; quiz 653
Felippe Goncalves-de-Albuquerque C, Ribeiro Silva A, Ignacio da Silva C, Caire Castro-Faria-Neto H, Burth P (2017) Na/K pump and beyond: Na/K-ATPase as a modulator of apoptosis and autophagy. Molecules 22(4). https://doi.org/10.3390/molecules22040578
Friedberg JW (2017) How I treat double-hit lymphoma. Blood 130(5):590–596
Funderburk SF, Wang QJ, Yue Z (2010) The Beclin 1-VPS34 complex—at the crossroads of autophagy and beyond. Trends Cell Biol 20(6):355–362
Galluzzi L, Vicencio JM, Kepp O, Tasdemir E, Maiuri MC, Kroemer G (2008) To die or not to die: that is the autophagic question. Curr Mol Med 8(2):78–91
Gambacorti Passerini C, Farina F, Stasia A, Redaelli S, Ceccon M, Mologni L, Messa C, Guerra L, Giudici G, Sala E, Mussolin L, Deeren D, King MH, Steurer M, Ordemann R, Cohen AM, Grube M, Bernard L, Chiriano G, Antolini L, Piazza R (2014) Crizotinib in advanced, chemoresistant anaplastic lymphoma kinase-positive lymphoma patients. J Natl Cancer Inst 106(2):djt378
Germic N, Frangez Z, Yousefi S, Simon HU (2019) Regulation of the innate immune system by autophagy: monocytes, macrophages, dendritic cells and antigen presentation. Cell Death Differ 26(4):715–727
Guo JY, Chen HY, Mathew R, Fan J, Strohecker AM, Karsli-Uzunbas G, Kamphorst JJ, Chen G, Lemons JM, Karantza V, Coller HA, Dipaola RS, Gelinas C, Rabinowitz JD, White E (2011) Activated Ras requires autophagy to maintain oxidative metabolism and tumorigenesis. Genes Dev 25(5):460–470
Guo JY, Karsli-Uzunbas G, Mathew R, Aisner SC, Kamphorst JJ, Strohecker AM, Chen G, Price S, Lu W, Teng X, Snyder E, Santanam U, Dipaola RS, Jacks T, Rabinowitz JD, White E (2013) Autophagy suppresses progression of K-ras-induced lung tumors to oncocytomas and maintains lipid homeostasis. Genes Dev 27(13):1447–1461
Hamurcu Z, Delibasi N, Gecene S, Sener EF, Donmez-Altuntas H, Ozkul Y, Canatan H, Ozpolat B (2018) Targeting LC3 and Beclin-1 autophagy genes suppresses proliferation, survival, migration and invasion by inhibition of Cyclin-D1 and uPAR/Integrin beta1/ Src signaling in triple negative breast cancer cells. J Cancer Res Clin Oncol 144(3):415–430
Han Y, Fan S, Qin T, Yang J, Sun Y, Lu Y, Mao J, Li L (2018) Role of autophagy in breast cancer and breast cancer stem cells (Review). Int J Oncol 52(4):1057–1070

He C, Klionsky DJ (2009) Regulation mechanisms and signaling pathways of autophagy. Annu Rev Genet 43(1):67–93

Heintz AP, Odicino F, Maisonneuve P, Quinn MA, Benedet JL, Creasman WT, Ngan HY, Pecorelli S, Beller U (2006) Carcinoma of the ovary. FIGO 26th annual report on the results of treatment in gynecological cancer. Int J Gynaecol Obstet 95(Suppl 1):S161–S192

Hinzman CP, Aljehane L, Brown-Clay JD, Kallakury B, Sonahara F, Goel A, Trevino J, Banerjee PP (2018) Aberrant expression of PDZ-binding kinase/T-LAK cell-originated protein kinase modulates the invasive ability of human pancreatic cancer cells via the stabilization of oncoprotein c-MYC. Carcinogenesis 39(12):1548–1559

Huang JJ, Zhu YJ, Lin TY, Jiang WQ, Huang HQ, Li ZM (2011) Beclin 1 expression predicts favorable clinical outcome in patients with diffuse large B-cell lymphoma treated with R-CHOP. Hum Pathol 42(10):1459–1466

Iwadate R, Inoue J, Tsuda H, Takano M, Furuya K, Hirasawa A, Aoki D, Inazawa J (2014) High expression of SQSTM1/p62 protein is associated with poor prognosis in epithelial ovarian cancer. Acta Histochem Cytochem 47(6):295–301

Janku F, McConkey DJ, Hong DS, Kurzrock R (2011) Autophagy as a target for anticancer therapy. Nat Rev Clin Oncol 8(9):528–539

Jemal A, Siegel R, Xu J, Ward E (2010) Cancer statistics, 2010. CA Cancer J Clin 60(5):277–300

Joel M, Mughal AA, Grieg Z, Murrell W, Palmero S, Mikkelsen B, Fjerdingstad HB, Sandberg CJ, Behnan J, Glover JC, Langmoen IA, Stangeland B (2015) Targeting PBK/TOPK decreases growth and survival of glioma initiating cells in vitro and attenuates tumor growth in vivo. Mol Cancer 14:121

Johnson L, Mercer K, Greenbaum D, Bronson RT, Crowley D, Tuveson DA, Jacks T (2001) Somatic activation of the K-ras oncogene causes early onset lung cancer in mice. Nature 410(6832):1111–1116

Kaza N, Kohli L, Roth KA (2012) Autophagy in brain tumors: a new target for therapeutic intervention. Brain Pathol 22(1):89–98

Kiffin R, Christian C, Knecht E, Cuervo AM (2004) Activation of chaperone-mediated autophagy during oxidative stress. Mol Biol Cell 15(11):4829–4840

Kim JY, Cho CH, Song HS (2017) Targeted therapy of ovarian cancer including immune check point inhibitor. Korean J Intern Med 32(5):798–804

Kim KW, Hwang M, Moretti L, Jaboin JJ, Cha YI, Lu B (2008) Autophagy upregulation by inhibitors of caspase-3 and mTOR enhances radiotherapy in a mouse model of lung cancer. Autophagy 4(5):659–668

Kimmelman AC, White E (2017) Autophagy and tumor metabolism. Cell Metab 25(5):1037–1043

Klarer AC, O'Neal J, Imbert-Fernandez Y, Clem A, Ellis SR, Clark J, Clem B, Chesney J, Telang S (2014) Inhibition of 6-phosphofructo-2-kinase (PFKFB3) induces autophagy as a survival mechanism. Cancer Metab 2(1):2

Kohler BA, Ward E, McCarthy BJ, Schymura MJ, Ries LA, Eheman C, Jemal A, Anderson RN, Ajani UA, Edwards BK (2011) Annual report to the nation on the status of cancer, 1975–2007, featuring tumors of the brain and other nervous system. J Natl Cancer Inst 103(9):714–736

Kondo Y, Kanzawa T, Sawaya R, Kondo S (2005) The role of autophagy in cancer development and response to therapy. Nat Rev Cancer 5(9):726–734

Konecny G, Pauletti G, Pegram M, Untch M, Dandekar S, Aguilar Z, Wilson C, Rong HM, Bauerfeind I, Felber M, Wang HJ, Beryt M, Seshadri R, Hepp H, Slamon DJ (2003) Quantitative association between HER-2/neu and steroid hormone receptors in hormone receptor-positive primary breast cancer. J Natl Cancer Inst 95(2):142–153

Kong D, Ma S, Liang B, Yi H, Zhao Y, Xin R, Cui L, Jia L, Liu X, Liu X (2012) The different regulatory effects of p53 status on multidrug resistance are determined by autophagy in ovarian cancer cells. Biomed Pharmacother 66(4):271–278

Lee IH, Cao L, Mostoslavsky R, Lombard DB, Liu J, Bruns NE, Tsokos M, Alt FW, Finkel T (2008) A role for the NAD-dependent deacetylase Sirt1 in the regulation of autophagy. Proc Natl Acad Sci U S A 105(9):3374–3379

Lee MH, Koh D, Na H, Ka NL, Kim S, Kim HJ, Hong S, Shin YK, Seong JK, Lee MO (2018) MTA1 is a novel regulator of autophagy that induces tamoxifen resistance in breast cancer cells. Autophagy 14(5):812–824

Levine B, Kroemer G (2008) Autophagy in the pathogenesis of disease. Cell 132(1):27–42

Li YJ, Lei YH, Yao N, Wang CR, Hu N, Ye WC, Zhang DM, Chen ZS (2017) Autophagy and multidrug resistance in cancer. Chin J Cancer 36(1):52

Li D, Xie K, Wolff R, Abbruzzese JL (2004) Pancreatic cancer. Lancet 363(9414):1049–1057

Li Y, Zhou X, Zhang Y, Yang J, Xu Y, Zhao Y, Wang X (2019) CUL4B regulates autophagy via JNK signaling in diffuse large B-cell lymphoma. Cell Cycle 18(4):379–394

Lin Y, Kuang W, Wu B, Xie C, Liu C, Tu Z (2017) IL-12 induces autophagy in human breast cancer cells through AMPK and the PI3K/Akt pathway. Mol Med Rep 16(4):4113–4118

Lin J, Xia L, Liang J, Han Y, Wang H, Oyang L, Tan S, Tian Y, Rao S, Chen X, Tang Y, Su M, Luo X, Wang Y, Wang H, Zhou Y, Liao Q (2019) The roles of glucose metabolic reprogramming in chemo- and radio-resistance. J Exp Clin Cancer Res 38(1):218

Liu C, Sun L, Yang J, Liu T, Yang Y, Kim SM, Ou X, Wang Y, Sun L, Zaidi M, New MI, Yuen T, Guo Q (2018) FSIP1 regulates autophagy in breast cancer. Proc Natl Acad Sci U S A 115(51):13075–13080

Lock R, Roy S, Kenific CM, Su JS, Salas E, Ronen SM, Debnath J (2011) Autophagy facilitates glycolysis during Ras-mediated oncogenic transformation. Mol Biol Cell 22(2):165–178

Lohinai Z, Klikovits T, Moldvay J, Ostoros G, Raso E, Timar J, Fabian K, Kovalszky I, Kenessey I, Aigner C, Renyi-Vamos F, Klepetko W, Dome B, Hegedus B (2017) KRAS-mutation incidence and prognostic value are metastatic site-specific in lung adenocarcinoma: poor prognosis in patients with KRAS mutation and bone metastasis. Sci Rep 7:39721

Lozy F, Karantza V (2012) Autophagy and cancer cell metabolism. Semin Cell Dev Biol 23(4):395–401

Lu Z, Luo RZ, Lu Y, Zhang X, Yu Q, Khare S, Kondo S, Kondo Y, Yu Y, Mills GB, Liao WS, Bast RC Jr (2008) The tumor suppressor gene ARHI regulates autophagy and tumor dormancy in human ovarian cancer cells. J Clin Invest 118(12):3917–3929

Lv L, Li D, Zhao D, Lin R, Chu Y, Zhang H, Zha Z, Liu Y, Li Z, Xu Y, Wang G, Huang Y, Xiong Y, Guan KL, Lei QY (2011) Acetylation targets the M2 isoform of pyruvate kinase for degradation through chaperone-mediated autophagy and promotes tumor growth. Mol Cell 42(6):719–730

Ma R, Li X, Liu H, Jiang R, Yang M, Zhang M, Wang Y, Zhao Y, Li H (2019a) GATA6-upregulating autophagy promotes TKI resistance in nonsmall cell lung cancer. Cancer Biol Ther 20(9):1206–1212

Ma H, Li Y, Wang X, Wu H, Qi G, Li R, Yang N, Gao M, Yan S, Yuan C, Kong B (2019b) PBK, targeted by EVI1, promotes metastasis and confers cisplatin resistance through inducing autophagy in high-grade serous ovarian carcinoma. Cell Death Dis 10(3):166

Ma L, Maruwge W, Strambi A, D'Arcy P, Pellegrini P, Kis L, de Milito A, Lain S, Brodin B (2014) SIRT1 and SIRT2 inhibition impairs pediatric soft tissue sarcoma growth. Cell Death Dis 5:e1483

Mammucari C, Milan G, Romanello V, Masiero E, Rudolf R, Del Piccolo P, Burden SJ, Di Lisi R, Sandri C, Zhao J, Goldberg AL, Schiaffino S, Sandri M (2007) FoxO3 controls autophagy in skeletal muscle in vivo. Cell Metab 6(6):458–471

Mannava S, Grachtchouk V, Wheeler LJ, Im M, Zhuang D, Slavina EG, Mathews CK, Shewach DS, Nikiforov MA (2008) Direct role of nucleotide metabolism in C-MYC-dependent proliferation of melanoma cells. Cell Cycle 7(15):2392–2400

Marzec M, Kasprzycka M, Liu X, El-Salem M, Halasa K, Raghunath PN, Bucki R, Wlodarski P, Wasik MA (2007) Oncogenic tyrosine kinase NPM/ALK induces activation of the rapamycin-sensitive mTOR signaling pathway. Oncogene 26(38):5606–5614

McDermott U, Iafrate AJ, Gray NS, Shioda T, Classon M, Maheswaran S, Zhou W, Choi HG, Smith SL, Dowell L, Ulkus LE, Kuhlmann G, Greninger P, Christensen JG, Haber DA, Settleman J (2008) Genomic alterations of anaplastic lymphoma kinase may sensitize tumors to anaplastic lymphoma kinase inhibitors. Cancer Res 68(9):3389–3395

Menotti M, Ambrogio C, Cheong TC, Pighi C, Mota I, Cassel SH, Compagno M, Wang Q, Dall'Olio R, Minero VG, Poggio T, Sharma GG, Patrucco E, Mastini C, Choudhari R, Pich A, Zamo A, Piva R, Giliani S, Mologni L, Collings CK, Kadoch C, Gambacorti-Passerini C, Notarangelo LD, Anton IM, Voena C, Chiarle R (2019) Wiskott-Aldrich syndrome protein (WASP) is a tumor suppressor in T cell lymphoma. Nat Med 25(1):130–140

Mitou G, Frentzel J, Desquesnes A, Le Gonidec S, AlSaati T, Beau I, Lamant L, Meggetto F, Espinos E, Codogno P, Brousset P, Giuriato S (2015) Targeting autophagy enhances the anti-tumoral action of crizotinib in ALK-positive anaplastic large cell lymphoma. Oncotarget 6(30):30149–30164

Mizushima N, Komatsu M (2011) Autophagy: renovation of cells and tissues. Cell 147(4):728–741

Mizushima N, Levine B, Cuervo AM, Klionsky DJ (2008) Autophagy fights disease through cellular self-digestion. Nature 451(7182):1069–1075

Monk BJ, Coleman RL (2009) Changing the paradigm in the treatment of platinum-sensitive recurrent ovarian cancer: from platinum doublets to nonplatinum doublets and adding antiangiogenesis compounds. Int J Gynecol Cancer 19(Suppl 2):S63–S67

Mu N, Lei Y, Wang Y, Wang Y, Duan Q, Ma G, Liu X, Su L (2019) Inhibition of SIRT1/2 upregulates HSPA5 acetylation and induces pro-survival autophagy via ATF4-DDIT4-mTORC1 axis in human lung cancer cells. Apoptosis 4(9–10):798–811

Murakami T, Nishiyama T, Shirotani T, Shinohara Y, Kan M, Ishii K, Kanai F, Nakazuru S, Ebina Y (1992) Identification of two enhancer elements in the gene encoding the type 1 glucose transporter from the mouse which are responsive to serum, growth factor, and oncogenes. J Biol Chem 267(13):9300–9306

Nagelkerke A, Sieuwerts AM, Bussink J, Sweep FC, Look MP, Foekens JA, Martens JW, Span PN (2014) LAMP3 is involved in tamoxifen resistance in breast cancer cells through the modulation of autophagy. Endocr Relat Cancer 21(1):101–112

Nicotra G, Mercalli F, Peracchio C, Castino R, Follo C, Valente G, Isidoro C (2010) Autophagy-active beclin-1 correlates with favourable clinical outcome in non-Hodgkin lymphomas. Mod Pathol 23(7):937–950

Oh S, Xiaofei E, Ni D, Pirooz SD, Lee JY, Lee D, Zhao Z, Lee S, Lee H, Ku B, Kowalik T, Martin SE, Oh BH, Jung JU, Liang C (2011) Downregulation of autophagy by Bcl-2 promotes MCF7 breast cancer cell growth independent of its inhibition of apoptosis. Cell Death Differ 18(3):452–464

Osthus RC, Shim H, Kim S, Li Q, Reddy R, Mukherjee M, Xu Y, Wonsey D, Lee LA, Dang CV (2000) Deregulation of glucose transporter 1 and glycolytic gene expression by c-Myc. J Biol Chem 275(29):21797–21800

Pandareesh MD, Kandikattu HK, Razack S, Amruta N, Choudhari R, Vikram A, Doddapattar P (2018) Nutrition and nutraceuticals in neuroinflammatory and brain metabolic stress: implications for neurodegenerative disorders. CNS Neurol Disord Drug Targets 17(9):680–688

Pavlova NN, Thompson CB (2016) The emerging hallmarks of cancer metabolism. Cell Metab 23(1):27–47

Perera RM, Stoykova S, Nicolay BN, Ross KN, Fitamant J, Boukhali M, Lengrand J, Deshpande V, Selig MK, Ferrone CR, Settleman J, Stephanopoulos G, Dyson NJ, Zoncu R, Ramaswamy S, Haas W, Bardeesy N (2015) Transcriptional control of autophagy-lysosome function drives pancreatic cancer metabolism. Nature 524(7565):361–365

Qadir MA, Kwok B, Dragowska WH, To KH, Le D, Bally MB, Gorski SM (2008) Macroautophagy inhibition sensitizes tamoxifen-resistant breast cancer cells and enhances mitochondrial depolarization. Breast Cancer Res Treat 112(3):389–403

Qu X, Yu J, Bhagat G, Furuya N, Hibshoosh H, Troxel A, Rosen J, Eskelinen EL, Mizushima N, Ohsumi Y, Cattoretti G, Levine B (2003) Promotion of tumorigenesis by heterozygous disruption of the beclin 1 autophagy gene. J Clin Invest 112(12):1809–1820

Qu X, Zou Z, Sun Q, Luby-Phelps K, Cheng P, Hogan RN, Gilpin C, Levine B (2007) Autophagy gene-dependent clearance of apoptotic cells during embryonic development. Cell 128(5):931–946

Racanelli AC, Kikkers SA, Choi AMK, Cloonan SM (2018) Autophagy and inflammation in chronic respiratory disease. Autophagy 14(2):221–232

Ren YA, Mullany LK, Liu Z, Herron AJ, Wong KK, Richards JS (2016) Mutant p53 promotes epithelial ovarian cancer by regulating tumor differentiation, metastasis, and responsiveness to steroid hormones. Cancer Res 76(8):2206–2218

Rikiishi H (2010) Possible role of autophagy in the treatment of pancreatic cancer with histone deacetylase inhibitors. Cancers (Basel) 2(4):2026–2043

Roberts DJ, Tan-Sah VP, Ding EY, Smith JM, Miyamoto S (2014) Hexokinase-II positively regulates glucose starvation-induced autophagy through TORC1 inhibition. Mol Cell 53(4):521–533

Rosenfeldt MT, O'Prey J, Morton JP, Nixon C, MacKay G, Mrowinska A, Au A, Rai TS, Zheng L, Ridgway R, Adams PD, Anderson KI, Gottlieb E, Sansom OJ, Ryan KM (2013) p53 status determines the role of autophagy in pancreatic tumour development. Nature 504(7479):296–300

Ryan DP, Hong TS, Bardeesy N (2014) Pancreatic adenocarcinoma. N Engl J Med 371(11):1039–1049

Sahu R, Kaushik S, Clement CC, Cannizzo ES, Scharf B, Follenzi A, Potolicchio I, Nieves E, Cuervo AM, Santambrogio L (2011) Microautophagy of cytosolic proteins by late endosomes. Dev Cell 20(1):131–139

Samaddar JS, Gaddy VT, Duplantier J, Thandavan SP, Shah M, Smith MJ, Browning D, Rawson J, Smith SB, Barrett JT, Schoenlein PV (2008) A role for macroautophagy in protection against 4-hydroxytamoxifen-induced cell death and the development of antiestrogen resistance. Mol Cancer Ther 7(9):2977–2987

Semenza GL (2010) HIF-1: upstream and downstream of cancer metabolism. Curr Opin Genet Dev 20(1):51–56

Shandilya J, Swaminathan V, Gadad SS, Choudhari R, Kodaganur GS, Kundu TK (2009) Acetylated NPM1 localizes in the nucleoplasm and regulates transcriptional activation of genes implicated in oral cancer manifestation. Mol Cell Biol 29(18):5115–5127

Shen Y, Li DD, Wang LL, Deng R, Zhu XF (2008) Decreased expression of autophagy-related proteins in malignant epithelial ovarian cancer. Autophagy 4(8):1067–1068

Shi WY, Xiao D, Wang L, Dong LH, Yan ZX, Shen ZX, Chen SJ, Chen Y, Zhao WL (2012) Therapeutic metformin/AMPK activation blocked lymphoma cell growth via inhibition of mTOR pathway and induction of autophagy. Cell Death Dis 3:e275

Shintani T, Klionsky DJ (2004) Autophagy in health and disease: a double-edged sword. Science 306(5698):990–995

Siegel RL, Miller KD, Jemal A (2019) Cancer statistics, 2019. CA Cancer J Clin 69(1):7–34

Son J, Lyssiotis CA, Ying H, Wang X, Hua S, Ligorio M, Perera RM, Ferrone CR, Mullarky E, Shyh-Chang N, Kang Y, Fleming JB, Bardeesy N, Asara JM, Haigis MC, DePinho RA, Cantley LC, Kimmelman AC (2013) Glutamine supports pancreatic cancer growth through a KRAS-regulated metabolic pathway. Nature 496(7443):101–105

Strohecker AM, Guo JY, Karsli-Uzunbas G, Price SM, Chen GJ, Mathew R, McMahon M, White E (2013) Autophagy sustains mitochondrial glutamine metabolism and growth of BrafV600E-driven lung tumors. Cancer Discov 3(11):1272–1285

Sun M, Gadad SS, Kim DS, Kraus WL (2015) Discovery, annotation, and functional analysis of long noncoding RNAs controlling cell-cycle gene expression and proliferation in breast cancer cells. Mol Cell 59(4):698–711

Sun H, Huang Z, Sheng W, Xu MD (2018a) Emerging roles of long non-coding RNAs in tumor metabolism. J Hematol Oncol 11(1):106

Sun WL, Wang L, Luo J, Zhu HW, Cai ZW (2018b) Ambra1 modulates the sensitivity of breast cancer cells to epirubicin by regulating autophagy via ATG12. Cancer Sci 109(10):3129–3138

Tanaka K, Sasayama T, Irino Y, Takata K, Nagashima H, Satoh N, Kyotani K, Mizowaki T, Imahori T, Ejima Y, Masui K, Gini B, Yang H, Hosoda K, Sasaki R, Mischel PS, Kohmura E (2015) Compensatory glutamine metabolism promotes glioblastoma resistance to mTOR inhibitor treatment. J Clin Invest 125(4):1591–1602

Thumm M, Egner R, Koch B, Schlumpberger M, Straub M, Veenhuis M, Wolf DH (1994) Isolation of autophagocytosis mutants of Saccharomyces cerevisiae. FEBS Lett 349(2):275–280

Torre LA, Trabert B, DeSantis CE, Miller KD, Samimi G, Runowicz CD, Gaudet MM, Jemal A, Siegel RL (2018) Ovarian cancer statistics, 2018. CA Cancer J Clin 68(4):284–296

Trenti A, Grumati P, Cusinato F, Orso G, Bonaldo P, Trevisi L (2014) Cardiac glycoside ouabain induces autophagic cell death in non-small cell lung cancer cells via a JNK-dependent decrease of Bcl-2. Biochem Pharmacol 89(2):197–209

True O, Matthias P (2012) Interplay between histone deacetylases and autophagy—from cancer therapy to neurodegeneration. Immunol Cell Biol 90(1):78–84

Van Cutsem E, van de Velde H, Karasek P, Oettle H, Vervenne WL, Szawlowski A, Schoffski P, Post S, Verslype C, Neumann H, Safran H, Humblet Y, Perez Ruixo J, Ma Y, Von Hoff D (2004) Phase III trial of gemcitabine plus tipifarnib compared with gemcitabine plus placebo in advanced pancreatic cancer. J Clin Oncol 22(8):1430–1438

Van Meir EG, Hadjipanayis CG, Norden AD, Shu HK, Wen PY, Olson JJ (2010) Exciting new advances in neuro-oncology: the avenue to a cure for malignant glioma. CA Cancer J Clin 60(3):166–193

Vander Heiden MG, Cantley LC, Thompson CB (2009) Understanding the Warburg effect: the metabolic requirements of cell proliferation. Science 324(5930):1029–1033

Vander Heiden MG, DeBerardinis RJ (2017) Understanding the intersections between metabolism and cancer biology. Cell 168(4):657–669

Verhaak RG, Hoadley KA, Purdom E, Wang V, Qi Y, Wilkerson MD, Miller CR, Ding L, Golub T, Mesirov JP, Alexe G, Lawrence M, O'Kelly M, Tamayo P, Weir BA, Gabriel S, Winckler W, Gupta S, Jakkula L, Feiler HS, Hodgson JG, James CD, Sarkaria JN, Brennan C, Kahn A, Spellman PT, Wilson RK, Speed TP, Gray JW, Meyerson M, Getz G, Perou CM, Hayes DN, Cancer Genome Atlas Research Network (2010) Integrated genomic analysis identifies clinically relevant subtypes of glioblastoma characterized by abnormalities in PDGFRA, IDH1, EGFR, and NF1. Cancer Cell 17(1):98–110

Wang C, Jiang J, Ji J, Cai Q, Chen X, Yu Y, Zhu Z, Zhang J (2017a) PKM2 promotes cell migration and inhibits autophagy by mediating PI3K/AKT activation and contributes to the malignant development of gastric cancer. Sci Rep 7(1):2886

Wang M, Zhang J, Huang Y, Ji S, Shao G, Feng S, Chen D, Zhao K, Wang Z, Wu A (2017b) Cancer-associated fibroblasts autophagy enhances progression of triple-negative breast cancer cells. Med Sci Monit 23:3904–3912

Wei Y, Pattingre S, Sinha S, Bassik M, Levine B (2008) JNK1-mediated phosphorylation of Bcl-2 regulates starvation-induced autophagy. Mol Cell 30(6):678–688

Weinberg SE, Chandel NS (2015) Targeting mitochondria metabolism for cancer therapy. Nat Chem Biol 11(1):9–15

Wen ZP, Zeng WJ, Chen YH, Li H, Wang JY, Cheng Q, Yu J, Zhou HH, Liu ZZ, Xiao J, Chen XP (2019) Knockdown ATG4C inhibits gliomas progression and promotes temozolomide chemosensitivity by suppressing autophagic flux. J Exp Clin Cancer Res 38(1):298

White E (2012) Deconvoluting the context-dependent role for autophagy in cancer. Nat Rev Cancer 12(6):401–410

Williams T, Forsberg LJ, Viollet B, Brenman JE (2009) Basal autophagy induction without AMP-activated protein kinase under low glucose conditions. Autophagy 5(8):1155–1165

Wise DR, DeBerardinis RJ, Mancuso A, Sayed N, Zhang XY, Pfeiffer HK, Nissim I, Daikhin E, Yudkoff M, McMahon SB, Thompson CB (2008) Myc regulates a transcriptional program that stimulates mitochondrial glutaminolysis and leads to glutamine addiction. Proc Natl Acad Sci U S A 105(48):18782–18787

Wojtkowiak JW, Rothberg JM, Kumar V, Schramm KJ, Haller E, Proemsey JB, Lloyd MC, Sloane BF, Gillies RJ (2012) Chronic autophagy is a cellular adaptation to tumor acidic pH microenvironments. Cancer Res 72(16):3938–3947

Xu L, Zhang X, Li Y, Lu S, Lu S, Li J, Wang Y, Tian X, Wei JJ, Shao C, Liu Z (2016) Neferine induces autophagy of human ovarian cancer cells via p38 MAPK/ JNK activation. Tumour Biol 37(7):8721–8729

Yan J, Zhang J, Zhang X, Li X, Li L, Li Z, Chen R, Zhang L, Wu J, Wang X, Sun Z, Fu X, Chang Y, Nan F, Yu H, Wu X, Feng X, Li W, Zhang M (2018) AEG-1 is involved in hypoxia-induced autophagy and decreases chemosensitivity in T-cell lymphoma. Mol Med 24(1):35

Yang ZJ, Chee CE, Huang S, Sinicrope FA (2011a) The role of autophagy in cancer: therapeutic implications. Mol Cancer Ther 10(9):1533–1541

Yang S, Imamura Y, Jenkins RW, Canadas I, Kitajima S, Aref A, Brannon A, Oki E, Castoreno A, Zhu Z, Thai T, Reibel J, Qian Z, Ogino S, Wong KK, Baba H, Kimmelman AC, Pasca Di Magliano M, Barbie DA (2016) Autophagy inhibition dysregulates TBK1 signaling and promotes pancreatic inflammation. Cancer Immunol Res 4(6):520–530

Yang A, Rajeshkumar NV, Wang X, Yabuuchi S, Alexander BM, Chu GC, Von Hoff DD, Maitra A, Kimmelman AC (2014) Autophagy is critical for pancreatic tumor growth and progression in tumors with p53 alterations. Cancer Discov 4(8):905–913

Yang S, Wang X, Contino G, Liesa M, Sahin E, Ying H, Bause A, Li Y, Stommel JM, Dell'antonio G, Mautner J, Tonon G, Haigis M, Shirihai OS, Doglioni C, Bardeesy N, Kimmelman AC (2011b) Pancreatic cancers require autophagy for tumor growth. Genes Dev 25(7):717–729

Ying H, Qu D, Liu C, Ying T, Lv J, Jin S, Xu H (2015) Chemoresistance is associated with Beclin-1 and PTEN expression in epithelial ovarian cancers. Oncol Lett 9(4):1759–1763

Ying H, Dey P, Yao W, Kimmelman AC, Draetta GF, Maitra A, DePinho RA (2016) Genetics and biology of pancreatic ductal adenocarcinoma. Genes Dev 30(4):355–385

Youle RJ, Narendra DP (2011) Mechanisms of mitophagy. Nat Rev Mol Cell Biol 12(1):9–14

Yu L, Alva A, Su H, Dutt P, Freundt E, Welsh S, Baehrecke EH, Lenardo MJ (2004) Regulation of an ATG7-beclin 1 program of autophagic cell death by caspase-8. Science 304(5676):1500–1502

Zhan L, Zhang Y, Wang W, Song E, Fan Y, Li J, Wei B (2016) Autophagy as an emerging therapy target for ovarian carcinoma. Oncotarget 7(50):83476–83487

Zhang L, Ma T, Brozick J, Babalola K, Budiu R, Tseng G, Vlad AM (2016) Effects of Kras activation and Pten deletion alone or in combination on MUC1 biology and epithelial-to-mesenchymal transition in ovarian cancer. Oncogene 35(38):5010–5020

Zhang Q, Zhang Y, Zhang P, Chao Z, Xia F, Jiang C, Zhang X, Jiang Z, Liu H (2014) Hexokinase II inhibitor, 3-BrPA induced autophagy by stimulating ROS formation in human breast cancer cells. Genes Cancer 5(3–4):100–112

Zi D, Zhou ZW, Yang YJ, Huang L, Zhou ZL, He SM, He ZX, Zhou SF (2015) Danusertib induces apoptosis, cell cycle arrest, and autophagy but inhibits epithelial to mesenchymal transition involving PI3K/Akt/mTOR signaling pathway in human ovarian cancer cells. Int J Mol Sci 16(11):27228–27251

Role of c-Met/HGF Axis in Altered Cancer Metabolism

7

Vaishali Chandel, Sibi Raj, Ramesh Choudhari,
and Dhruv Kumar

Abstract

c-Met (mesenchymal–epithelial transition factor) is a receptor tyrosine kinase that belongs to the Met family and is majorly expressed on the surfaces of epithelial cells. Hepatocyte growth factor (HGF) is the receptor specific to c-Met. HGF binding to c-Met leads to the initiation of series of cascade mediating wound healing and embryogenesis. However, in cancer cells, mutation in c-Met stimulates various downstream signalling pathways such as PI3K/AKT, Ras/MAPK, and JAK/STAT, causing aberrant c-Met/HGF axis activation and resulting in development and progression through migration, invasion, and metabolic reprogramming in cancer. c-Met/HGF axis modulates glucose metabolism in cancer by altering major enzymes and transporters such as hexokinase, phosphofructokinase, lactate dehydrogenase, and glucose transporters and shifts the reliance of cancer cells on glucose rather than oxidative phosphorylation even in the presence of oxygen (Warburg phenomena). In addition, c-Met/HGF axis modulates and interferes with other pathways such as pentose phosphate pathway, amino acid metabolism, and TCA cycle leading to its aggressive phenotypes. Therefore, understanding the association between c-Met/ HGF axis and signalling pathways is critical and clinically important to develop

The original version of this chapter was revised with the correction received from the author. The correction to this chapter can be found at https://doi.org/10.1007/978-981-15-1991-8_12

V. Chandel · S. Raj · D. Kumar (✉)
Amity Institute of Molecular Medicine & Stem Cell Research (AIMMSCR), Amity University Uttar Pradesh (AUUP), Noida, Uttar Pradesh, India
e-mail: dkumar13@amity.edu

R. Choudhari
Center of Emphasis in Cancer Research, Department of Molecular and Translational Medicine, Paul L. Foster School of Medicine, Texas Tech University Health Sciences Center El Paso, El Paso, TX, USA

Shri B. M. Patil Medical College, Hospital and Research Centre, BLDE (Deemed to be University), Vijayapur, India

D. Kumar (ed.), *Cancer Cell Metabolism: A Potential Target for Cancer Therapy*,
https://doi.org/10.1007/978-981-15-1991-8_7

therapeutic drugs. In this chapter, we discuss the molecular structure of HGF and c-Met and the mechanism through which this axis interacts and activates other signalling pathways involved in metabolic reprogramming of cancer cells.

Keywords
HGF · c-Met · PI3K · Akt · Cancer metabolism

7.1 Introduction

c-Met (mesenchymal–epithelial transition factor) belongs to the family of MET and is a receptor tyrosine kinase which is expressed on the surfaces of various epithelial cells. Hepatocyte growth factor (HGF) is the ligand for c-Met (Fu et al. 2017; Salgia 2017). HGF is a member of plasminogen-related growth factor and belongs to the family of cytokines. It acts through a paracrine mechanism and synthesized majorly by fibroblasts, mesenchymal cells, and smooth muscle cells to activate the c-Met/HGF signalling pathway to exert various biological functions (Rucki et al. 2018). Tumor-associated factors (TAF) are the major source of HGF in the tumor microenvironment. c-Met, a proto-oncogene, is responsible for mediating the development and progression of majority cancers such as lung, colon, liver, prostate, ovarian, gastric, and pancreatic carcinomas through migration, invasion, and metabolic reprogramming in cancer cells (Bender et al. 2016; Kim et al. 2016). The c-Met/HGF axis cooperates synergistically with other tyrosine kinases to induce downstream signalling pathways, including PI3K/AKT/mTOR, Ras/MAPK, and STAT3 (Imura et al. 2016; Liang et al. 2017) responsible for metabolic reprogramming in cancer cells to modulate glycolytic enzymes, amino acid metabolism, pentose phosphate pathway (PPP), etc. Additionally, these signalling pathways provide an advantage to cancer cells for proliferation, migration, invasion, metastasis, epithelial–mesenchymal transition, and angiogenesis (Hughes et al. 2016; Kuang et al. 2017; Leung et al. 2016; Qamsari et al. 2017). It has been reported that higher c-Met expression is directly related to poor prognosis in cancer patients (Yan et al. 2015). The metabolic shift from oxidative phosphorylation (OXPHOS) to anaerobic glycolysis is a major hallmark of cancer cells in order to meet their energy demands and biosynthetic intermediates for the rapid cell proliferation (Coppock et al. 2013; Gillies et al. 2008; Hamanaka and Chandel 2012; Noch and Khalili 2012). Cancer cells utilize glucose even in the presence of oxygen (Warburg phenomena). Glycolysis provides an added advantage to cancer cells for survival, independent supply of oxygen and potential to detoxify chemotherapeutic drugs and free radicals. Also, glycolytic pathway products such as pyruvate and lactate have been shown to promote and confer radio resistance (Kumar 2017).

Studies have shown that c-Met is the major proto-oncogene involved in resistance to targeted therapies and the drugs that target the associated signalling pathways altering metabolism in cancer. Therefore, it is very important to understand c-Met/HGF axis in cancer metabolism to treat the difficulty associated with tumor treatment (Caenepeel et al. 2017; Zhu et al. 2016).

7.2 c-Met and HGF Structure

MET, the gene encoding c-Met, includes 20 introns and 21 exons and is located on chromosome 7 (7q21-q31) (Zhang et al. 2018). c-Met is a single pass tyrosine kinase receptor consisting of an alpha subunit (45 kDa) and a beta subunit (145-kDa) linked via disulfide bonds (Hartmann et al. 2016; Zhang et al. 2018). The transmembrane chain consists of a sema homology region (SEMA), a plexin-semaphorin-integrin (PSI) domain, four immunoglobulin-like regions in plexins and transcription factors (IPT) domains, a transmembrane domain, a juxtamembrane domain, a tyrosine kinase domain (TK) domain, and a C-terminal docking site (carboxyl terminal; CT) (Zhang et al. 2018). HGF binds to SEMA site on c-Met and PSI is responsible for the stabilization of this interaction (Zhang et al. 2018). At the juxtamembrane domain, Ser-975 and Tyr-1003 sites play a key role in the negative regulation of c-Met (Hass et al. 2017; Qamsari et al. 2017; Yin et al. 2017). HGF binding to c-Met leads to the dimerization and further autophosphorylation of three tyrosine residues (Y1230, Y1234, Y1235) (Ferracinis et al. 1991). This initial phosphorylation cascade causes the phosphorylation of two other tyrosine residues (Y1349, Y1356) in the C-terminal docking site. This serves as the docking sites for downstream signalling pathways such as PI3K/Akt/mTOR, Ras/Raf, STAT3, and Wnt/β-catenin (Hartmann et al. 2016; Hughes et al. 2016; Wu et al. 2016). The HGF encodes a protein consisting of six domains of 728 KDa located on human chromosome 7 and consists of 17 introns and 18 exons. HGF is a heterodimer consisting of an α chain (69 kDa) and a β chain (34 kDa) linked by a disulfide bond (Zhang et al. 2018) (Fig. 7.1).

7.3 c-Met/HGF Signalling Cascade in Cancer Metabolism

HGF binding to c-Met initiates various downstream signalling pathways resulting in metabolic reprogramming in cancer cells (Fig. 7.2).

7.3.1 c-Met/HGF and PI3K Signalling

The activation of c-Met by HGF binding causes autophosphorylation of c-Met and acts as a docking site for phosphatidylinositol-3-kinase (PI3K-p85) subunit. The p85 subunit binds to SH2/SH3 domain, an adaptor protein at the same phosphorylated site. Recruitment of more activated receptors by PI3K initiates a cascade of many phosphatidylinositol intermediates. PI3K is responsible for converting phosphatidylinositol-4, 5-diphosphate (PIP2) to phosphatidylinositol-3,4,5-trisphosphate (PIP3) in tumor-associated signalling cascade. The association between signalling proteins and PIP3 having a PH domain known as Akt (protein kinase B) and PDK1 leads to the phosphorylation of Akt at Ser-473 and at Thr-308 by PDK1 (Birchmeier and Rosa 2003). Akt activation causes its translocation to cell nucleus, altering the downstream transcription factors, for example, Bcl-2 and NF-κB to inhibit the

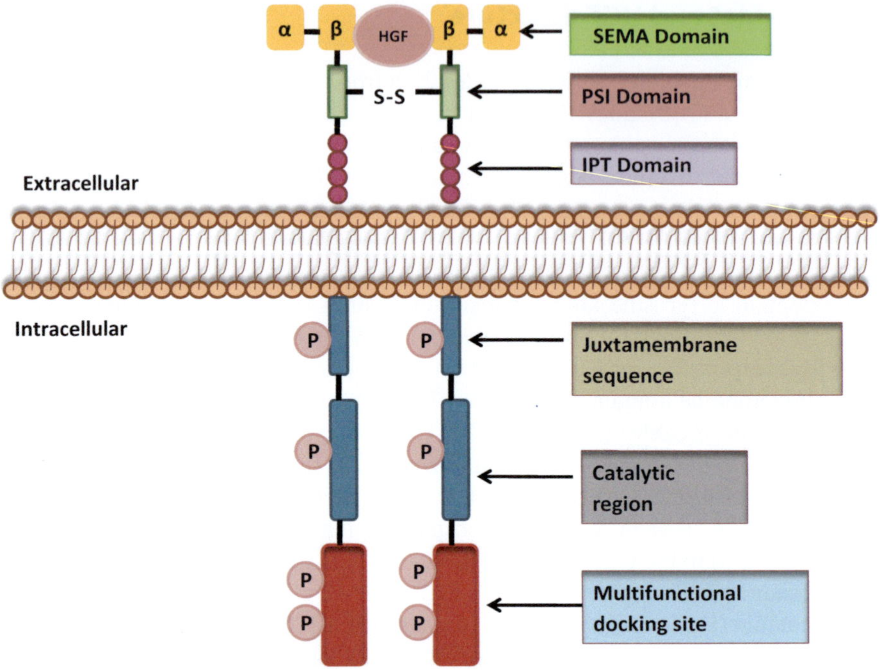

Fig. 7.1 Structure of c-Met and HGF. c-Met is a single pass tyrosine kinase receptor consisting of an extracellular α subunit and transmembrane β subunit linked via disulfide bonds. The β subunit consists of a SEMA domain, a PSI domain, four IPT domains, a transmembrane domain, a juxtamembrane domain, a tyrosine kinase domain, and a C-terminal tail region. HGF is a heterodimer consisting of an α subunit and a β subunit. HGF binds to SEMA site on c-Met and PSI stabilizes this interaction. *c-Met* mesenchymal–epithelial transition, *SEMA* sema homology region, *PSI* plexin-semaphorin-integrin, *IPT* immunoglobulin-like regions in plexins and transcription factors, *HGF* hepatocyte growth factor

expression of tumor suppressor genes. Additionally, Akt phosphorylates glycogen synthase kinase 3 (GSK-3) and mammalian target of rapamycin (mTOR) that plays an important role in various cellular processes during cell cycle and metabolic alteration, causing tumorigenesis (Shaw and Cantley 2006). Furthermore, RTKs are also responsible for activating PI3K/Akt pathway via Ras. c-Met/HGF driven PI3K signalling pathway plays a major role in various cellular processes such as cell survival, inflammation, metabolism, motility, and progression of cancer (Vanhaesebroeck et al. 2010). Studies have shown that PI3K signalling pathway regulates the uptake of glucose via Akt activation, and enhances the expression of glucose transporters (GLUT) and captures glucose inside the cell and stimulates the activity of phosphofructokinase (PFK). DeBerardinis et al. (2008) suggested that c-Met/HGF signalling activated PI3K causes cancer cells to become more reliant on higher levels of glucose. Furthermore, c-Met activated PI3K signalling inhibits pyruvate kinase preventing the entry of pyruvate to mitochondria to initiate TCA cycle (Martini et al. 2014), causing increased glycolysis in cancer cells and

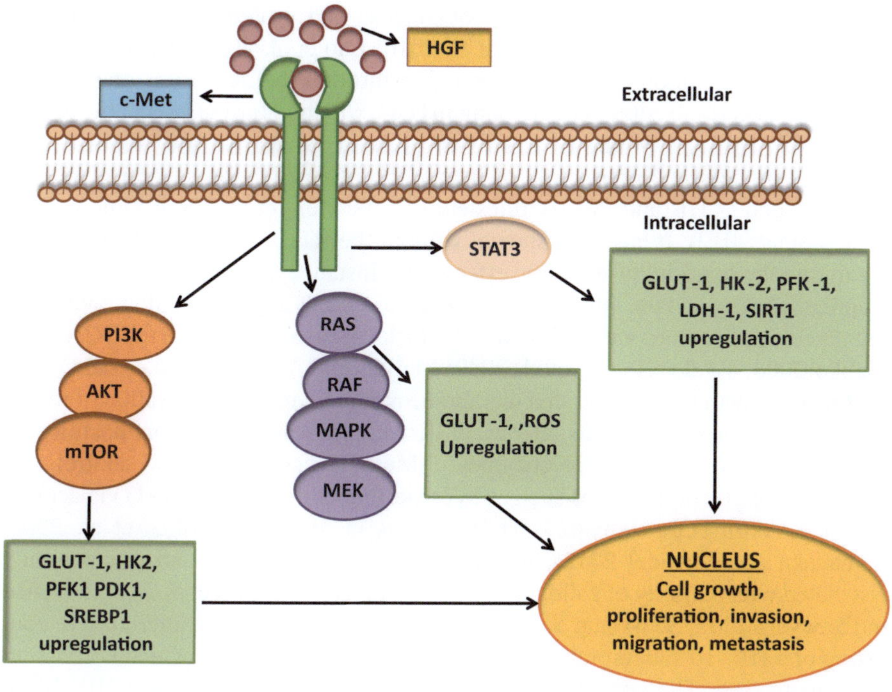

Fig. 7.2 c-Met/HGF signalling axis. HGF binding to c-Met activates PI3K/Akt/mTOR, Ras/MAPK, and STAT3 signalling pathways involved in metabolic reprogramming of cancer cells. The activation of these pathways upregulates several enzymes, transporters, and factors (GLUT1, HKII, PFK1, PDK1, SREBP1, ROS, MDH-1, SIRT-1) involved in modulating cancer metabolism resulting in progression and development of cancer through proliferation, migration, and invasion. *HGF* hepatocyte growth factor, *c-Met* mesenchymal–epithelial transition, *GLUT1* glucose transporter 1, *HKII* hexokinase II, *PFK1* phosphofructokinase, *PDK1* pyruvate dehydrogenase kinase 1, *SREBP1* sterol response element-binding protein, *ROS* reactive oxygen species, *SIRT1* silent mating type information regulation 2 homolog

following Warburg phenomena. Activation of Akt by c-Met is responsible in regulating cell cycle progression, cell death, and growth as well as influencing the rate of glucose uptake into the cell through GLUT1 transporter. Previously reports have shown that upregulated Akt levels and its activation have a direct correlation with increased glycolysis in cancer cells compared to normal cells (Simons et al. 2011). Akt also influences glycolysis by modulating various substrates involved in glycolysis such as HKII and PFK (Dang 2012). Additionally, Akt causes the activation of Forkhead box protein O (FOXO) to disrupt apoptosis and increase OXPHOS to support growing cell by the generation of ATP (Dang 2012). Therefore c-Met activated PI3K/Atk signalling causes modulation in glycolytic process and alters metabolism (Hein et al. 2009).

Hexokinase is the first rate-limiting enzyme mediating the conversion of glucose to glucose 6-phosphate (G6P). In the cytosol, Akt leads to the phosphorylation of mammalian target of rapamycin (mTOR) and phosphorylate tuberous sclerosis

(TSC) factor 2 activating metabolism of glucose and protein translation (Cairns et al. 2011; Goetze et al. 2011; Lien et al. 2016; Luo et al. 2015). In addition, Akt promotes the activation of lactate production through the activation of PFK and HK. Akt is also responsible for activating mTOR, which in turn results in the activation of HIF-1. It also promotes activity of glucose transporter and stimulates the glycolytic process and production of lactate through activating several glycolytic enzymes such as HK and PFK (Gillies et al. 2008; Hein et al. 2009; Simons et al. 2011; Zheng 2012). It has been shown, without the RTKs activation, lactate alone can mimic the majority of the same effects. For instance, the expression of HIF-1α is upregulated by lactate, which in turn enhances GLUT expression along with several glycolytic enzymes and PDK1, which blocks pyruvate entry into the TCA cycle (Denko 2008; Vander Heiden et al. 2009; Meijer et al. 2012; Semenza 2011). The binding of growth factor to plasma membrane receptors initiates activation of receptor tyrosine kinases (RTKs) to activate PI3K/Akt pathway. In addition, posttranslational regulation of glycolytic enzymes, c-Met/HGF signalling also controls the expression of glycolytic genes such as hypoxia-inducible factor (HIF-1) via activating PI3K/Akt/mTOR signalling (DeBerardinis et al. 2008; Gillies et al. 2008; Hamanaka and Chandel 2012). Increased level of HIF-1α protein is commonly associated with majority of solid tumors (Cai et al. 2017; Brown et al. 2001; Vivanco and Sawyers 2002; Sen-xiang Yan et al. 2013). HIF-1 is a heterodimer protein consisting of a HIF-1α subunit regulated by O_2 and a HIF-1β subunit which is constitutively expressed. The stability of the subunits of HIF-1 (HIF-1α and HIF-1β) is regulated by prolyl hydroxylase domain (PHD) protein family (Gillies et al. 2008). Under normoxia, HIF-1α is rapidly degraded because of hydroxylation of HIF-1α by prolyl hydroxylase domain 2 (PHD2) creating a binding site for a tumor suppressor protein von Hippel-Lindau (VHL), an E3 ubiquitin ligase complex that promotes rapid degradation of HIF-1α (Meijer et al. 2012). Under the hypoxic condition, the activity of PHD is inhibited by mutations in PI3K/Akt/mTOR pathway as well as von Hippel-Lindau protein; thus inhibiting proteasomal degradation of HIF-1α by reactive oxygen and nitrogen species leads to the stabilization and accumulation of HIF-1α. Post the stabilization of HIF-1α complex, it binds specifically to the hypoxia response elements (HRE) present in the promoter region of target genes which activates transcription of multiple genes involved in glycolytic metabolism such as HK, GLUT1 and GLUT3, LDH, phosphoglycerate kinase as well as for pH regulation such as carbonic anhydrase IX (CAIX) and Na+/H+ exchanger 1 (NHE1) (Gillies et al. 2008; Krupar et al. 2014; Sandulache and Myers 2012; Semenza 2011; Xu et al. 2005). c-Met/HGF signalling activated PI3K/Akt/mTOR network not only is responsible for stimulating the Warburg phenomena mediating aerobic glycolysis but also coordinates synergistically with its downstream anabolic processes for metabolite synthesis required for malignant growth and proliferation enhancing tumorigenesis (Kim et al. 2016; Zhang et al. 2018).

Pentose phosphate pathway (PPP) branches off from glycolysis and uses glucose-6-phosphate dehydrogenase (G6PD), the intermediate to generate nicotinamide adenine dinucleotide phosphate (NADPH) which is responsible for generating nucleotides for tumor cell survival and proliferation. mTOR activation upregulates the expression of several genes such as G6PD, ribulose 5-phosphate isomerase (RPIA), 6-phosphogluconate dehydrogenase (PGD), ribulose 5-phosphate epimerase (RPE), and transaldolase 1 (TALDO1) (Duvel et al. 2010). Amino acids stimulate mTOR and activate the synthesis of protein via its translation effects and biogenesis of ribosomes (Noch and Khalili 2012). The majority of nonessential amino acids are generated through the transamination reactions. Aggressive tumor cells utilize glutamine generated from transamination reaction for proliferation (Hensley et al. 2013). Together, a large glutamate pool is generated for the synthesis of nonessential amino acid. Both the glutaminase activity and glutamine uptake are stimulated by activation of mTOR, providing glutamate for the maintenance of TCA cycle and contributing the synthesis of amino acids to tumor cells. Fatty acid synthesis is regulated by transcription of Sterol Response Element-Binding Protein (SREBP-1) (Horton et al. 2002). SREBP-1 is responsible for regulating enzymes required for conversion of acetyl-coA into fatty acids as well as the enzymes involved in PPP. Cancer cells constitutively express enhanced rate of fatty acids. c-Met/HGF activated mTOR signalling through its effector S6 kinase activates SREBP-1 and SREBP-2 regulates the transcription of genes involved in sterol biosynthesis involved in cellular proliferation and aggressiveness (Duvel et al. 2010).

7.3.2 c-Met/HGF and the Ras Signalling

Interaction of HGF with receptor tyrosine kinase, c-Met induces structural changes, which leads to the activation and autophosphorylation of intracellular tyrosine kinase domain, resulting in the exposure of multisubstrate docking site (MDS), further directing the Grb2 protein to recruit at MDS site (Birchmeier and Rosa 2003). After autophosphorylation, the SH2/SH3 domain binds to Grb2 leading to the subsequent recruitment of other downstream factors such as guanine nucleotide exchange factors (GEFs). Furthermore, these GEFs, for example, SOS, are responsible for recruiting Ras-GDP from the matrix of the cell membrane and convert it to active Ras-GTP. Ras mediates the activation of Raf, MEK, MAPKs, JNK, ERK, and p38 (HOG), and then the activated MAPKs enter the nucleus of the cell to activate the transcription factors such as c-Myc, Etsl, and Elk1 through phosphorylation (Yin et al. 2017). Further, leads to the interference with various cellular processes including cellular transformation, metabolic reprogramming promoting carcinogenesis (Caenepeel et al. 2017; Kuang et al. 2017). MAPKs are also responsible for the degradation of matrix proteins, enhancing cell migration and sustaining proliferation of the tumor (Liebmann 2001; Wang et al. 2017). Various studies have been reported that the mutated RAS increases the expression of GLUT1 along with HK, a rate-limiting enzyme in glycolysis and LDH which converts pyruvate to lactate. It has also been shown that mutated KRAS maintains the growth of the tumor by mediating the uptake of glucose and channelling the intermediates of glycolysis into the PPP by ribose production and hexosamine biosynthesis pathway (HBP) by promoting glycosylation of protein (Ying et al. 2012). It has been demonstrated that knockdown of PPP gene (*Rpia* or *Rpe* and HBP *Gfpt1*) causes the inhibition of Ras-dependent growth of the tumor in vivo, suggesting that they can be used as a potential therapeutic target (Kawada et al. 2017). In colorectal carcinoma, mutation in KRAS enhanced the transport of glucose associated with increased production of lactate, although OXPHOS was not hampered (Yun et al. 2010). A glycolytic inhibitor known as 3-bromopyruvate (3-BrPA) was shown to be highly effective on the xenografts derived from colorectal carcinoma cells, suggesting that glycolytic inhibitors can be used to retard tumor growth at doses which are nontoxic to the normal tissues (Kawada et al. 2017). Son et al. (2013) reported that mutation in KRAS in pancreatic ductal cell adenocarcinoma regulates the metabolism of glutamine via its conversion to aspartate, therefore maintaining the redox balance in cells and supporting growth in PDCA mouse models (Son et al. 2013). c-Met/HGF driven signalling through oncogenic KRAS is responsible for maintaining redox balance through NADPH biosynthesis (Kimmelman 2016). KRAS is responsible for regulating the flux whereby mitochondrial aspartate aminotransferase (GOT2) is converted to oxaloacetate by the catalyzation of aspartate aminotransferase (GOT1) (Zhou et al. 2018). Oxaloacetate is then converted to malate dehydrogenase (MDH1) which is then produced to pyruvate and NADPH using malic enzyme (Lyssiotis et al. 2013; Son et al. 2013). Thus, the NADPH produced in this pathway mediates the redox balance in these cells. Another mechanism by which c-Met/HGF axis promotes the redox alteration in cancer is by downregulating NRF2 which is a transcription factor playing a key role in the antioxidant response (Denicola et al. 2012) through KRAS. This causes the metabolic reprogramming in cancer cells by the generation of reactive oxygen species.

7.3.3 c-Met/HGF and STAT3

Signal transducer and activator of transcription (STAT) proteins are a family of transcription factors which are activated by phosphorylation of conserved tyrosine residues in response cytokines and growth factors. The STAT dimers after phosphorylation translocate into the nucleus of the cell activating target genes responsible for various cellular processes such as cell proliferation and development (Williams 2000), abnormal tumorigenesis (Bowman et al. 2000; Bromberg 2002), and metabolic reprogramming and immune response suppression in the tumor microenvironment (Yu et al. 2007). *STAT3* is the most important member of the STAT family responsible for tumorigenesis (Bowman et al. 2000; Bromberg 2002). c-Met/HGF axis activates STAT3 and has been implicated in HGF-induced invasive behavior, metabolic alteration, and morphogenesis (Cheng et al. 2009; Cramer et al. 2005; Tamagnone et al. 2019). HGF promoter region has a STAT3 binding site and is important in STAT3 mediated activation of transcription of HGF (Hung and Elliott 2001; Wojcik et al. 2006). The transcriptional activity of STAT3 has been shown to regulate the metabolic switch in cancer by upregulating the glycolytic enzymes such HK, PFK, and LDH. Thus, enhancing glycolysis, mitochondrial activation, and OXPHOS mimics the Warburg phenomena (Giorgi et al. 2010). c-Met/

HGF signalling axis alters glycolysis through activation of STAT3 by increasing the expression of HIF-1α in the majority of cancers such as kidney, breast, ovary, melanoma, and prostate (Anglesio et al. 2011; Cho et al. 2014; Poliaková et al. 2018; Xu et al. 2005). Sirtuins (NAD^+ dependent deacetylases) also regulate the metabolic activity by c-Met/HGF driven STAT3 signalling. SIRT1 in particular regulates acetylation of STAT3 (Bernier et al. 2011). STAT3 upregulates glycolysis by inhibiting the PRPCK1 and g6pase transcription (Inoue et al. 2006), thereby suppressing gluconeogenesis.

Therefore, it is utmost important to understand the c-Met/HGF axis and its association with PI3K/Akt/mTOR, RAS, STAT pathways which play a major role in the metabolic flexibility and influence response to therapy. Since metabolic rewiring is shaped by mutations in c-Met, understanding the role of these specific signalling pathways affecting various metabolic fluxes will be crucial for the development of novel targeted therapies.

7.4 Targeting c-Met/HGF Axis in Cancer Metabolism

To understand c-Met/HGF signalling and its role in tumor aggressiveness, metastasis, carcinogenesis, altered metabolism, and several therapeutic approaches and agents have been developed to target this axis (Table 7.1).

In an NSCLC model, Met inhibition by PHA-665752 resulted in HKII downregulation which is the rate-limiting enzyme for the initiation of glycolysis (Guo et al. 2010; Poliaková et al. 2018). In addition, inhibition of Met significantly decreased phosphorylated pyruvate kinase isozyme (p-PKM2), a major factor responsible for maintaining the Warburg phenomena in cancer cells (Warburg et al. 1927). Met inhibitor PHA-665752 is also responsible for reducing the expression of glycolysis-related mitochondrial enzymes such as adenine nucleotide translocase 2 (ANT2) and voltage-dependent anion-selective channel protein 1 (VDAC1) in gastric cancer cell lines (Guo et al. 2010). It was previously reported that TIGAR is responsible for inhibiting the regulation of cellular NADPH and apoptosis via the regulation of the pentose phosphate pathway (PPP) (Lui et al. 2011). Lui et al. (2011) showed that in HK1-LMP1 and CNE-2 the two nasopharyngeal cancer cell lines, TP53-induced glycolysis and apoptotic regulator (TIGAR) which regulates glycolysis and apoptosis was downregulated after the treatment with two MET tyrosine kinase inhibitors (AM7) which binds to the kinase linker region and (SU11274) (Lui et al. 2011). Met inhibition impact on glycolysis was confirmed in H1975 NSCLC cancer cells and was monitored in vivo using FDG-PET scanning [56]. In addition, MET inhibitor SU11274 treated xenografts showed a 45% reduction in metabolism of glucose compared to untreated cells (Tang et al. 2008). Tivantinib (ARQ197) which is a small molecule inhibitor targets c-Met in hepatocellular carcinoma promotes apoptosis. A small molecule inhibitor known as Crizotinib (PF-02341066) has been shown to reduce HNSCC growth in vitro and in vivo models (Kumar et al. 2018). Crizotinib is a competitive inhibitor of ATP, and it induces apoptosis and inhibits the proliferation, migration, and invasion of cells in

Table 7.1 Therapeutic agents targeting c-Met

Inhibitor	Target	Major finding	References
PHA-665752	Hexokinase (HKII)	In NSCLC model, downregulation of HKII mediating reduced glycolysis expression	Guo et al. (2010) and Poliaková et al. (2018)
PHA-665752	Adenine nucleotide translocase 2 (ANT2) and voltage-dependent anion selective channel protein 1 (VDAC1)	Reducing the expression of glycolysis-related mitochondrial enzymes	Guo et al. (2010)
AM7	TP53-induced glycolysis and apoptotic regulator (TIGAR)	Downregulation of TIGAR in nasopharyngeal cancer cell lines	Lui et al. (2011)
SU11274	Hexokinase, lactate dehydrogenase, phosphofructokinase	SU11274-treated xenografts showed a 45% reduction in metabolism of glucose compared to untreated cells as control	Tang et al. (2008)
Tivantinib	Colchicine binding pocket	Promotion of angiogenesis in hepatocellular carcinoma	Mossenta et al. (2019)
Crizotinib	CAF-induced hexokinase-2 (HK2)	Reduced CAF-induced hexokinase-2 (HK2) levels and downregulation of HGF-induced lactate secretion from HNSCC	Kumar et al. (2018)
SU11274	Interleukin 8 (IL8)	Inhibitition of Met activation, wound closure, and IL8 secretion	
Ficlatuzumab	Tumor-associated fibroblast (TAF)	Inhibits TAF-facilitated cell proliferation, migration, and invasion. Inhibits Met activation in HGF-treated cells	Kumar et al. (2015)

preclinical cancer models. Kumar et al. (2018) showed that inhibition of c-Met with Crizotinib resulted in the reduction of glycolysis in HNSCC. In addition, c-Met inhibitor Crizotinib reduced CAF-induced hexokinase-2 (HK2) levels and decreased HGF-induced lactate secretion from HNSCC (Lui et al. 2011).

7.5 Conclusion

c-Met/HGF axis correlates with poor prognosis and increased recurrence rates in patients suffering from cancer. c-Met/HGF axis activates series of downstream signalling pathways, which leads to aggressive phenotype by metabolic reprogramming in cancer. This clearly indicates that understanding the association between c-Met/HGF and its activated pathways provides an insight and is a rationale for the development of novel therapeutic target for the treatment of cancer.

Acknowledgments We sincerely thank all authors for their valuable inputs and carefully reading the manuscript.

Conflicts of interest: The authors declare no conflict of interest.

References

Anglesio MS et al (2011) IL6-STAT3-HIF signaling and therapeutic response to the angiogenesis inhibitor sunitinib in ovarian clear cell cancer. Clin Cancer Res 17(8):2538–2548

Bender S et al (2016) Recurrent MET fusion genes represent a drug target in pediatric glioblastoma. Nat Med 22(11):1314–1320

Bernier M et al (2011) Negative regulation of STAT3 protein-mediated cellular respiration by SIRT1 protein. J Biol Chem 286(22):19270–19279

Birchmeier W, Rosa M (2003) How to make tubes: signaling by the Met receptor tyrosine kinase. Trends Cell Biol 13(6):328–335

Bowman T, Garcia R, Turkson J, Jove R (2000) STATs in oncogenesis. Oncogene 19(21):2474–2488

Bromberg J (2002) JAK-STAT signaling in human disease Stat proteins and oncogenesis. J Clin Invest 109(9):1139–1142

Brown et al (2001) In vivo measurement of gene expression, angiogenesis and physiological function in tumors using multiphoton laser scanning microscopy. Nat Med 7(7):864–868

Caenepeel S et al (2017) MAPK pathway inhibition induces MET and GAB1 levels, priming BRAF mutant melanoma for rescue by hepatocyte growth factor. Oncotarget 8(11):17795–17809

Cai Y, Dodhia S, Su GH (2017) Dysregulations in the PI3K pathway and targeted therapies for head and neck squamous cell carcinoma. Oncotarget 8(13):22203–22217

Cairns RA, Harris IS, Mak TW (2011) Regulation of cancer cell metabolism. Nat Rev Cancer 11(2):85–95

Cheng N et al (2009) TGF-β signaling deficient fibroblasts enhance hepatocyte growth factor signaling in mammary carcinoma cells to promote scattering and invasion. Mol Cancer Res 6(10):1521–1533

Cho KH et al (2014) A ROS/STAT3/HIF-1 a signaling cascade mediates EGF-induced TWIST1 expression and prostate cancer cell invasion. Prostate 74(5):528–536

Coppock JD et al (2013) Improved clearance during treatment of HPV-positive head and neck cancer. Neoplasia 15(6):620–630

Cramer A et al (2005) Activation of the c-Met receptor complex in fibroblasts drives invasive cell behavior by signaling through transcription factor STAT3. J Cell Biochem 816:805–816

Dang CV (2012) Links between metabolism and cancer. Genes Dev 26(9):877–890

DeBerardinis RJ, Lum JJ, Hatzivassiliou G, Thompson CB (2008) The biology of cancer: metabolic reprogramming fuels cell growth and proliferation. Cell Metab 7(1):11–20

Denicola GM et al (2012) Oncogene-induced Nrf2 transcription promotes ROS detoxification and tumorigenesis. Nature 475(7354):106–109

Denko NC (2008) Hypoxia, HIF1 and glucose metabolism in the solid tumour. Nat Rev Cancer 8(9):705–713

Duvel K et al (2010) Activation of a metabolic gene regulatory network downstream of mTOR complex 1. Mol Cell 39(2):171–183

Ferracinis R, Longati P, Naldini L, Vigna E (1991) Identification of the major autophosphorylation site of the Met/hepatocyte growth factor receptor tyrosine kinase. J Biochem 266(29):19558–19564

Fu Y-t et al (2017) Valproic acid, targets papillary thyroid cancer through inhibition of c-Met signalling pathway. Am J Transl Res 9(6):3138–3147

Gillies RJ, Robey I, Gatenby RA (2008) Causes and consequences of increased glucose metabolism of cancers. J Nucl Med 49(6):24–43

Giorgi C et al (2010) STAT3 – mediated metabolic switch is involved in tumour transformation and STAT3 addiction. Aging (Albany NY) 2(1):823–842

Goetze K et al (2011) Lactate enhances motility of tumor cells and inhibits monocyte migration and cytokine release. Int J Oncol 39(2):453–463
Guo T et al (2010) Quantitative proteomics discloses MET expression in mitochondria as a direct target of MET kinase inhibitor in cancer cells. Mol Cell Proteomics 9(12):2629–2641
Hamanaka RB, Chandel NS (2012) Targeting glucose metabolism for cancer therapy: figure 1. J Exp Med 209(2):211–215
Hartmann S, Bhola NE, Grandis JR (2016) HGF/Met signaling in head and neck cancer: impact on the tumor microenvironment. Clin Cancer Res 22(16):4005–4014
Hass R, Jennek S, Yang Y, Friedrich K (2017) c-Met expression and activity in urogenital cancers – novel aspects of signal transduction and medical implications. Cell Commun Signal 15(1):1–9
Hein O et al (2009) The Warburg effect returns to the cancer stage. Semin Cancer Biol 19(1):1–3
Hensley CT, Wasti AT, Deberardinis RJ (2013) Glutamine and cancer: cell biology, physiology, and clinical opportunities. J Clin Invest 123(9):3678–3684
Horton JD, Goldstein JL, Brown MS (2002) SREBPs: activators of the complete program of cholesterol and fatty acid synthesis in the liver. J Clin Invest 109(9):1125–1131
Hughes PE et al (2016) In vitro and in vivo activity of AMG 337, a potent and selective MET kinase inhibitor in MET-dependent cancer models. Mol Cancer Ther 15(7):1568–1580
Hung W, Elliott B (2001) Co-operative effect of c-Src tyrosine kinase and Stat3 in activation of hepatocyte growth factor expression in mammary carcinoma cells. J Biol Chem 276(15):12395–12403
Imura Y et al (2016) Functional and therapeutic relevance of hepatocyte growth factor/c-Met signaling in synovial sarcoma. Cancer Sci 107(12):1867–1876
Inoue H et al (2006) Role of hepatic STAT3 in brain-insulin action on hepatic glucose production. Cell Metab 3(4):267–275
Kawada K, Toda K, Sakai Y (2017) Targeting metabolic reprogramming in KRAS - driven cancers. Int J Clin Oncol 22(4):651–659
Kim B et al (2016) Apigenin inhibits cancer stem cell-like phenotypes in human glioblastoma cells via suppression of c-Met signaling. Phytother Res 30(11):1833–1840
Kimmelman AC (2016) Metabolic dependencies in *RAS*-driven cancers. Clin Cancer Res 21(8):1828–1834
Krupar R et al (2014) Immunologic and metabolic characteristics of HPV-negative and HPV-positive head and neck squamous cell carcinomas are strikingly different. Virchows Arch 465(3):299–312
Kuang W et al (2017) Hepatocyte growth factor induces breast cancer cell invasion via the PI3K/Akt and P38 MAPK signaling pathways to up-regulate the expression of COX2. Am J Transl Res 9(8):3816–3826
Kumar et al (2015) Mitigation of tumor-associated fibroblast-facilitated head and neck cancer progression with anti–hepatocyte growth factor antibody Ficlatuzumab. JAMA Otolaryngol Head Neck Surg 141(12):1133
Kumar D (2017) Regulation of glycolysis in head and neck squamous cell carcinoma. Postdoc J 5(1):14–28
Kumar et al (2018) Cancer-associated fibroblasts drive glycolysis in a targetable signaling loop implicated in head and neck squamous cell carcinoma progression. Cancer Res 78(14):3769–3782
Leung E et al (2016) Blood vessel endothelium-directed tumor cell streaming in breast tumors requires the HGF/c-Met signaling pathway. Oncogene 36(19):2680–2692
Liang Y, Liu J, Liu T, Yang X (2017) Anti-c-Met antibody bioconjugated with hollow gold nanospheres as a novel nanomaterial for targeted radiation ablation of human cervical cancer cell. Oncol Lett 14(2):2254–2260
Liebmann C (2001) Regulation of MAP kinase activity by peptide receptor signalling pathway: paradigms of multiplicity. Cell Signal 13:777–785
Lien EC, Lyssiotis CA, Cantley LC (2016) Metabolic reprogramming by the PI3K-Akt-MTOR pathway in cancer. Recent Results Cancer Res 207:39–72

Lui et al (2011) Inhibition of c-Met downregulates TIGAR expression and reduces NADPH production leading to cell death. Oncogene 30(9):1127–1134
Luo X-m et al (2015) Co-inhibition of GLUT-1 expression and the PI3K/Akt signaling pathway to enhance the radiosensitivity of laryngeal carcinoma xenografts in vivo. PLoS One 10(11):1–15
Lyssiotis CA, Son J, Cantley LC, Kimmelman AC (2013) Pancreatic cancers rely on a novel glutamine metabolism pathway to maintain redox balance. Cell Cycle 12(13):1987–1988
Martini et al (2014) PI3K/AKT signaling pathway and cancer: an updated review. Ann Med 46(6):372–383
Meijer TWH, Kaanders JHAM, Span PN, Bussink J (2012) Targeting hypoxia, HIF-1, and tumor glucose metabolism to improve radiotherapy efficacy. Clin Cancer Res 18(20):5585–5595
Mossenta et al (2019) New insight into therapies targeting angiogenesis in hepatocellular carcinoma. Cancers 11(8):1086
Noch E, Khalili K (2012) Oncogenic viruses and tumor glucose metabolism: like kids in a candy store. Mol Cancer Ther 11(1):14–23
Poliaková M, Aebersold DM, Zimmer Y, Medová M (2018) The relevance of tyrosine kinase inhibitors for global metabolic pathways in cancer. Mol Cancer 17(1):1–12
Qamsari ES et al (2017) The c-Met receptor: implication for targeted therapies in colorectal cancer. Tumor Biol 39(5):1–13
Rucki AA et al (2018) Role of AnnexinA2, Sema3D and PlexinD1 in mediating perineural invasion as a mechanism of metastasis in pancreatic ductal adenocarcinoma. Cancer Res 16(11):2399–2409
Salgia R (2017) MET in lung cancer: biomarker selection based on scientific rationale. Mol Cancer Ther 16(4):555–566
Sandulache VC, Myers JN (2012) Altered metabolism in head and neck squamous cell carcinoma: an opportunity for identification of novel biomarkers and drug targets. Head Neck 34(2):282–290
Semenza GL (2011) HIF-1 – upstream and downstream of cancer metabolism. Curr Opin Genet Dev 20(1):1–10
Shaw RJ, Cantley LC (2006) Ras, PI(3)K and MTOR signalling controls tumour cell growth. Nature 441(7092):424–430
Simons AL et al (2011) The role of Akt pathway signaling in glucose metabolism and metabolic oxidative stress. In: Oxidative stress in cancer biology and therapy. Humana Press, Totowa, NJ, pp 21–46
Son J et al (2013) Glutamine supports pancreatic cancer growth through a KRAS-regulated metabolic pathway. Nature 496(7443):101–105
Tamagnone L et al (2019) Induction of epithelial tubules by growth factor HGF depends on the STAT pathway. Nature 391(6664):285–288
Tang Z et al (2008) Dual MET – EGFR combinatorial inhibition against T790M-EGFR-mediated erlotinib-resistant lung cancer. Br J Cancer 99(6):911–922
Vander Heiden M, Cantley L, Thompson C (2009) Understanding the Warburg effect: the metabolic requirements of cell proliferation. Science 324(5930):1029–1033
Vanhaesebroeck B, Guibert JG, Graupera M (2010) The emerging mechanisms of isoform-specific PI3K signalling. Nat Rev 11(5):329–341
Vivanco I, Sawyers CL (2002) The phosphatidylinositol 3-kinase–AKT pathway in human cancer. Nat Rev 2(7):489–501
Wang M et al (2017) Role of tumor microenvironment in tumorigenesis. J Cancer 8(5):761–773
Warburg O, Wind F, Negelein E (1927) The metabolism of tumors in the body. J Gen Physiol 8(6):519–530
Williams JG (2000) STAT signalling in cell proliferation and in development. Curr Opin Genet Dev 10(5):503–507
Wojcik EJ et al (2006) A novel activating function of C-Src and Stat3 on HGF transcription in mammary carcinoma cells. Oncogene 25(19):2773–2784
Wu J-c, Wang C-t, Hung H-c, Wu W-j (2016) Heteronemin is a novel c-Met/STAT3 inhibitor against advanced prostate cancer cells. Prostate 76(16):1469–1483

Xu Q et al (2005) Targeting Stat3 blocks both HIF-1 and VEGF expression induced by multiple oncogenic growth signaling pathways. Oncogene 24(36):5552–5560

Yan S, Jiao X, Zou H, Li K (2015) Prognostic significance of c-Met in breast cancer: a meta-analysis of 6010 cases. Diagn Pathol 10(62):1–10

Yan S-x et al (2013) Effect of antisense oligodeoxynucleotides glucose transporter-1 on enhancement of radiosensitivity of laryngeal carcinoma. Int J Med Sci 10(10):1375–1386

Yin B et al (2017) RON and c-Met facilitate metastasis through the ERK signaling pathway in prostate cancer cells. Oncol Rep 37(6):3209–3218

Ying H et al (2012) Oncogenic Kras maintains pancreatic tumors through regulation of anabolic glucose metabolism. Cell 149(3):656–670

Yu H, Kortylewski M, Pardoll D (2007) Crosstalk between cancer and immune cells: role of STAT3 in the tumour microenvironment. Nat Rev 7(1):41–51

Yun J et al (2010) Glucose deprivation contributes to the development of KRAS pathway mutations in tumor cells. Science 325(5947):1555–1559

Zhang Y et al (2018) Function of the c-Met receptor tyrosine kinase in carcinogenesis and associated therapeutic opportunities. Mol Cancer 17(1):1–14

Zheng JIE (2012) Energy metabolism of cancer: glycolysis versus oxidative phosphorylation (review). Oncol Lett 4(6):1151–1157

Zhou X et al (2018) Inhibition of glutamate oxaloacetate transaminase 1 in cancer cell lines results in altered metabolism with increased dependency of glucose. BMC Cancer 18(1):559

Zhu L et al (2016) Acid sphingomyelinase/ASM is required for cell surface presentation of Met receptor tyrosine kinase in cancer cells. J Cell Sci 129(22):4238–4251

Recent Advances in Drug Development Targeting Cancer Metabolism

8

Narayan Sugandha, Lovika Mittal, Amit Awasthi, and Shailendra Asthana

Abstract

Cancer cell proliferation and their adaptation to tough environments depend critically on metabolic pathways. The pathological, phenotypic, and structural level understanding of metabolic reprogramming that actually takes place in the tumor microenvironment is known to provide an essential understanding of the strategies of anticancer drug development. Here, the different metabolic pathways, their key targets, and treatments are highlighted for the implementation of interdisciplinary approaches to understand the cancer metabolism pathways as well as the discovery-to-development process of anticancer drugs. In recent years, there have been advancements in metabolomics, proteomics, and in silico tools and techniques having higher sensitivity and prediction accuracy for the determination of various pharmacodynamic, pharmacokinetic properties, and metabolic pathways in the early drug discovery stages. Hence, they are more efficient to identify and validate the cancer proteins and characterize their structural–dynamical–functional relationships in an economically, fast, and less tedious process. Here, we review the available pathways, therapeutic targets, and the therapeutically active compounds reported to date which are known to modulate cancerous targets and reached into the clinical trials and/or approved by the FDA are highlighted. Some novel anticancer modulating mechanisms and targets reported recently and streamlined in the discovery phase are also discussed.

Keywords

Cancer metabolism · Drug targets · Metabolic pathways · Drug discovery

Narayan Sugandha and Lovika Mittal equally contributed to this work.

N. Sugandha · L. Mittal · A. Awasthi · S. Asthana (✉)
Translational Health Science and Technology Institute, NCR Biotech Science Cluster, Faridabad, Haryana, India
e-mail: aawasthi@thsti.res.in; sasthana@thsti.res.in

D. Kumar (ed.), *Cancer Cell Metabolism: A Potential Target for Cancer Therapy*,
https://doi.org/10.1007/978-981-15-1991-8_8

Abbreviations

AML	Acute myeloid leukemia
BCR-ABL	Breakpoint cluster region protein-Abelson murine leukemia viral oncogene homolog
BPTES	Bis-2-(5-phenylacetamido-1,2,4-thiadiazol-2-yl) ethyl sulfide
CPT1	Carnitine *O*-palmitoyltransferase 1
DLBCL	Diffuse large-B cell lymphoma
EGFR	Epidermal growth factor receptor
ERK	Extracellular-signal-regulated kinase
$GABA_A$	Gamma-aminobutyric acid
HER2	Human epidermal growth factor receptor 2
HIF-1	Hypoxia-inducible factor 1
HMGCR	3-Hydroxy-3-methylglutaryl-CoA reductase
HSP90	Heat shock protein 90
IDO	Indoleamine-2,3-dioxygenase
LDH	Lactate dehydrogenase
MRS	Magnetic resonance spectroscopy
MTH1	MutT homolog-1
mTOR	Mammalian Target of Rapamycin
NAD	Nicotinamide adenine dinucleotide
NADH	Nicotinamide adenine dinucleotide
Nmnat	Nicotinamide/nicotinic acid mononucleotide adenylyltransferase
NMR	Nuclear magnetic resonance spectroscopy
NRF2	Nuclear factor E2-related factor 2
OXPHOS	Oxidative phosphorylation
PARP	Poly (ADP-ribose) polymerase
PDGFR	Platelet-derived growth factor receptor
PDH	Pyruvate dehydrogenase
PI3K	Phosphoinositide 3-kinase
PKM2	Pyruvate kinase M2
RAS	Rat sarcoma
STAT3	Signal transducer and activator of transcription 3
VEGFR	Vascular endothelial growth factor receptor

8.1 Introduction

Cancer cells are known to proliferate from an abnormal cell to more than ~10^9 cells and for their sustained proliferation activation of the metabolic pathways is required as they generate energy from different sources of nutrients (Vazquez et al. 2016). So, identifying and targeting the various cancer metabolic pathways that aid in their survival and progression will help in the development of anticancer agents that can be used as cytotoxic drugs. Important among them are antimitotic agents, alkylating agents, topoisomerase inhibitors, and DNA/RNA antimetabolites. While some are targeted drugs namely inhibitors of tyrosine receptor kinases, Wnt signaling, RAS signaling, and mTOR signaling (Kim 2015). In the last two decades, the major focus of cancer therapy is on targeting growth signaling pathways such as receptor tyrosine kinases (EGFR, VEGFR, PDGFR), downstream kinases of these pathways (PI3K, AKT, ERK), and final downstream signaling of biomolecule synthesis such as mTOR (Engelman et al. 2006; Kim 2015). However, it is noticed that the blockade of a signaling pathway opens other routes or mechanisms for cancer survival. Therefore, possible remedial approaches are required to block such opportunities for cancer cells. One such alternative is exploring and targeting cancer metabolic pathways to overcome the drawbacks in cancer therapy (Kim 2015). Since, the dry mass of mammalian cells is mainly composed of proteins, lipids, and nucleotides synthesized from metabolic precursors such as amino acids, acetyl-CoA, and purines and pyrimidines, respectively (Vazquez et al. 2016). The cancer cells also take advantage of these sources for their survival. Therefore, once a correct druggable target, as well as the metabolic pathway, is identified in a disease progression, it would be effortless to arrest the cancer cell growth without affecting the normal cells.

A number of druggable targets such as proteins, transcription factors, etc. are being identified at an accelerating pace targeting cancer metabolism along with a better understanding of the cancer metabolic pathways. Researchers are scrutinizing various approaches for the identification of metabolic therapeutic targets, biomarkers, diagnostic kits, drugs, natural products, etc. with combined effects of in silico and experimental approaches (Kang et al. 2018; Wang et al. 2018; Anand et al. 2018; Bordel 2018; Shen et al. 2018; Guerra et al. 2018; Mehta et al. 2015). Different cancer metabolic pathways are being targeted such as glycolysis (Neugent et al. 2018), glutamine metabolism (Choi and Park 2018), lactate metabolism, pentose phosphate pathway (Cho et al. 2018), pyruvate metabolism, ketone bodies and fatty acid metabolism, nucleic acid synthesis, amino acid metabolism, lipid synthesis, and mitochondrial synthesis. Therapeutic strategies in cancer metabolism can be targeted along with immunity (Van Dang and Kim 2018). Cancer epigenetics is closely associated with cancer metabolism in many cases (Kim and Yeom 2018). NRF2 is a transcription factor and important genetic factor that mediates cancer metabolism (Jung et al. 2018). Several oncogenes such as RAS, MYC, and EGFR also mediate metabolic regulation (Min and Lee 2018). Glucose and glutamine are the most abundant and consumed nutrients in the cells (Vazquez et al. 2016). In this chapter, we focus only on the development of drugs targeting cancer metabolic pathways and novel advancements related to it.

8.2 Drugs, Drug Targets, and Novel Advancements

Several therapeutic targets and strategies have been identified in cancer metabolic pathways and that led to the development of their modulators (Tables 8.1 and 8.2).

Table 8.1 List of cancer metabolism therapeutics

Metabolic pathways	Metabolic targets	Compound names	Developmental phase	References
Glycolysis	GLUT1	STF-31 WZB117 BAY-876 Fasentin Apigenin Genistein	Investigational Phase II Phase II	Granchi et al. (2014), Akins et al. (2018), Ma et al. (2018) and Qian (2014)
	GLUT4	BAY-876 Silibinin Ritonavir	Investigational Phase I/II Phase I	Ma et al. (2018) and Qian (2014)
	GLUT3	BAY-876 GSK-3 inhibitors	Investigational	Ma et al. (2018) and Qian (2014)
	GLUT2	Phloretin Quercetin	Investigational Phase I	Qian (2014)
	Hexokinase2 (HK-II)	2-Deoxyglucose Lonidamine 3-Bromopyruvate	Phase I/II Phase II/III Investigational	Galluzzi et al. (2013), Akins et al. (2018)
	Phosphofructokinase 2	3PO N4A YZ9	Investigational	Qian (2014)
	LDHA	PSTMB (1-(phenylseleno)-4-(trifluoromethyl) benzene FX11 Quinoline 3-sulfonamides	Investigational	Kim et al. (2019) and Qian (2014)
Beta oxidation	CPT1 (Carnitine O-palmitoyl-transferase1)	Etomoxir Oxfenicine Perhexiline	Phase-II-discontinued	Samudio et al. (2010) and Galluzzi et al. (2013)
		RNAi	Approved	
Mitochondrial respiration	OXPHOS	Metformin Phenformin	Approved Investigational	El-Mir et al. (2000) and Galluzzi et al. (2013)

(continued)

Table 8.1 (continued)

Metabolic pathways	Metabolic targets	Compound names	Developmental phase	References
Glutamine metabolism	GLS1	CB-839	Phase I/II	Akins et al. (2018) and Muthu and Nordström (2019)
		BPTES	Investigational	
		968	Investigational	
	SLC1A5	GPNA γ- FBP Benzylserine	Investigational	
	GLUD	EGCG	Investigational	
		R162	Investigational	
	Aminotransferase	Amino oxyacetate (AOA)	Investigational	Korangath et al. (2015)
Kreb's cycle	MCT1	AZD3965 Syrosingopine	Phase-I/II Investigational	Benjamin et al. (2018) and Muthu and Nordström (2019)
	MCT2	AZD3965	Investigational	Afonso et al. (2019)
	MCT4	AZ93 Syrosingopine Bindarit	Investigational	Benjamin et al. (2018) and Fisel et al. (2018)
	PDK1	Dichloroacetate	Approved	Michelakis et al. (2008)
	PDK	VER-246608	Investigational	Moore et al. (2014)
	PDK2	AZD7545		
	IDH2	Enasidenib (AG-221) IDH305 AG-120 AG-881	Approved Phase I/II	Dugan and Pollyea (2018) and Muthu and Nordström (2019)
	IDH1	AG-120	Phase I	Akins et al. (2018)

(continued)

Table 8.1 (continued)

Metabolic pathways	Metabolic targets	Compound names	Developmental phase	References
	α-Ketoglutarate dehydrogenase complex	CPI-613	Phase II	Muthu and Nordström (2019)
Fatty acid synthesis	FASN	TVB-2640	Phase II	Muthu and Nordström (2019)
Lipid metabolism	Choline kinase	CK37 TCD-717 RNAi	Phase I	Galluzzi et al. (2013) and Kall et al. (2018)
	MGLL	ABX-1431 JZL184 RNAi	Investigational	Galluzzi et al. (2013)
	Acetyl-coenzyme A acetyltransferase 1 (ACAT1)	ATR-101 Avasimibe	Approved	Raal et al. (2003)
Mevalonate pathway	HMGCR	Statins	Approved	Cao et al. (2011) and Galluzzi et al. (2013)
Pentose phosphate pathway	PGAM1	N-Xanthone benzenesulfonamides PGMI-004A MJE3	Investigational	Wang et al. (2018) and Qian (2014)
	G6PD	6-Aminonicotinamide	Investigational	Qian (2014)
	PKM2	TLN-232 TT-232 Shikonin/alkannin ML265 (TEPP-46) SAICAR Serine	Discontinued Investigational	Qian (2014)
Hypoxic responses	HIF-1 alpha	PX-478 Acriflavine	Phase-I Investigational	Tibes et al. (2010) and Galluzzi et al. (2013)
	Carbonic anhydrase (CA9)	Indisulam SLC-0111	Phase-II-discontinued Phase Ib/II	Supuran (2018)

(continued)

Table 8.1 (continued)

Metabolic pathways	Metabolic targets	Compound names	Developmental phase	References
Cell growth autophagy	mTOR	Rapalogues Torins	Approved	Sabatini (2006) and Galluzzi et al. (2013)
	Ribosomal protein S6 kinase beta-1 (S6K1)	Metformin Rapamycin	Phase II Investigational	Muthu and Nordström (2019) and Choo et al. (2008)
	PI3K	GDC-0941 (Pictilisib)	Phase I	Sarker et al. (2015)
	Eukaryotic translation initiation factor 4E (eIF4E)-binding protein 1 (4E-BP1)	Metformin Rapamycin	Phase II Investigational	Muthu and Nordström (2019) and Choo et al. (2008)
	AKT	Perifosine	Phase I/II	Richards et al. (2010) and Becher et al. (2017)
	mTORC1	Temsirolimus (CCI-779)	Approved	Wan et al. (2006)
	AMPK	A-769662 Acadesine Dorsomorphin Phenformin Bempedoic acid EX229 PF-06409577 MK-3903 Metformin	Phase II	Muthu and Nordström (2019)
Cell growth	Cyclogenase2	Aspirin		Hawley et al. (2012)
Nucleic acid biosynthesis	Dihydrofolate reductase (DHFR)	Methotrexate Pemetrexed	Approved	Muthu and Nordström (2019)
	5-Phosphoribosyl-1-pyrophosphatase (PRPP) amidotransferase	6-Mercaptopurine (6-MP) 6-Thioguanine (6-TG)	Approved	Muthu and Nordström (2019)

(continued)

Table 8.1 (continued)

Metabolic pathways	Metabolic targets	Compound names	Developmental phase	References
	Thymidylate synthase (TS)	5-Fluorouracil (5-FU) Capecitabine	Approved	Muthu and Nordström (2019)
	DNA polymerase/ ribonucleotide reductase (RnR)	Gemcitabine Cytarabine	Approved	Muthu and Nordström (2019)
Amino acid biosynthesis	Circulating asparagine	L-Asparaginase	Approved	Muthu and Nordström (2019)
Amino acid biosynthesis	Dihydroorotate dehydrogenase (DHODH)	Leflunomide	Phase II/III	Muthu and Nordström (2019)
Amino acid biosynthesis	Arginine Deiminase	ADI-PEG 20	Phase I/II/III	Muthu and Nordström (2019)

Table 8.2 List of immunometabolic drugs

Modulating agent	Target	Developmental stage	References
Epacadostat	IDO1	Phase III	Mullard (2016)
CB-839	GLS1	Phase I/II	Mullard (2016)
CB-1158	Arginase	Phase I	Mullard (2016)
CPI-444	Adenosine A2a receptor	Phase I	Mullard (2016)
FK866/APO866 LSN3154567 CHS 828/ GMX-1778 GMX1777 GNE-617 GNE-618	NAMPT	Investigational	Chen et al. (2017) and Zhao et al. (2017)
BZ-423	Mitochondrial FoF1-ATP synthase	Investigational	Starke et al. (2018)

8.2.1 Drugs Targeting Glycolysis Pathway

Cancer cells have a unique way of glucose metabolism as compared to that of normal cells. Glucose transport into the cells is the first step in the metabolism of glucose. There have been several therapeutic targets identified in glycolysis pathway such as glucose transport proteins (GLUTs), hexokinases (HKs), Phosphofructokinase 2 (PFK2), and LDHA, and against them small molecule inhibitors are being developed (Granchi et al. 2014; Akins et al. 2018; Ma et al. 2018; Qian 2014). There are 14 glucose transport proteins (GLUTs) present in humans and they are observed to be overexpressed by cancer cells. Inhibition of GLUTs became the primary focus for the development of inhibitors such as STF-31 and WZB117 targeting GLUT1;

Phloretin and quercetin (GLUT2); BAY-876 and GSK-3 inhibitors (GLUT3); and silibinin and ritonavir (GLUT4). Apigenin and Genistein, inhibitors for GLUT1, silibinin for GLUT4 are currently under phase II clinical trials (Table 8.1). Hexokinase catalyzes the first reaction step of glycolysis by converting glucose to glucose-6-phosphate (G-6-P). The hexokinase-II inhibitors namely lonidamine, 3-bromopyruvate, and 2-deoxyglucose are currently under clinical trials (Table 8.1). Phosphofructokinases phosphorylate fructose-6-phosphate to fructose-1,6-bisphosphate in glycolysis. Currently, its inhibitors are investigated in preclinical stages (Table 8.1).

8.2.2 Drugs Targeting Glutamine Metabolism

Glutamine acts as a substrate for hexosamine, nucleotide biosynthesis, and can be metabolized via TCA cycle for fatty acid synthesis in hypoxic cells (HIF-1 activated cells). Hence, it becomes essential for cell proliferation and its de novo synthesis is observed in tumor cells (Marin-Valencia et al. 2012; Metallo et al. 2011). It is important for the glutathione synthesis whose abundance as an antioxidant in the cancer cells helps in their survival in the oxidative stress environment (Diehn et al. 2009). It also acts as an alternative to glucose for lipid synthesis (Metallo et al. 2011). An example of glutaminase inhibitor is BPTES that is known to possess anticancer effects in several tumor models showing increased glutaminase activity in the cells (Xiang et al. 2015) (Table 8.1). CB-839 is currently under clinical trials for patients suffering from solid and hematological malignancies (Gross et al. 2014) (Table 8.1). Recently a study reported that NK cells do not use glutamine as a source of energy, so glutamine metabolism can be targeted in tumor cells as these drugs will not hinder cancer killing NK cells' mechanism (Loftus et al. 2018).

8.2.3 Drugs Targeting Lactate Metabolism

Cancer cells use lactate as their energy source for assistance in the regulation of mitochondrial metabolism and also for their growth and proliferation (Martinez-Outschoorn et al. 2012). Alanine and glutamate generation requires lactate as a substrate (Kennedy et al. 2013). Aerobic cancer cells make use of lactate produced by hypoxic cells in tumor by plasma membrane monocarboxylate transporters (MCTs) by the transportation of lactate and thus, the blockade of lactate transportation bagged the attention as a potential therapeutic approach. AZD3965 (MCT1 inhibitor), is recently in clinical phases (Marchiq and Pouysségur 2016) (Table 8.1). Since the lactate transportation is observed in both cancerous and noncancerous cells, there is a need to study the effects of drugs targeting lactate transportation in noncancerous tissues also (Halestrap 2013; Pellerin and Magistretti 2012). Lactate dehydrogenase (LDH) is another therapeutic target that converts pyruvate into lactate to generate energy for the cancer cells under hypoxic conditions. However, there are no clinical trials testing anticancer molecules that inhibit LDH. However, the LDHA inhibitors are at preclinical stages as anticancer agents that are mentioned in Table 8.1 (Rani and Kumar 2016). However, none of these compounds is under oncology clinical trials.

Carbonic anhydrases regulate acid–base balance inside the cells in tumor setup whose disruption causes anticancer effects, e.g., indisulam (CA9 inhibitor) is being tested in clinical trials (Bailey et al. 2012). The transcription factor HIF-1 activates CA9, a HIF-1 transcription target and inhibition of HIF-1 is reported to reduce lactate production and expression of CA9 in tumor cells. The inhibitors of HIF-1 are under clinical phases (Table 8.1).

8.2.4 Drugs Targeting Pyruvate Metabolism

Pyruvate increases the mitochondrial metabolism that aids in the proliferation of cells (Diers et al. 2012). It has been observed in breast cancer cells that the presence of pyruvate makes cancer cells become more invasive as compared to the presence of glucose and lactate (Diers et al. 2012). It is a validated pathway for the development of anticancer therapies and the inhibitors designed for targets such as MCTs, PKM2, LDHA, and modulators of the TCA cycle, which are involved in this pathway are under investigation (Table 8.1). The efficacy and side effects of these inhibitors should be speculated in clinical trials with regard to rate of altered pyruvate concentrations.

8.2.5 Drugs Targeting Acetyl-CoA Metabolism

Cancer cells meet their cholesterol and fatty acid requirements using acetyl-CoA, which is generated from glucose, glutamine, or acetate (Vazquez et al. 2016). The therapeutic targets identified from such metabolisms are PDH (Metallo et al. 2011), AKT expression in cancer cells, or stimulation of HER2 or EGFR. It is noticed that downstream metabolic pathways of pyruvate get affected by the activation of other signaling pathways and thus a better therapeutic strategy would be to target the pyruvate metabolism. In a recent study, aspirin is found to reduce the synthesis and transfer of acetyl-CoA into the mitochondria of *Saccharomyces cerevisiae* cells deficient in manganese superoxide dismutase (MnSOD) (Farrugia et al. 2019). Another study has reported that prolyl isomerase (Pin1) expression level is increased in most malignant tissues and is found to bind and stabilize the acetyl-CoA expression in cells by decreasing its degradation by lysosomal pathway. Therefore, Pin1 also appears to be a potential target for anticancer effects by development of inhibitors against it (Ueda et al. 2019).

8.2.6 Drugs Targeting Ketone Bodies and Fatty Acids

Fatty acid metabolism helps in the generation of energy and some important biological molecules such as ketone bodies, hormones, and triglycerides. The studies of inhibitors that modulate the enzymes involved in fatty acid oxidation (FAO) are very limited. The inhibition of CPT1 enzyme, an enzyme involved in FAO has shown anticancer activity both in in vitro and in vivo experiments (Pike et al. 2011). Perhexiline and oxfenicine are approved antianginal drugs and their anticancer properties by inhibiting CPT1 are being determined (Table 8.1). Nevertheless, Etomoxir, a CPT1 inhibitor was withdrawn from clinical trials due to major side effects observed in patients (Holubarsch et al. 2007) (Table 8.1). Various combination treatments or repurposing of drugs can be promising strategies to treat metabolism in cancer cells (Woyach et al. 2014; Bertolini et al. 2015).

8.2.7 Drugs Targeting Nucleic Acid Synthesis

Antimetabolites that interfere with nucleic acid synthesis, were known to be the first effective chemotherapeutic drugs, e.g., an antifolate drug, aminopterin (Farber and Diamond 1948). Other anticancer drugs or antifolates are methotrexate, pralatrexate, and pemetrexed, and are in clinical practice (Table 8.1). They interfere with cellular proliferation by inhibition of tetrahydrofolate (THF) production. The antipyrimidine, 5-fluorouracil (5-FU), inhibits thymidylate synthetase and is being widely used in cancer therapy.

8.2.8 Drugs Targeting Amino Acid Metabolism

Amino acid deprivation is already well studied and documented as an anticancer therapy. L-Asparaginase is an FDA approved drug as a standard therapy of acute lymphoblastic leukemia (Table 8.1). It causes the breakdown of L-asparagine (essential for protein synthesis) to ammonia and aspartic acid (one-carbon metabolism), thus interferes with the protein synthesis in cells. In addition, providing pegylated arginine deiminases which converts circulating arginine into citrulline have shown encouraging results by depleting plasma arginine in the clinical trials on several solid malignancies (Ascierto et al. 2005). IDO is the rate-limiting enzyme in tryptophan catabolism and it was observed to be overexpressed in many cancer cell types. The inhibitors of IDO (e.g., epacadostat and indoximod) are in clinical trials as immunotherapies for cancer patients, to enhance efficacy of other anticancer agents (Joyce and Fearon 2015) (Table 8.2).

8.2.9 Drugs Targeting Lipid Synthesis

The enzymes that are involved in de novo generation of lipids and steroids are also known to be involved in tumor development and progression. For example, choline kinase activity is observed to be overexpressed by cancer cells during proliferation stages. Inhibitors of choline kinase are under different developmental stages for evaluation of their anticancer effects in humans (Glunde et al. 2011). Statins are reported antagonists of HMGCR and cholesterol synthesis, and received approval for the cardiovascular disease therapies, and are also being tested under many clinical trials for their anticancer activities (Kubatka et al. 2014) (Table 8.1).

8.2.10 Drugs Targeting Mitochondrial Metabolism

The potential anticancer drugs that inhibit NADH–coenzyme Q oxidoreductase (complex I) and Q-cytochrome-c oxidoreductase (complex III) and thus eventually inhibiting OXPHOS are metformin and arsenic trioxide, respectively. It is reported that high mitochondrial membrane potential comprising cancer cells tends to have higher accumulation of a cyanine dye analogue, MKT-007 and observed reduction of mitochondrial metabolism that inhibits tumor growth. However, MKT-077 treatment comes with major side effects such as renal toxicities due to which it is discontinued from clinical development (Propper et al. 1999). Mitochondrial metabolic enzymes are known to be attractive targets for anticancer treatment. Dichloroacetate (DCA), a pyruvate analogue, is observed to change the metabolic flux in cancer cells with defective mitochondrial activity (OXPHOS) and also cause apoptosis in mitochondria (Table 8.1). There are no severe adverse effects observed during the clinical trials of DCA in patients with glioma. The conversion of isocitrate to α-ketoglutarate is catalyzed by IDH enzymes and it is also involved in other roles such as epigenetic modulation of gene expression, hypoxic response, and mTOR regulation. The inhibitors of mutant IDH are being tested in clinical trials in patients with glioma or AML (Fathi et al. 2015) (Table 8.1).

8.2.11 Drugs Targeting Mitoribosomes

Human mitochondrial ribosome (mitoribosomes) plays an important role in the synthesis of 13 key subunits in the mitochondrial OXPHOS electron transport system (Beckmann and Herrmann 2015). Occurrences of the upregulation of mitochondrial protein translation have been observed in some types of human malignancies and preclinical studies have proven that the inhibition of this aforementioned mitochondrial protein translation takes part in anticancer activity. Aminoglycosides are antagonist drugs which interfere with the binding of bacterial ribosomes to the 30S subunit. Their function also includes the inhibition of mitochondrial protein synthesis, which is carried out by binding to the small subunit of the human mitoribosome (O'Sullivan et al. 2017). Nevertheless, their binding to mitochondrial ribosomes can cause side effects such as hearing loss and kidney damage (O'Sullivan et al. 2017). Oxazolidinone antibiotics, such as linezolid, also influences mitoribosomes but only the larger (mito) ribosomal subunits (Soriano et al. 2005). The rational design of small molecules that could specifically inhibit the mitochondrial protein translation can be possible with the availability of atomic structures (Greber et al. 2015).

8.2.12 Drugs Targeting Transcription Factors

HIF-1 is a transcription factor that regulates the body's response to low oxygen in cellular environment, thereby, helps in maintaining homeostasis to increase vascularization under hypoxic conditions such as in localized ischemia and tumors. Many inhibitors of HIF-1 are being tested on cancer patients in different clinical phases (Table 8.1). Topoisomerase 1 (TOP1) causes HIF-1α translation and the inhibitors of HIF-1α (e.g., topotecan and irinotecan) are efficient to reduce HIF-1α expression. They are in developmental phases but their anticancer efficacy is still not revealed. Some examples of the inhibitors that are being clinically evaluated in different phases are digoxin (peptide inhibitor of HIF-1α translation), the HSP90 inhibitor ganetespib (HIF-1α stability gets reduced), and the proteasome inhibitor bortezomib (inhibition of HIF-1α transactivation) (Semenza 2012). However, the development of prognosis of responses and toxicity will be required to increase the success rate of anti HIF-1 therapies.

MYC is another key transcription factor that is responsible to enhance the catabolic process and it gets deregulated in many human cancers. To block the interaction of MYC with other proteins, inhibitors such as INCB054329 and CPI-0610, are being clinically evaluated (Stine et al. 2015; Chen et al. 2014). NRF2 is a transcription factor and is also known as a nuclear factor (erythroid-derived 2)-like 2 (NFE2L2) (Jung et al. 2018). It helps in maintaining redox homeostasis in antioxidant defense mechanisms by stimulating the expression of a wide array of genes (Jung et al. 2018). The activation of NRF2 is reported to be critically associated with proliferation, growth, and survival of tumor cells (Jia et al. 2016; Jung et al. 2018) and its activation might cause resistance to chemotherapies and radiotherapies (Jung et al. 2018). Therefore, it is supposed to be an efficient approach for the development of anti-NRF2 molecules to be used in mono- or combination therapies for cancer. However, none of the NRF2 inhibitors are FDA approved and not under any clinical phases in spite of having many investigational NRF2 inhibitors with promising therapeutic efficacy (Jung et al. 2018). NRF2 also appears to be activated in cancer by the presence of KEAP1-NRF2 disrupting proteins (such as p62, CDK20 (cyclin-dependent kinase 20), sequestosome 1 (SQSTM1), dipeptidyl-peptidase 3 (DPP3) and p21) and metabolites (e.g., oncometabolite fumarate) (Jung et al. 2018). Some natural compounds such as flavonoids and alkaloids, novel synthetic compounds (such as ML385, ARE expression modulator 1 (AEM1)), as well as some vitamins and commercial drugs (such as ascorbic acid, all-trans retinoic acid, metformin, and glucocorticoids) are also reported to act as NRF2 inhibitors (Jung et al. 2018). To overcome the unmet medical requirements in the current scenario by considering the risks and tedious process of anticancer drug development, a drug repurposing strategy can be employed to develop NRF2 inhibitors for anticancer treatments (Jung et al. 2018).

8.2.13 Targeting Cancer Metabolism by Nmnat

Recently, it was reported that Nmnat2 and Nmapt are inhibited by vacor adenine dinucleotide (VAD) (Buonvicino et al. 2018). Tiazofurin is an analog of NAD that is known to induce cell death in the overexpressed Nmnat2 colorectal cancer cells. Tiazofurin is converted into thiazole-4-carboxamide adenine dinucleotide by the enzymatic action of Nmnat2 for gyanylate synthesis in the cancer cells (Kusumanchi et al. 2013).

8.2.14 CK2 Inhibitors for Medulloblastoma

Medulloblastoma is an aggressive brain tumor in children, which is driven by the sonic hedgehog (SHH) pathway. Most of its subtypes are resistant to currently available drugs. Smoothened (SMO) inhibitors can able to suppress this pathway and are currently used to treat medulloblastoma. It is been reported that kinase, CK2 is essential for driving SHH signaling in medulloblastoma. The inhibitors of CK2 kinase have been proven to effectively block the growth of SMO inhibitor–resistant, SHH-type mouse and human medulloblastoma cells, and also resulted in the extended the survival of tumor-bearing mice (Purzner et al. 2018). Currently a clinical trial is testing a CK2 inhibitor in pediatric patients (Ferrarelli 2018) whose outcome is much awaited for further clinical benefits.

8.2.15 Exosome-Derived MicroRNAs Play an Important Role in Cancer Metabolism

It was observed that tumor cells secrete exosomes to target neighboring or adjacent cells by either, autocrine, paracrine, or endocrine effects and these exosome help in cancer cell growth, angiogenesis, activation of stromal fibroblasts, suppression of host immune responses, etc. Exosomes consists of mRNA, microRNAs, pro-inflammatory proteins, and help to stimulate the cell proliferation. Exosomal-derived miRNAs (miRs) are being used for diagnostics (acting as prognostic biomarkers) and cancer therapy by reprogramming the metabolic processes in cancer cells. They hold promising efficacy due to their high stability, tissue specificity and secretion into body fluids. Exosomes derived from MSCs have also been used as a cargo to deliver antitumor miRNAs and may be combined with some surface moieties to target specificity to reach the "diseased sites" and to pass the normal clearance mechanisms of the body.

8.2.16 Salicylate Enhances the Prostate Cancer Therapeutic Response to Radiotherapy by Activating the Metabolic Stress Sensor AMPK

Prostate cancer is effectively treated using radiotherapy (RT). However, the resistance developed by prostate cancer to radiotherapy is calling for the dose escalation, which is resulting in the side effects such as bladder and rectal toxicity. In the clinical prostate cancer cases, the use of Aspirin which is a prodrug of salicylate (SAL) has resulted in the improved RT responses, but its mechanism of action is still not clear. SAL activates AMP-activated protein kinase (AMPK), which is the metabolic stress sensor. The activated AMPK resulting in the inhibition of protein synthesis and de novo lipogenesis via inhibition of mTOR and Acetyl-CoA Carboxylase (ACC), respectively. However, RT has also proven to activate AMPK using different mechanisms from the one used by SAL. Thus, to reduce PrCa, the combination of two therapies will be having synergistic effects by inhibiting the survival and proliferation of tumor cells. RT activates the mTOR pathway and AMPK and results in inhibitory phosphorylation of ACC and also activates some genotoxic stress markers. SAL has proven to enhance the therapeutic effects of RT on ACC and AMPK, and also shown to block the mTOR activation (Broadfield et al. 2019).

8.2.17 Nanoparticles of Sodium Bicarbonate Modulating Tumor pH

Cancer metabolism is related to the acidic pH in the tumor microenvironment (TME). Acidic pH prevents the drugs from penetrating into the tumor cells by creating a physiological barrier. Doxorubicin (ionizable weak-base drug) freely permeates membranes in its uncharged form but in the acidic TME it becomes charged due to which its cellular permeability gets retarded (Abumanhal-Masarweh et al. 2019). Therefore, in such cases, adjuvants such as sodium bicarbonate-containing liposomes with size approximately 100 nm can be used to elevate the tumor pH (Abumanhal-Masarweh et al. 2019). It is observed that, treatment of triple-negative breast cancer cells along with sodium bicarbonate and doxorubicin has resulted in increased drug uptake and effective anticancer activity (Abumanhal-Masarweh et al. 2019).

8.2.18 STAT3 as a Therapeutic Target for Cancer

Over the years it has been observed that many cancer cell types undergo "metabolic shift" to OXPHOS to obtain energy for their survival and in some cases drug-resistant oncogenes too rely on OXPHOS in tumors (Lee et al. 2018; Bourgeais et al. 2013). It has been revealed that presence of STAT3 (Signal transducer and activator of transcription factor 3) in mitochondria provides a biological link between cancer cell metabolism and oncogene-induced signaling mechanisms (Lee et al. 2018). Therefore, STAT3 and OXPHOS are being looked upon as promising targets to combat drug-resistance issues in different tumor types (Lee et al. 2018). There have been certain drugs repurposed as inhibitors for OXPHOS such as Metformin and Phenformin and many novel molecules are in developmental phases exhibiting promising results (Table 8.1). STAT3 is highly involved in many oncogenic signaling pathways as observed in different cancer types (Lee et al. 2018). STAT3 is also found to modulate the mitochondrial respiration and is specifically associated with GRIM-19 that generate energy by OXPHOS (Lee et al. 2018). There have been several strategies employed to target STAT3 signaling pathway either through direct inhibition of STAT3 protein itself, inhibition of upstream tyrosine kinases, or the DNA-binding complexes. Different inhibitors of STAT3 signaling pathway are under clinical phases such as OPB-51602 (that binds with high affinity to the STAT3-SH2 domain) interfering with mitochondrial STAT3 (mSTAT3) (Lee et al. 2018).

8.2.19 Zebra Fish as a Powerful Tool to Identify Novel Therapies

Cancer cells and glioblastoma (GBM) in particular depend on effective antioxidant defense systems and enzymes that detoxify oxidized bases such as MTH1 to prevent DNA damage and subsequent cell death. The development of novel therapies against GBM is, among other reasons, hampered by the lack of orthotopic animal models that support large drug discovery screens. During the last decade, the zebra fish has been introduced as a clinically relevant model for human malignancies including cancer. Owing its biological and technical advantages, the zebra fish is the only vertebrate animal suitable for automated drug discovery screens to facilitate the identification and validation of novel cancer therapies. It has been demonstrated that the cellular redox environment and activation of the hypoxia signaling axis determines sensitivity to MTH1 inhibition in vitro and in vivo, thus suggesting that inhibition of MTH1 would be a promising strategy to treat cancers. Additionally, an orthotopic animal model may be developed for GBM that could readily be implemented in fully automatable drug discovery screens in order to accelerate the identification and development of novel therapies against GBM (Pudelko 2018).

8.2.20 Immunometabolism Modulating Advancements

Immunometabolism is an emerging field of investigation that corresponds to immuno-suppressive and immune-boosting roles that metabolites play in the microenvironment (Mullard 2016). Many companies working in the therapeutic domain of cancer metabolism are now shifting their interest toward immunometabolism-modulating drugs. The unique therapeutic approach of these drugs by improving the immune cell survival and modification of cancer cell interaction with immune cells proving them as promising drug candidates. For example, indoleamine 2,3-dioxygenase I (IDOI) inhibitor epacadostat manufactured by Incyte, controls tryptophan metabolism by nurturing immune cell activity (Table 8.2). Thus, the drug developers have shifted their focus on modulating the interplay between cancer cells and immune cells in the tumor microenvironment using metabolites. The development programme of the drug CB-839 targeting GLS1 has changed the course of cancer metabolic drug development research (Mullard 2016) (Table 8.2). Metabolic pathways play an important role in controlling the activity and anticancer responses of T cells, B cells, NK cells, and other immune cells. Rapid switching of T cells from oxidative phosphorylation to glycolysis is a common phenomenon during hypoxia and low nutrient conditions. Also antitumor function of CD8+ T-cell is affected by changes in lipid metabolism while acetyl CoA acetyltransferase 1 (ACAT1) inhibition results in enhanced effector CD8+ T cell function. PD-1 plays an important role in T cell development. In recent research, Patsoukis et al. (2015) stated that PD-1 promotes FAO via carnitine palmitoyltransferase (CPT1A) thus contributing to T cell development. Many compounds modulating immunometabolism have proven to give promising results and several have undergone preclinical stage studies, the inhibitor of lipogenic enzymes is notable among them. The recent example is the mouse melanoma study using combinatorial approach with anti-PD-1 and ACAT1 inhibitors, which gave positive results. Currently for atherosclerosis, Avasimibe, an ACAT1 inhibitor, is widely used with high human safety profile.

Targeting Myeloid-Derived Suppressor Cells (MDSCs) depending on the amino acids and fatty acids metabolism: MDSCs are the cell lines derived from bone marrow which form the major cell population infiltrating into tumor microenvironment under inflammatory conditions. The major metabolic fuel of MDSCs is FAO which is essential for the production and release of inhibitory cytokines. Thus, FAO is a major clinical target to inhibit the suppressive function of MDSCs. The FDA approved FAO inhibitor, Raloxizine is successfully used to interfere MDSCs function and growth in immunogenic preclinical models (Mathis and Shoelson 2011).

Immunomodulatory drugs targeting Mitochondrial FoF1-ATP Synthase: The non-anxiolytic 1,4-benzodiazepine drug, Bz-423, blocks respiratory chain function and generates superoxide thus affects the survival of malignant B cells (Boitano et al. 2003), targeting the mitochondrial F1Fo ATPase (Starke et al. 2018) (Table 8.2). Pathogenic T cells with depleted antioxidants level becomes selectively susceptible to Bz-423 induced enhanced ROS production. Also, Bz-423 is reported to play an important role in rescuing the mice from graft-versus-host disease (GVHD). While there is no report on adverse effects regarding the repopulation of lymphocytes, donor thymocytes, and granulocytes (Norata et al. 2015).

Nicotinamide phosphoribosyltransferase (Nampt) as a therapeutic target and diagnostic tool in cancer metabolism: A pleiotropic molecule, Nampt (called visfatin) helps in regulating the cell growth and may act as an enzyme or as a cytokine. Recent research is supporting the association of Nampt with number of malignancies. It is upregulated in obesity-associated cancer leading to its worst prognosis. Thus, Nampt level of serum can be used as a potential biomarker in cancer diagnostic and prognostic research. There is a great demand for pharmacologic agents that inhibit Nampt by decreasing its levels, affecting the Nampt downstream signaling pathways and medications that can neutralize Nampt are gaining importance. The inhibitors of Nampt are successfully used as anticancer therapeutics both as monotherapy or as a combination therapy and have shown promising outcomes in vivo and in vitro. Both intracellular Nampt (iNampt) and extracellular Nampt (eNampt) have been reported to show neoplastic actions. Thus, inhibition of Nampt by biochemical way or by interfering the eNampt receptor or using antibody neutralization or antisense oligonucleotides is gaining importance for the effective cancer treatment perspective. Inhibition of Nampt works mainly by exhausting the intracellular NAD and downregulating inflammatory TME. The current major focus is to elucidate the structure of Nampt receptor and the signaling pathways induced by it, which would help to target the downstream signaling molecules of Nampt pathway as a promising cancer therapeutics. Currently there are few competitive Nampt inhibitors namely GMX1777 (EB1627), APO 866 (also known as FK866 or WK175), CHS-828 (GMX1778), the soluble pro-drug of GMX1778 have successfully entered into clinical trials and recently, Nampt inhibitors such as GNE-617 and GNE-618 were published in the patent and medical literature (Table 8.2). STF-1, an anti-GLUT-1 drug candidate (Table 8.1) is also observed to show inhibitory effects against NAMPT. It was also reported that for normal physiological functioning of the cells, some amount of Nampt is also required, thus the inhibitors of Nampt might cause some side effects that should also be considered during designing and development stages. The best way to target cancer cells and preserve normal cells from harmful side effects of Nampt inhibitors is combined use of Nampt inhibitor along with nicotinic acid (NA). As normal cells express both Naprt and Nampt, the simultaneous use of NA would help to maintain NAD levels through NA-Naprt pathway. The cancer cells lacking Naprt were observed to have reduction in the NAD and ATP levels due to dysfunctional glycolysis mechanism by the treatment of Nampt inhibitor. Thus, it leads to the death of cancer cells without harming the normal cells (Cole et al. 2017). Thus, the level of Naprt can be used as a critical biomarker to predict the success of cancer treatment using Nampt inhibitors. IDH mutation in tumors can be used as a good biomarker for suitability of Nampt inhibitor therapy. As IDH-mutated cells have low Naprt levels that make them susceptible to Nampt inhibitors due to depletion of NAD levels. IDH mutant cells treated with FK866 exhibits a decreased NAD levels and a reduction in ATP production due to suppress in the TCA cycle flux, finally leading to the death of autophagic cells (Tateishi et al. 2015).

Chemotherapy along with combination therapeutics will form an efficient cancer treatment strategy. Nampt inhibitors can be used along with other chemotherapeutic and radiation drugs all of which are targeted to cause damage to DNA thus leading to activation of PARP-1. The genomic instability and DNA damage caused by extensive therapy lead to high PARP levels in cancer cells, which makes them vulnerable to NAD depletion caused by high energy consumption. Nampt inhibitor can be used along with other chemotherapeutic agents forming the best treatment option for cancer by inducing "synthetic lethality." However, some of the recent studies have reported toxicity effect of combination therapy of Nampt inhibitors particularly with 5-FU, β-lapachone, melphalan, fludarabine, pemetrexed, and temozolomide. A recent research article has reported successful combination therapy of Nampt inhibitors and olaparib (PARP-I/II inhibitor) for treating triple-negative breast cancer patients (Dalamaga et al. 2018).

8.2.21 Advancements with Gut Microbiota Reshaping

Among the broad-spectrum natural anticancer reagents, PTX (paclitaxel) is the most widely used therapeutic drug but it needs to be improved to enhance its efficacy as it comes with certain drawbacks of drug resistance and severe side effects. SGP, a polysaccharide from spore of *Ganoderma. lucidum* is a potent agent of Tc-based tumor immune surveillance and also studies have reported they play an important role in reshaping the gut microbiota. Combination therapy using PTX and SGP has shown the restoration of PTX-induced gut dysbiosis, this reshaped the gut microbiota community and also regulated gut microbiome function (Su et al. 2018). However, the combination therapy of PTX and SGP can be used to treat breast cancer depends on the basis of regulation of tumor metabolism and the gut microbiota (Su et al. 2018).

8.3 Concluding Remarks

The dynamic and volatile behavior of metabolic pathways has been a dramatic problem for drug discovery in academia as well as in the pharmaceutical industry. The investigation of crucial factors involved in cancer progression due to the reprogramming of cellular metabolism and their prioritization will be helpful in the development of anticancer strategies. The systemic, proteomic, metabolomic, and lipidomic preferences and their in-depth analysis will be required to reveal essential properties constituting the cancer cells and their tissue of origin as well as their interactions within TME. The recent advances in computational and analytical methods support the research investigations of cellular metabolism. This has served as a boon for further advancements in the drug development paradigms targeting the cancer metabolic pathways. The multidisciplinary approaches using a combination of cancer metabolomics as well as other high-throughput -omics platform, have helped researchers in understanding the underlying metabolic rewiring observed in cancer and normal cells. In order to make complete use of all acquired knowledge on cellular metabolism further refinements of the currently available techniques are essential. In fact, reusing (repurposing) of the existing drugs or the drugs that are either in clinical trials or withdrawn from the trials could also be screened or tested on other targets to reduce the time of drug development process. An in-depth study of TME and continued focus on recent developments targeting tumor metabolomics is essential for furthering our understanding of cancer metabolism at molecular level so that these molecular insights can be translated to inform of therapeutics. As such, the recent development of computational methodologies, ex vivo metabolite tracing, lipidomics, and patient tumor-derived organoid modeling would pave a way for future anticancer drug discoveries and enhancements in therapeutic interventions.

References

Abumanhal-Masarweh H, Koren L, Zinger A, Yaari Z, Krinsky N, Kaneti G, Dahan N et al (2019) Sodium bicarbonate nanoparticles modulate the tumor pH and enhance the cellular uptake of doxorubicin. J Control Release 296:1–13

Afonso J, Pinto T, Simões-Sousa S, Schmitt F, Longatto-Filho A, Pinheiro C, Marques H, Baltazar F (2019) Clinical significance of metabolism-related biomarkers in non-Hodgkin lymphoma – MCT1 as potential target in diffuse large B cell lymphoma. Cell Oncol 42(3):303–318

Akins NS, Nielson TC, Le HV (2018) Inhibition of glycolysis and glutaminolysis: an emerging drug discovery approach to combat cancer. Curr Top Med Chem 18(6):494–504

Anand R, Sarmah DT, Chatterjee S (2018) Extracting proteins involved in disease progression using temporally connected networks. BMC Syst Biol 12(1):78

Ascierto PA, Scala S, Castello G, Daponte A, Simeone E, Ottaiano A, Beneduce G et al (2005) Pegylated arginine deiminase treatment of patients with metastatic melanoma: results from phase I and II studies. J Clin Oncol Off J Am Soc Clin Oncol 23(30):7660–7668

Bailey KM, Wojtkowiak JW, Hashim AI, Gillies RJ (2012) Targeting the metabolic microenvironment of tumors. Adv Pharmacol 65:63–107

Becher OJ, Millard NE, Modak S, Kushner BH, Haque S, Spasojevic I, Trippett TM et al (2017) A phase I study of single-agent perifosine for recurrent or refractory pediatric CNS and solid tumors. PLoS One 12(6):e0178593

Beckmann R, Herrmann JM (2015) Structural biology. Mitoribosome oddities. Science 348(6232):288–289

Benjamin D, Robay D, Hindupur SK, Pohlmann J, Colombi M, El-Shemerly MY, Maira S-M, Moroni C, Lane HA, Hall MN (2018) Dual inhibition of the lactate transporters MCT1 and MCT4 is synthetic lethal with metformin due to NAD depletion in cancer cells. Cell Rep. https://doi.org/10.1016/j.celrep.2018.11.043

Bertolini F, Sukhatme VP, Bouche G (2015) Drug repurposing in oncology—patient and health systems opportunities. Nat Rev Clin Oncol 12(12):732–742

Boitano A, Ellman JA, Glick GD, Opipari AW Jr (2003) The proapoptotic benzodiazepine Bz-423 affects the growth and survival of malignant B cells. Cancer Res 63(20):6870–6876

Bordel S (2018) Constraint based modeling of metabolism allows finding metabolic cancer hallmarks and identifying personalized therapeutic windows. Oncotarget 9(28):19716–19729

Bourgeais J, Gouilleux-Gruart V, Gouilleux F (2013) Oxidative metabolism in cancer. JAK-STAT. https://doi.org/10.4161/jkst.25764

Broadfield LA, Marcinko K, Tsakiridis E, Zacharidis PG, Villani L, Lally JSV, Menjolian G et al (2019) Salicylate enhances the response of prostate cancer to radiotherapy. Prostate. https://doi.org/10.1002/pros.23755

Buonvicino D, Mazzola F, Zamporlini F, Resta F, Ranieri G, Camaioni E, Muzzi M et al (2018) Identification of the nicotinamide salvage pathway as a new toxification route for antimetabolites. Cell Chem Biol 25(4):471–82.e7

Cao Z, Fan-Minogue H, Bellovin DI, Yevtodiyenko A, Arzeno J, Yang Q, Gambhir SS, Felsher DW (2011) MYC phosphorylation, activation, and tumorigenic potential in hepatocellular carcinoma are regulated by HMG-CoA reductase. Cancer Res 71(6):2286–2297

Chen C-X, Huang J, Ga-Qi T, Jia-Tong L, Xie X, Zhao B, Ming W et al (2017) NAMPT inhibitor protects ischemic neuronal injury in rat brain via anti-neuroinflammation. Neuroscience. https://doi.org/10.1016/j.neuroscience.2017.05.022

Chen B-J, Wu Y-L, Tanaka Y, Zhang W (2014) Small molecules targeting c-Myc oncogene: promising anti-cancer therapeutics. Int J Biol Sci 10(10):1084–1096

Cho ES, Cha YH, Kim HS, Kim NH, In Yook J (2018) The pentose phosphate pathway as a potential target for cancer therapy. Biomol Ther 26(1):29–38

Choi Y-K, Park K-G (2018) Targeting glutamine metabolism for cancer treatment. Biomol Ther 26(1):19–28

Choo AY, Yoon S-O, Kim SG, Roux PP, Blenis J (2008) Rapamycin differentially inhibits S6Ks and 4E-BP1 to mediate cell-type-specific repression of mRNA translation. Proc Natl Acad Sci U S A 105(45):17414–17419

Cole J, Guiot M-C, Gravel M, Bernier C, Shore GC, Roulston A (2017) Novel NAPRT specific antibody identifies small cell lung cancer and neuronal cancers as promising clinical indications for a NAMPT inhibitor/niacin co-administration strategy. Oncotarget 8(44):77846–77859

Dalamaga M, Christodoulatos GS, Mantzoros CS (2018) The role of extracellular and intracellular nicotinamide phosphoribosyl-transferase in cancer: diagnostic and therapeutic perspectives and challenges. Metab Clin Exp 82:72–87

Diehn M, Cho RW, Lobo NA, Kalisky T, Dorie MJ, Kulp AN, Qian D et al (2009) Association of reactive oxygen species levels and radioresistance in cancer stem cells. Nature 458(7239):780–783

Diers AR, Broniowska KA, Chang C-F, Hogg N (2012) Pyruvate fuels mitochondrial respiration and proliferation of breast cancer cells: effect of monocarboxylate transporter inhibition. Biochem J 444(3):561–571

Dugan J, Pollyea D (2018) Enasidenib for the treatment of acute myeloid leukemia. Expert Rev Clin Pharmacol 11(8):755–760

El-Mir MY, Nogueira V, Fontaine E, Avéret N, Rigoulet M, Leverve X (2000) Dimethylbiguanide inhibits cell respiration via an indirect effect targeted on the respiratory chain complex I. J Biol Chem 275(1):223–228

Engelman E, Salengros JC, Chr Paquot M, Barvais L (2006) The acute pain service (APS): how we should have done it. Acta Anaesthesiol Belg 57(3):233–238

Farber S, Diamond LK (1948) Temporary remissions in acute Leukemia in children produced by folic acid antagonist, 4-aminopteroyl-glutamic acid. N Engl J Med 238(23):787–793

Farrugia G, Azzopardi M, Saliba C, Grech G, Gross AS, Pistolic J, Benes V et al (2019) Aspirin impairs acetyl-coenzyme a metabolism in redox-compromised yeast cells. Sci Rep 9(1):6152

Fathi AT, Wander SA, Faramand R, Emadi A (2015) Biochemical, epigenetic, and metabolic approaches to target IDH mutations in acute myeloid leukemia. Semin Hematol 52(3):165–171

Ferrarelli LK (2018) A target for medulloblastoma. Science 361(6407):1083–1085

Fisel P, Schaeffeler E, Schwab M (2018) Clinical and functional relevance of the monocarboxylate transporter family in disease pathophysiology and drug therapy. Clin Transl Sci 11(4):352–364

Galluzzi L, Kepp O, Vander Heiden MG, Kroemer G (2013) Metabolic targets for cancer therapy. Nat Rev Drug Discov 12(11):829–846

Glunde K, Bhujwalla ZM, Ronen SM (2011) Choline metabolism in malignant transformation. Nat Rev Cancer 11(12):835–848

Granchi C, Fancelli D, Minutolo F (2014) An update on therapeutic opportunities offered by cancer glycolytic metabolism. Bioorg Med Chem Lett 24(21):4915–4925

Greber BJ, Bieri P, Leibundgut M, Leitner A, Aebersold R, Boehringer D, Ban N (2015) Ribosome. The complete structure of the 55S mammalian mitochondrial ribosome. Science 348(6232):303–308

Gross MI, Demo SD, Dennison JB, Chen L, Chernov-Rogan T, Goyal B, Janes JR et al (2014) Antitumor activity of the glutaminase inhibitor CB-839 in triple-negative breast cancer. Mol Cancer Ther 13(4):890–901

Guerra AR, Duarte MF, Duarte IF (2018) Targeting tumor metabolism with plant-derived natural products: emerging trends in cancer therapy. J Agric Food Chem. https://doi.org/10.1021/acs.jafc.8b04104

Halestrap AP (2013) Monocarboxylic acid transport. Compr Physiol 3(4):1611–1643

Hawley SA, Fullerton MD, Ross FA, Schertzer JD, Chevtzoff C, Walker KJ, Peggie MW et al (2012) The ancient drug salicylate directly activates AMP-activated protein kinase. Science 336(6083):918–922

Holubarsch CJF, Rohrbach M, Karrasch M, Boehm E, Polonski L, Ponikowski P, Rhein S (2007) A double-blind randomized multicentre clinical trial to evaluate the efficacy and safety of two doses of etomoxir in comparison with placebo in patients with moderate congestive heart failure: the ERGO (etomoxir for the recovery of glucose oxidation) study. Clin Sci 113(4):205–212

Jia Y, Wang H, Wang Q, Ding H, Wu H, Pan H (2016) Silencing Nrf2 impairs glioma cell proliferation via AMPK-activated mTOR inhibition. Biochem Biophys Res Commun. https://doi.org/10.1016/j.bbrc.2015.12.034

Joyce JA, Fearon DT (2015) T cell exclusion, immune privilege, and the tumor microenvironment. Science 348(6230):74–80

Jung B-J, Yoo H-S, Shin S, Park Y-J, Jeon S-M (2018) Dysregulation of NRF2 in cancer: from molecular mechanisms to therapeutic opportunities. Biomol Ther 26(1):57–68

Kall SL, Delikatny EJ, Lavie A (2018) Identification of a unique inhibitor-binding site on choline kinase α. Biochemistry 57(8):1316–1325

Kang YP, Ward NP, DeNicola GM (2018) Recent advances in cancer metabolism: a technological perspective. Exp Mol Med 50(4):31

Kennedy KM, Scarbrough PM, Ribeiro A, Richardson R, Yuan H, Sonveaux P, Landon CD et al (2013) Catabolism of exogenous lactate reveals it as a legitimate metabolic substrate in breast cancer. PLoS One 8(9):e75154

Kim S-Y (2015) Cancer metabolism: strategic diversion from targeting cancer drivers to targeting cancer suppliers. Biomol Ther 23(2):99–109

Kim E-Y, Chung T-W, Han CW, Park SY, Park KH, Jang SB, Ha K-T (2019) A novel lactate dehydrogenase inhibitor, 1-(phenylseleno)-4-(trifluoromethyl) benzene, suppresses tumor growth through apoptotic cell death. Sci Rep 9(1):3969

Kim J-A, Yeom YI (2018) Metabolic signaling to epigenetic alterations in cancer. Biomol Ther. https://doi.org/10.4062/biomolther.2017.185

Korangath P, Teo WW, Sadik H, Han L, Mori N, Huijts CM, Wildes F et al (2015) Targeting glutamine metabolism in breast cancer with aminooxyacetate. Clin Cancer Res 21(14):3263–3273

Kubatka P, Kruzliak P, Rotrekl V, Jelinkova S, Mladosievicova B (2014) Statins in oncological research: from experimental studies to clinical practice. Crit Rev Oncol Hematol 92(3):296–311

Kusumanchi P, Zhang Y, Jani MB, Jayaram NH, Khan RA, Tang Y, Antony AC, Jayaram HN (2013) Nicotinamide mononucleotide adenylyltransferase2 overexpression enhances colorectal cancer cell-kill by tiazofurin. Cancer Gene Ther 20(7):403–412

Lee M, Hirpara JL, Jie-Qing E, Sethi G, Wang L, Goh B-C, Wong AL (2018) Targeting STAT3 and oxidative phosphorylation in oncogene-addicted tumors. Redox Biol 25:101073

Loftus RM, Assmann N, Kedia-Mehta N, O'Brien KL, Garcia A, Gillespie C, Hukelmann JL et al (2018) Amino acid-dependent cMyc expression is essential for NK cell metabolic and functional responses in mice. Nat Commun 9(1):2341

Ma Y, Wang W, Idowu MO, Unsong O, Wang X-Y, Temkin SM, Fang X (2018) Ovarian cancer relies on glucose transporter 1 to fuel glycolysis and growth: anti-tumor activity of BAY-876. Cancers (Basel) 11(1). https://doi.org/10.3390/cancers11010033

Marchiq I, Pouysségur J (2016) Hypoxia, cancer metabolism and the therapeutic benefit of targeting lactate/H(+) symporters. J Mol Med 94(2):155–171

Marin-Valencia I, Yang C, Mashimo T, Cho S, Baek H, Yang X-L, Rajagopalan KN et al (2012) Analysis of tumor metabolism reveals mitochondrial glucose oxidation in genetically diverse human glioblastomas in the mouse brain in vivo. Cell Metab 15(6):827–837

Martinez-Outschoorn UE, Sotgia F, Lisanti MP (2012) Power surge: supporting cells 'fuel' cancer cell mitochondria. Cell Metab 15:4–5

Mathis D, Shoelson SE (2011) Immunometabolism: an emerging frontier. Nat Rev Immunol 11(2):81

Mehta J, Asthana S, Mandal CC, Saxena S (2015) A molecular analysis provides novel insights into androgen receptor signalling in breast cancer. PLoS One 10(3):e0120622

Metallo CM, Gameiro PA, Bell EL, Mattaini KR, Yang J, Hiller K, Jewell CM et al (2011) Reductive glutamine metabolism by IDH1 mediates lipogenesis under hypoxia. Nature 481(7381):380–384

Michelakis ED, Webster L, Mackey JR (2008) Dichloroacetate (DCA) as a potential metabolic-targeting therapy for cancer. Br J Cancer 99(7):989–994

Min H-Y, Lee H-Y (2018) Oncogene-driven metabolic alterations in cancer. Biomol Ther 26(1):45–56

Moore JD, Staniszewska A, Shaw T, D'Alessandro J, Davis B, Surgenor A, Baker L et al (2014) VER-246608, a novel pan-isoform ATP competitive inhibitor of pyruvate dehydrogenase kinase, disrupts Warburg metabolism and induces context-dependent cytostasis in cancer cells. Oncotarget 5(24). https://doi.org/10.18632/oncotarget.2656

Mullard A (2016) Cancer metabolism pipeline breaks new ground. Nat Rev Drug Discov 15(11):735–737

Muthu M, Nordström A (2019) Current status and future prospects of clinically exploiting cancer-specific metabolism—why is tumor metabolism not more extensively translated into clinical targets and biomarkers? Int J Mol Sci. https://doi.org/10.3390/ijms20061385

Neugent ML, Goodwin J, Sankaranarayanan I, Yetkin CE, Hsieh M-H, Kim J-W (2018) A new perspective on the heterogeneity of cancer glycolysis. Biomol Ther (Seoul). https://doi.org/10.4062/biomolther.2017.210

Norata GD, Caligiuri G, Chavakis T, Matarese G, Netea MG, Nicoletti A, O'Neill LAJ, Marelli-Berg FM (2015) The cellular and molecular basis of translational immunometabolism. Immunity 43(3):421–434

O'Sullivan ME, Perez A, Lin R, Sajjadi A, Ricci AJ, Cheng AG (2017) Towards the prevention of aminoglycoside-related hearing loss. Front Cell Neurosci 11:325

Patsoukis N, Bardhan K, Chatterjee P, Sari D, Liu B, Bell LN, Karoly ED et al (2015) PD-1 alters T-cell metabolic reprogramming by inhibiting glycolysis and promoting lipolysis and fatty acid oxidation. Nat Commun 6:6692

Pellerin L, Magistretti PJ (2012) Sweet sixteen for ANLS. J Cereb Blood Flow Metab 32(7):1152–1166

Pike LS, Smift AL, Croteau NJ, Ferrick DA, Wu M (2011) Inhibition of fatty acid oxidation by etomoxir impairs NADPH production and increases reactive oxygen species resulting in ATP depletion and cell death in human glioblastoma cells. Biochim Biophys Acta 1807(6):726–734

Propper DJ, Braybrooke JP, Taylor DJ, Lodi R, Styles P, Cramer JA, Collins WCJ et al (1999) Phase I trial of the selective mitochondrial toxin MKT 077 in chemo-resistant solid tumours. Ann Oncol 10(8):923–927

Pudelko L (2018) Fishing for cures: The zebrafish as a powerful tool to identify novel therapies against glioblastoma by targeting MTH1 and beyond. Thesis

Purzner T, Purzner J, Buckstaff T, Cozza G, Gholamin S, Rusert JM, Hartl TA et al (2018) Developmental phosphoproteomics identifies the kinase CK2 as a driver of hedgehog signaling and a therapeutic target in medulloblastoma. Sci Signal. https://doi.org/10.1126/scisignal.aau5147

Qian Y (2014) Inhibitors of glucose transport and glycolysis as novel anticancer therapeutics. World J Transl Med. https://doi.org/10.5528/wjtm.v3.i2.37

Raal FJ, Marais AD, Klepack E, Lovalvo J, McLain R, Heinonen T (2003) Avasimibe, an ACAT inhibitor, enhances the lipid lowering effect of atorvastatin in subjects with homozygous familial hypercholesterolemia. Atherosclerosis. https://doi.org/10.1016/j.atherosclerosis.2003.07.011

Rani R, Kumar V (2016) Recent update on human lactate dehydrogenase enzyme 5 (hLDH5) inhibitors: a promising approach for cancer chemotherapy. J Med Chem 59(2):487–496

Richards DA, Nemunaitis JJ, Vukelja SJ, Hagenstad CT, Campos LT, Letzer JP, Hermann RC, Sportelli P, Gardner LR, Bendell JC (2010) Final results of a randomized phase II study of perifosine in combination with capecitabine (P-CAP) versus placebo plus capecitabine (CAP) in patients (pts) with second- or third-line metastatic colorectal cancer (mCRC). J Clin Oncol. https://doi.org/10.1200/jco.2010.28.15_suppl.3531

Sabatini DM (2006) mTOR and cancer: insights into a complex relationship. Nat Rev Cancer 6(9):729–734

Samudio I, Harmancey R, Fiegl M, Kantarjian H, Konopleva M, Korchin B, Kaluarachchi K et al (2010) Pharmacologic inhibition of fatty acid oxidation sensitizes human leukemia cells to apoptosis induction. J Clin Invest 120(1):142–156

Sarker D, Ang JE, Baird R, Kristeleit R, Shah K, Moreno V, Clarke PA et al (2015) First-in-human phase I study of pictilisib (GDC-0941), a potent pan-class I phosphatidylinositol-3-kinase (PI3K) inhibitor, in patients with advanced solid tumors. Clin Cancer Res 21(1):77–86

Semenza GL (2012) Hypoxia-inducible factors: mediators of cancer progression and targets for cancer therapy. Trends Pharmacol Sci 33(4):207–214

Shen W-J, Asthana S, Kraemer FB, Azhar S (2018) Scavenger receptor B type 1: expression, molecular regulation, and cholesterol transport function. J Lipid Res. https://doi.org/10.1194/jlr.r083121

Soriano A, Miró O, Mensa J (2005) Mitochondrial toxicity associated with linezolid. N Engl J Med 353(21):2305–2306

Starke I, Glick GD, Börsch M (2018) Visualizing mitochondrial FoF1-ATP synthase as the target of the immunomodulatory drug Bz-423. Front Physiol. https://doi.org/10.3389/fphys.2018.00803

Stine ZE, Walton ZE, Altman BJ, Hsieh AL, Dang CV (2015) MYC, metabolism, and cancer. Cancer Discov 5(10):1024–1039

Su J, Li D, Chen Q, Li M, Lu S, Luo T, Liang D et al (2018) Anti-breast cancer enhancement of a polysaccharide from spore of ganoderma lucidum with paclitaxel: suppression on tumor metabolism with gut microbiota reshaping. Front Microbiol. https://doi.org/10.3389/fmicb.2018.03099

Supuran CT (2018) Carbonic anhydrase inhibitors as emerging agents for the treatment and imaging of hypoxic tumors. Expert Opin Investig Drugs 27(12):963–970

Tateishi K, Wakimoto H, Iafrate AJ, Tanaka S, Loebel F, Lelic N, Wiederschain D et al (2015) Extreme vulnerability of IDH1 mutant cancers to NAD+ depletion. Cancer Cell 28(6):773–784

Tibes R, Falchook GS, Von Hoff DD, Weiss GJ, Iyengar T, Kurzrock R, Pestano L, Lowe AM, Herbst RS (2010) Results from a phase I, dose-escalation study of PX-478, an orally available inhibitor of HIF-1α. J Clin Oncol. https://doi.org/10.1200/jco.2010.28.15_suppl.3076

Ueda K, Nakatsu Y, Yamamotoya T, Ono H, Inoue Y, Inoue M-K, Mizuno Y et al (2019) Prolyl isomerase Pin1 binds to and stabilizes acetyl CoA carboxylase 1 protein, thereby supporting cancer cell proliferation. Oncotarget 10(17):1637–1648

Van Dang C, Kim J-W (2018) Convergence of cancer metabolism and immunity: an overview. Biomol Ther 26(1):4–9

Vazquez A, Kamphorst JJ, Markert EK, Schug ZT, Tardito S, Gottlieb E (2016) Cancer metabolism at a glance. J Cell Sci. https://doi.org/10.1242/jcs.181016

Wan X, Shen N, Mendoza A, Khanna C, Helman LJ (2006) CCI-779 inhibits rhabdomyosarcoma xenograft growth by an antiangiogenic mechanism linked to the targeting of mTOR/Hif-1alpha/VEGF signaling. Neoplasia 8(5):394–401

Wang P, Jiang L, Cao Y, Ye D, Zhou L (2018) The design and synthesis of N-xanthone benzenesulfonamides as novel phosphoglycerate mutase 1 (PGAM1) inhibitors. Molecules. https://doi.org/10.3390/molecules23061396

Wang L, Liu X, Yang Q (2018) Application of metabolomics in cancer research: as a powerful tool to screen biomarker for diagnosis, monitoring and prognosis of cancer. Biomarkers J. https://doi.org/10.21767/2472-1646.100050

Woyach JA, Furman RR, Liu T-M, Ozer HG, Zapatka M, Ruppert AS, Xue L et al (2014) Resistance mechanisms for the Bruton's tyrosine kinase inhibitor ibrutinib. N Engl J Med 370(24):2286–2294

Xiang Y, Stine ZE, Xia J, Yunqi L, O'Connor RS, Altman BJ, Hsieh AL et al (2015) Targeted inhibition of tumor-specific glutaminase diminishes cell-autonomous tumorigenesis. J Clin Invest 125(6):2293–2306

Zhao G, Green CF, Hui Y-H, Prieto L, Shepard R, Dong S, Wang T et al (2017) Discovery of a highly selective NAMPT inhibitor that demonstrates robust efficacy and improved retinal toxicity with nicotinic acid coadministration. Mol Cancer Ther 16(12):2677–2688

9 Clinical Relevance of "Biomarkers" in Cancer Metabolism

Niraj Kumar Jha, Saurabh Kumar Jha, Ankur Sharma, Rahul Yadav, Pratibha Pandey, Kavindra Kumar Kesari, Neeraj Kumar, Parma Nand, Mansi Agrahari, and Nancy Sanjay Gupta

Abstract

Nowadays, the field of biomarker discovery has become the topic of vivid research with the current emergence of novel technologies. Major progress in cancer control will be significantly aided by early detection for the diagnosis and treatment of cancer in its preinvasive state. Cancer being a diverse disease involves mutations in mostly three classes of genes such as oncogenes (proto-oncogenes), DNA repair genes, and tumor suppressor genes, presenting a wide range of opportunities for the development and formulation of various cancer biomarkers. Cancer biomarkers are used to follow up disease process before it becomes more severe and help in screening, thus greatly aid in cancer diagnosis and treatment. They also act as biochemical indicators to show the evidence of the presence of a tumor. There are various types of tumor biomarkers, which are classified on the basis of their functionalities. For instance, tumor diagnostic markers aid in predicting the occurrence of tumor during diagnosis, while tumor prognostic markers are clinical measures used to assist in bringing out an

N. K. Jha (✉) · S. K. Jha · P. Nand · N. S. Gupta
Department of Biotechnology, School of Engineering & Technology, Sharda University, Greater Noida, India
e-mail: niraj.jha@sharda.ac.in

A. Sharma · R. Yadav · M. Agrahari
Department of Life Science, School of Basic Science and Research (SBSR), Sharda University, Greater Noida, India

P. Pandey
Department of Biotechnology, Noida Institute of Engineering & Technology (NIET), Greater Noida, India

K. K. Kesari
Department of Applied Physics, Aalto University, Espoo, Finland

N. Kumar
Department of Chemistry, SRM University, Modi Nagar, Uttar Pradesh, India

D. Kumar (ed.), *Cancer Cell Metabolism: A Potential Target for Cancer Therapy*,
https://doi.org/10.1007/978-981-15-1991-8_9

individual patients risk of a future consequence including disease reoccurrence after primary treatment. Similarly, various biomarkers are accountable for serving as a potential biochemical indicator to examine the processes of disease progression and help in disease diagnosis. However, the precise roles of cancer biomarkers in contributing to examine the cancer progression remain uncertain. This chapter therefore recapitulates about the recent findings of current and emerging biomarkers in cancer with fundamental insight into different markers used in cancer detection. Further, biomarkers based on these strategies may lead to remarkable improvement in cancer screening, prognosis, and management of therapeutic response in cancer patients.

Keywords
Cancer · Biomarkers · Cancer Stem Cells (CSCs) · Micro RNAs (miRNAs) · Prostate-Specific Antigen (PSA) · Therapeutics

9.1 An Overview of the Promise of Tumor Biomarkers in Cancer Metabolism

Oncologists hope that tumor biomarkers can be used for true early detection of cancer. Many of todays detection methodologies avail imaging techniques that can detect a tumor only after it has been present many years, often as much as a decade or two. Conversely, tumor markers are used to follow up disease process before it becomes more severe and help in screening, thus greatly used in cancer diagnosis and treatment. They are biochemical indicators which show evidence of the presence of a tumor (Bhatt et al. 2010). Clinically, it refers to a molecule/substance that can be observed or detected in plasma and body fluids (Virji et al. 1988). There are various types of tumor biomarkers which have been classified on the basis of their functionalities. For instance, tumor diagnostic markers aid in predicting the occurrence of tumor during diagnosis, while tumor prognostic markers are clinical measures used to assist in bringing out an individual patients risk of a future consequence including disease reoccurrence after primary treatment (Bhatt et al. 2010). They are quantifiable biochemicals that are related to malignant cells and may be elevated when there is cancer in the body (Virji et al. 1988). They are either produced by tumor cells or by the body in response to tumor-associated cells and that are normally discharged or released into the main blood stream (circulation) and in consequence measured in the blood (Sotiriou et al. 2004). Additionally, they are also found in urine or body tissues that can be elevated by the occurrence of one or more types of cancer. Tumor markers also serve as an indicator of a particular disease process, and they are utilized in oncology to assist in identifying the presence of tumor. However, tumors, including colorectal and lung tumor, are often diagnosed at a late stage with poor progression (Bhatt et al. 2010; Virji et al. 1988; Sotiriou et al. 2004). Although tumor diagnostic markers remarkably improve diagnosis, the unpleasant, invasive, and problematic nature of current diagnostic procedures limits their application (Sotiriou et al. 2004; Nagpal et al. 2016). Therefore, there is a great need for identifying viral biomarkers of novel non-invasive biomarkers for early tumor detection. Indeed, they are not the key modalities for cancer diagnosis, rather they can be used as a laboratory test to assist in diagnosis (Bhatt et al. 2010). Notably, these markers are not very "specific" meaning non-cancer health issues can also cause them to be elevated. Most importantly, identification of biomarkers during cancer progression is very crucial, because imperfect selection of biomarkers causes economic burden and severe health concern to the patients (Fig. 9.1). However, the precise roles of tumor markers in contributing to the cancer diagnosis remain uncertain. This chapter thus consolidates recent findings regarding the clinical significance of biomarkers in *cancer metabolism.*

9.2 How Does Cancer Biomarker Aid in Disease Diagnosis?

Blood and tumor tissues are tested while diagnosing cancer. These tests facilitate to find out the characteristics of the tumor such as rate of growth, aggressiveness, and degree of abnormality. Numerous tests for tumor markers may be availed with other laboratory procedures, including X-rays to spot and diagnose some cancers. Tumor markers may be hormones, proteins, or antigens. Tumor marker tests are not used by themselves for cancer diagnosis because nearly all markers can be observed in elevated levels in people who have benign conditions, and because no tumor marker is specific to a particular cancer. They are most frequently measured in blood and urine. They can also be found in tumors and other tissues. Further, they are sent to a laboratory where a variety of methods are utilized to enumerate the levels. The marker is generally found by combining the sample with antibodies that react with

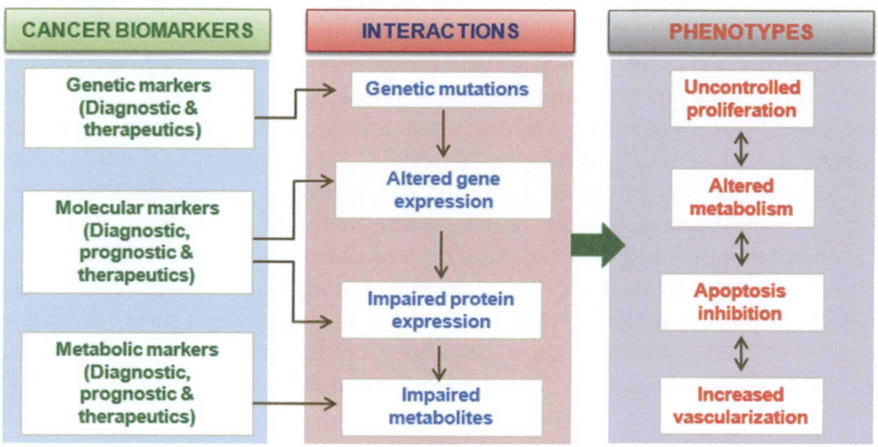

Fig. 9.1 Schematic representation showing the identification of various biomarkers during cancer prognosis

the tumor marker protein, thereby aiding in detecting tumor prognosis and occurrence (Chatterjee and Zetter 2005).

9.3 Are Cancer Biomarkers Authentic Indicators of Cancer?

Not every tumor will show an elevated expression in the diagnostic marker test, particularly in the early phases of cancer. Clinicians can make changes in tumor diagnostic marker levels to track the course of the disease, to validate the effect of treatment, and to verify for recurrence (Sharma 2009). They are not always reliable for the cancer diagnosis because: (1) the majority of tumor markers can be made by both normal and cancer cells, (2) they can be linked with non-cancerous conditions, (3) they are not always present in early-stage cancers, (4) people with cancer may never have elevated tumor markers, and (5) even when tumor marker levels are high, they are not precise enough to detect cancer. Further, authenticity of tumor markers also relies on test sensitivity and specificity. Tumor marker sensitivity refers to the test's ability to spot persons who have the disease. If a test is not very responsive or sensitive, there will be a lot of "false negative" results and persons with tumor will go undetected. A test that gives many false negative yields will evidently not be very good at serving diminishing cancer mortality. Moreover, tumor marker specificity refers to the test's ability to recognize or spot persons who do not have the disease. If a cancer test is not very specific or precise, it will give many "false positive" results where a person will test positive even though they are cancer free (Chatterjee and Zetter 2005).

9.4 How Is Cancer Biomarker Used in Cancer Care?

Since unusual biomarker levels may only advocate the presence of cancer, other scientific tests are generally needed before validating a cancer diagnosis. Physicians use numerous tests such as biopsies and the assessment of various tumor markers with some cancer types. A patient's history, physical exam, and other lab tests are also carefully considered. Tumor biomarkers are assessed over a period of time to observe if the levels are accelerating or reducing. They are primarily used to track persons who have already been diagnosed with cancer. In examining persons with cancer, tumor diagnostic markers can be cost-effective or less expensive and invasive than other diagnostic approaches. They can also assist doctors in finding out where a cancer started when the disease, when found, is already widespread. Tests include measuring tumor biomarkers to assist in diagnosing cancer, examining treatment effectiveness, and disease condition before, during and after therapies, and also assessing the risk of reappearance (Pellino et al. 2018; Puglisi et al. 2014).

9.5 Cancer Biomarker: A Potent Trafficator in Cancer Metabolism

Cancer biomarker plays a significant role in cancer metabolism as it helps in monitoring tumor cell growth and their prognosis. In this following section, we extensively discussed about the crucial role of various biomarkers that monitor the occurrence of tumor cells and early detection of cancer prognosis. Further, we have illustrated the diverse applications of biomarker in cancer metabolism in Fig. 9.2.

9.5.1 Cells as Biomarker

Monitoring the tumor cells in the bloodstream is easy, if the tumor cells are in the advance stage. The tumor and immune cells can be served for biomarker of prognosis. At the same time, as position of this in another tumor is nonetheless beneath assessment by the existing period and that can be achieved by advanced clinical and experimental practice in positive malignant cells. Further, some most imperative cells that serve as potential biomarkers of cancer are discussed here.

9.5.1.1 Regulatory T Cells

Regulatory T cells (T-regs) are notably observed by the experiments of FoxP3 (transcription factor), employing anti-FoxP3 antibodies. $FoxP3^+$ cells presence contained via tumors have been observed to forecast the metastasis, prognosis, and invasive capability about tumors by regulating the functionality of the immune system for targeting tumor cells or cancers (Schreiber 2007). T-regs consisting of $CD25^+$, $CD4^+$, and $Foxp3^+$ may function like a surrogate immune marker for the development of

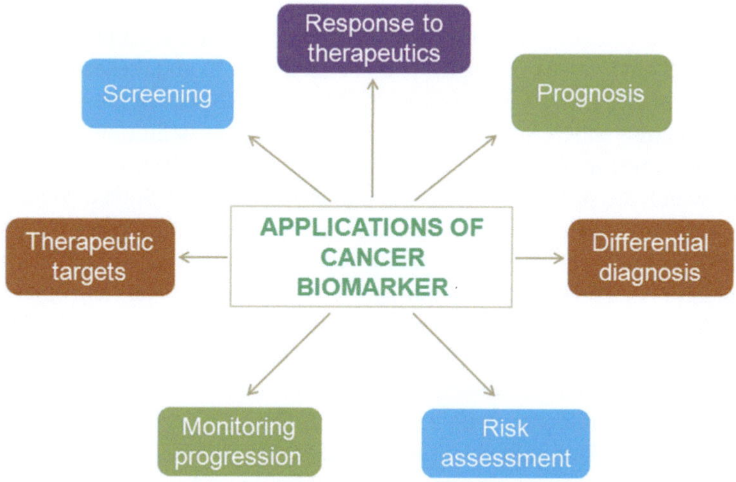

Fig. 9.2 Diverse applications of biomarker in cancer metabolism

most cancers (as well as perhaps diagnosis) and it appears to be stronger as a forecaster to remedy reaction (Schreiber 2007).

9.5.1.2 Circulating Tumor Cells

Circulating tumor cells (CTCs) are simple yet potential biomarker in cancer biology. The presence of CTCs has been appeared to forecast survival in metastatic breast cancer patients at many time points all through the course of therapy (Hall et al. 2016). In the metastatic breast cancer, the therapy which is the best for the diagnosis of this problem is CTCs. CTCs deliver systematic survival therapy and one of the reliable signals of disease prognosis. As the removal of CTCs unfolds therapy effectiveness, the increased CTCs during therapy at any time are a messenger of prognosis (Poveda et al. 2011; Hanahan and Weinberg 2000).

9.5.1.3 Cancer Stem Cells

Cancer stem cells (CSCs) have crucial implications for cancer metabolism and therapy, since it is expected that abolition of CSCs is the decisive determinant in attaining cure. It has been introduced that CSCs may be principally resistant to radiation therapy and chemotherapy as evident in a study with glioblastoma (Bao et al. 2006). $CD133^+$ cells were earlier recommended as the tumorigenic population in primary glioblastoma multiforme specimens; however, recent studies have reported that these are in fact more radioresistant compared with $CD133^-$ tumor cells, as their fraction enhances after irradiation which emerges to be principally accountable for the tumor regrowth (Singh et al. 2004; Bao et al. 2006). Hence, it is important to figure out and identify every character of CSCs to know about the tumor and its diagnosis, and the new ways of healing therapy windows would be discovered.

9.5.2 MicroRNAs as Biomarker

In the most recent cancer development, it is evident that a fraction of non-coding RNAs (19–25 nucleotides in length) is associated with it, and these nucleotides are naturally occurring and are called as microRNAs (miRNAs). In the various serious cancers, impaired miRNAs have been observed. In the definition of cancer, this miRNA tissue has an excellent potential. In a regular subject, it is found that 63 miRNAs which are new were absent. The analysis report of Solexa which is done on non-small cell lung carcinoma (NSCLC) patients regarding expression profile of serum miRNAs clearly shows it. Among these new miRNAs in NSCLC, various miRNAs have been recognized to be connected to the lung cancers and other tumors. As an instance, miR-23a, miR-27a, miR-24, miR-125b, miR-152, miR-128b, miR-222, miR-150, miR-205, etc. reported enlarged levels found in tissue testers analyzed with lung tumor or cancer, whereas the countenance ranges of miR-25, miR-29a, miR-92, miR-99a, miR-223, miR-221, etc. have been found in elevated amount in the tissues of colorectal tumors. Furthermore, it has been stated that lots of patients suffering and bearing pain by papillary thyroid cancers exerted elevated levels of miR-221, miR-146, and miR-222. Similarly, miR-221, miR-125b, and miR-222 have been recounted to be upregulated in the TRAIL-resistant larger cells of lung tumor cells (Chen et al. 2008). Importantly, miRNAs could also serve as an optimal cancer sensing group of blood-based biomarkers because: (1) countenance patterns of miRNAs in malignant tumor appear to be tissue-specific, (2) its expression is regularly altered in cancer, and (3) miRNAs have unusually high stability in formalin-fixed tissues. Further, miRNAs were relatively stable in serum/plasma clinical specimens. Additionally, miRNAs have also been suspected of having an effect on the cellular activity and biomedical physiology of the cancer by several miRNAs presented within the cancer tissues (Mitchell et al. 2017).

9.5.3 Virus as Biomarker

Many viruses have been found to serve as a potential marker for cancer diagnosis and prognosis. Hepatocellular carcinoma (HCC), which is among the world's most prevalent tumors, and is also among the most common death factors in developing nations, has been recorded among virally instated cancerous cells, with almost 80–85% (Chen et al. 2000). Chronic infections of hepatitis C virus (HCV) have even been identified in a small fraction (13–18%) of HCC, primarily because of an endogenous infection of hepatitis B virus (HBV) (Chen et al. 2000). In addition to immunoinflammatory reactions, HBV can also advance tumorigenesis through genetic instability mainly caused by its common integration in host DNA (Kirk et al. 2006). Further, numerous biomarkers have been implemented to know about the etiology and prognosis of HCC. Possibly, the most common is the plasma/serum markers of HBV or HCV infection (Kirk et al. 2006). These markers can also be used to evaluate the production of viral proteins/DNAs/antibodies toward viral proteins. The surface antigens of HBV (HBsAg) and HBeAg are most widely used for identifying and analyzing persistent infections including low and high viral replications, respectively. Antibodies, including anti-HBV core antigen, anti-HBsAg, and anti-HBeAg assay, are also essential groups of biomarkers in studies conducted with HCC (Chen et al. 2000; Kirk et al. 2006; Chisari et al. 2010). Thus, viral biomarkers are having prospective relevance in the identification, forecasting, estimation, and evaluation of therapy responses.

9.5.4 Antigen-Based Biomarkers

The tumor antigens or associated proteins contain information about every biomolecular functions that occur in tumor cell, tumor tissue microenvironment, and host-tumor cell interactions. In the process of proliferation, tumor cells release various proteins and subsequent macromolecules into the extracellular fluid which may qualify as biological markers and helpful in disease diagnosis. Notably, a few of these substances can ultimately become blood streamed serving as probable serum biomarkers. Table 9.1 summarizes a few of the most common cancer antigens used as diagnostic and prognostic biomarker for cancer.

Table 9.1 Various cancers and their corresponding clinically specific biomarkers and associated applications

S. No.	Name of cancer	Associated biomarkers	Clinical functionalities
1	Thyroid cancer	Calcitonin	• Diagnose early disease • Screening for at-risk individuals
		Thyroglobulin (Tg)	• Monitor progression • Monitor response to treatment
2	Testicular cancer	Human chorionic gonadotropin (HCG)	• Diagnose at-risk individuals • Monitor response to treatment • Detect metastases
		Alpha-fetoprotein (AFP)	• Diagnosis • Follow-up after treatment
3	Pancreatic cancer	CA 19-9	• Predict prognosis • Monitor response to treatment • Monitor progression
4	Ovarian cancer (epithelial)	CA 125	• Monitor response to treatment • Detect recurrence
5	Ovarian cancer (germ cell)	AFP	• Diagnosis • Follow-up after treatment
6	Prostate cancer	Prostate-specific antigen (PSA)	• Screening • Detect early-stage disease • Monitor progression
		Heat shock proteins (HSP27 and HSP70)	• Diagnostic • Prognostic
		Cancer stem cells (CSCs)	• Diagnostic • Prognostic • Therapeutic
		Prostatic acid phosphatase (PAP)	• Rarely used because PSA is more sensitive
		Membrane antigen (PSMA)	• Diagnostic • Prognostic

(continued)

Table 9.1 (continued)

S. No.	Name of cancer	Associated biomarkers	Clinical functionalities
7	Multiple myeloma	Bence Jones protein	• Diagnosis • Predict prognosis • Monitor progression • Monitor response to treatment
		Myeloma protein (M-protein or Mspike)	• Diagnosis • Predict prognosis
		Gamma globulin	• Predict prognosis
		Beta-2 microglobulin (β2M)	• Predict prognosis • Monitor progression
8	Melanoma skin cancer	TA 90	• Detect metastasis • Predict prognosis
9	Lymphoma	β2M	• Predict prognosis • Monitor progression
10	Lung cancer (NSCLC)	Carcinoembryonic antigen (CEA)	• Diagnosis (but not very important because lung cancer can be easily seen on X-rays)
11	Liver cancer	AFP	• Diagnose liver cancer in patients with chronic hepatitis • Follow-up after surgery for liver cancer
12	Colorectal cancer	CA 19-9	• Monitor response to treatment • Monitor progression
		CEA	• Predict prognosis • Detect recurrence • Monitor response to treatment

(continued)

Table 9.1 (continued)

S. No.	Name of cancer	Associated biomarkers	Clinical functionalities
13	Breast cancer	CEA	• Predict prognosis • Monitor response to treatment • Detect recurrence • Used in combination with CA 15-3
		CA 27-29	• Monitor response to treatment • Detect metastases
		CSCs	• Diagnostic • Prognostic • Therapeutic
		BRCA-1 and BRCA-2	• Diagnostic
		Circulating tumor cells (CTCs)	• Diagnostic • Prognostic
		CA 15-3	• Monitor response to treatment • Detect metastases • Diagnostic • Prognostic
14	Bladder cancer	Nuclear matrix protein (NMP 22)	• Predict prognosis • Detect recurrence
		CA 19-9	• Diagnostic • Prognostic
		Bladder tumor antigen (BTA)	• Detect recurrence
15	Germ cell tumors (ovarian and testicular)	HCG	• Diagnostic
16	Papillary and follicular thyroid cancer	Tg	• Diagnostic • Prognostic
17	Osteosarcomas, gastric, uterine and cervical cancer	HSP27 and HSP70	• Diagnostic • Prognostic
18	Malignant tumors	Transforming growth factor-β (TGF-β)	• Diagnostic • Prognostic
19	Acute myeloid leukemia (AML), chronic myeloid leukemia (CML) and Burkitt's lymphoma	Genetic translocations viz., Philadelphia chromosome, Bcl2, and other gene translocation fusion products	• Diagnostic
20	Adenocarcinoma, squamous cell carcinoma of the stomach, pancreas, thyroid, and ovary	APC gene	• Diagnostic • Prognostic

(continued)

Table 9.1 (continued)

S. No.	Name of cancer	Associated biomarkers	Clinical functionalities
21	AML, melanoma, and brain tumor	CSCs	• Diagnostic • Prognostic • Therapeutic
22	All cancers, general	Glucose metabolism	• Daignostic • Prognostic • Therapeutic
23	Papillary and follicular thyroid cancer	Tg	• Diagnostic • Prognostic
24	Ovarian cancer and fallopian tube cancer	CA 125	• Diagnostic • Prognostic
25	Hepatocellular carcinoma (HCC)	AFP	• Diagnostic • Prognostic
26	Oral squamous cell carcinoma (OSCC)	MRP14, CD59, Profilin-1 and catalase	• Diagnostic
27	Neuroblastoma	Neuron-specific enolase (NSE)	• Diagnostic • Prognostic

9.5.4.1 Prostate-Specific Antigen

Prostate-specific antigen (PSA) is a serine protease that comes from both healthy and neoplastic prostate epithelial cells in the "Kallikrein" gene family. It is also the most commonly discussed biomarker of prostate cancer (Stephan et al. 2002). As a protease, it occurs from an anomalous production of the growth factor binding proteins and catabolism of growth factor proteins that contribute to the initiation and intensification of prostatic tumor. It may also have a pivotal role in invasion and metastases through the degradation of collagen and laminin. The most successful procedure currently offered for the early diagnosis of prostate cancer is a serum blood test to determine PSA (Stephan et al. 2002).

9.5.4.2 Carcinoembryonic Antigen

Glycoprotein carcinoembryonic antigen (CEA) was first identified by Gold and Freeman by administering an extract of human colonic carcinoma with an antibody induced in rabbits (Gold and Freeman 1965). Higher CEA rates are recorded in colorectal, breast, lung, and pancreatic cancer patients as well as in smoking individuals (Alaoui-Jamali and Xu 2006; Khan et al. 2008). In many other tumors, including pancreas, kidney, lung, uterus, ovary, breast, bladder, and thyroid, blood levels of CEA are also raised (Alaoui-Jamali and Xu 2006; Khan et al. 2008). Postoperative normalization of serum CEA level has been found to be a favorable prognostic indicator in lung cancer. In addition, the identification of unusual pre- and postoperative serum CEA levels may be helpful in the postoperative surveillance of colorectal cancer patients (Wang et al. 2007).

9.5.4.3 Alpha-Fetoprotein

Alpha-fetoprotein (AFP) is recognized as the most essential mammalian serum protein in fetal development that the liver hepatocyte actively develops and releases it throughout the fetal existence. Endodermal sinus cancer, hepatoblastoma, neuroblastoma, and HCC are the main cancers that produce AFP. This is also a commonly used biomarker for diagnostic prediction that is being used to monitor diagnosis of HCC where it is produced in large quantities. A significant increase in the amounts of serum AFP is often observable in individuals with poorly differentiated or extremely malignant tumors (Abelev 1971).

9.5.4.4 Cancer Antigen 19-9

Cancer antigen 19-9 (CA 19-9) was the first effective tumor indicator used for the serological diagnosis of pancreatic cancer (Casetta et al. 1993; Koprowski et al. 1979). It belongs to the family of glycolipid and has unrecognized biological functions. In individuals with gastric cancer, CA 19-9 was used as a perioperative indicator. In the event of both metastatic and chronic cases and perhaps also those who receive curative operations, this tends to be an effective indicator (Căinap et al. 2015).

9.5.5 Proteins as Biomarker

Currently, screening of four different proteins in cancerous sample of saliva has been reported to be significant biomarkers of oral cancer which are having 83% specificity and 90% sensitivity rate for oral squamous cell carcinoma (OSCC). These proteins include (1) CD59, which is over-expressed on cancerous cells that enables them to escape from complement-dependent and antibody-mediated immune responses; (2) catalase, an enzyme of the antioxidant process whose concentrations are highly regulated in various human cancers and engaged in carcinogenesis and tumor prognosis; (3) Profilin-1, a protein involved in various signaling activities with nuclear and cytoplasmic ligands, mostly released into tumor microenvironments in the process of the early introductory stage of cancer cells; and (4) MRP-14 (a calcium-binding protein) identified for different human cancers and employed for tumor prediction. However, the validity of such potential biomarkers for detection of oral cancer needs long-term trials with a significant patient population with oral cancer and those at increased risks of developing oral cancer (Saxena et al. 2017).

9.5.6 Genetic and Epigenetic Biomarkers

Tumor is a genetic ailment initially occurred by any gene modifications including tumor suppressors and transcription genes that are accountable for modulating cell development, reproduction, and other biochemical processes in the cells. Loss or gain of gene functions is principally accountable for conversion of oncogenes.

Numerous proto-oncogenes are transformed into oncogenes forming a slight point mutation on a chromosome, therefore changing the amount of its product (protein). Similarly, several non-random mutations and translocations within the regulatory segment of the gene are also considered to be linked with particular types of malignancy. For instance, the "Philadelphia chromosome" is linked with chronic myelogenous leukemia (CML) due to a translocation between chromosomes 9 and 22. Likewise, translocations within the regulatory segment occur in follicular B-cell lymphomas and Burkitt's lymphoma. These translocations act as highly specific tumor biomarkers for exclusive medical diagnosis (Bhatt et al. 2010).

In tumor cells, genes and their functional products (proteins) are either modified by mutations or in the course of epigenetic modifications to chromosomes that impair gene expression patterns. DNA methylation directly involves in epigenetic modifications, while modifications of histones and other proteins around which DNA is wrapped to produce chromatin can even be achieved indirectly, via acetylation, phosphorylation, and methylation. The main epigenetic regulation in humans in the form of 5′-CpG-3′ dinucleotides is the methylation of DNA in the cytotic residues. Specifically, it is apparent that cancer initiates and evolves as genetic anomalies are probably induced by epigenetic activities, which eventually facilitates in the tumor prediction through hypo- and hyper-DNA methylation. Enzyme DNA methyltransferases (DNMTs) have also been documented in many research findings, which adds methyl units into DNA at the site of cytosine residue, transformed into cancerous cells and related to a number of biological development procedures (Bhatt et al. 2010).

9.5.7 Cytogenetic and Cytokinetic Markers

Organizational and quantitative chromosome modifications are standard cancer indicators since the correlation among chromosome abnormalities and transformation of neoplasms has been very well studied. Differences in chromosomal numbers contributing to both hypo-and hyper-diploidy are reported in malignant tumors and structural deformations resulted in exchange and translocation of sister chromatids which could be readily identified using diversified banding methods (Dwarakanath et al. 1994). Furthermore, in malignant cells which are an indicator of tumor prediction, double minutes and even stained-region sections (indicator of gene modulation) are commonly found (Whitfield et al. 2006). However, the biopathological results have been followed by the ploidy variations but there's been a poor interaction among histological, ploidy, and therapeutic phases in various cancers (Zarbo et al. 2000). Somatic mutations which have been reported in reporter genes, oncogenes, and tumor suppressor genes are promising biomarkers for cancer risk as these can capture genetic events that are associated with malignant transformation (Bishop 1987). Mounting evidences have also advocated about the association between specific polymorphism in certain genes with the risk of cancer prognosis (Dunning et al. 1999; Toru et al. 2008).

9.5.8 Mitochondrial and Metabolism-Based Biomarker

Mitochondria generally consist of multiple haploid sets of their own genome (16.5 kb), along with almost all significant translation, localization, and protein structure elements. At 1000–10,000 copies/cell, mitochondrial DNA (mtDNA) is found; at birth, many of the copies are very similar (homoplasmic). Numerous aberrations in the mtDNA, mainly in the D-loop segment (region), have been currently observed in colon, breast, esophageal, liver, lung, endometrial, head and neck, kidney, leukemia, melanoma, prostate, oral, and thyroid cancer (Jakupciak et al. 2005; Maitra et al. 2004). Furthermore, increased glucose consumption by cells is most frequent and most important alteration identified by Warburg in many cancerous tumors regardless of its histological sources or significance of alterations (Warburg 1956; Dang and Semenza 1999). Mechanisms that encompass this key change cancer proliferation, which includes mtDNA causing modification, oncogeneic alterations combined with enhanced glycolysis, enhanced metabolic activity, and hypoxic lesion sub-micro-milieu modification of solid tumors (Kim et al. 2006).

9.5.9 Hormone as Cancer Biomarker

Placenta usually produces reproductive hormones such as human chorionic gonadotropin (HCG). The higher levels of HCG in individuals with certain tumors, such as cervical, ovarian or testicular cancers, and choriocarcinoma are recorded in the bloodstreams (Cole 1997). Free βHCG and its substituents also have been synthesized from pelvic carcinomas like the intestine, uterus, urinary tract, ovarian, and vulvo-vagina (Cole 1997). Ironically, the occurrence of higher concentrations of HCG in blood and related derivatives is usually considered a bad indication, and βHCG could potentially affect tumor growth and thus contribute to an improper diagnosis. Free βHCG as a cancer biomarker is restricted to a few patients in the clinical trials due to quick renal clearance and a short half-life. Increased levels of HCG in blood are also found in urine of pregnant women and thus might not be feasible as an identifier under such circumstance (Kurtzman et al. 2001).

9.5.10 Glycoprotein as Biomarker

Thyroglobulin (Tg) is a glycoprotein which is found in the thyroid gland and serves as pro-hormone in the intra-thyroid synthesis of triiodothyronine (T3) and thyroxine (T4). This may be recognized for organ-specific cancer biomarkers mostly connected to individuals who have been involved with distinct thyroid cancer (follicular or papillary thyroid) which results in higher amounts of Tg in the bloodstream from follicle cells. The Tg test has been used primarily to measure the success of thyroid cancer therapies and also to track recurrent incidents (Mazzaferri et al. 2003).

9.5.11 Heat Shock Proteins as Biomarker

Heat shock proteins (HSPs) have been over-expressed in a variety of malignant tumors which include the transformation of the cancer cells, development, immune system recognitions, metastases, intrusion, and cell death. At present, it is not obvious whether HSPs are being over-expressed in cancer cells; another theory is that HSP initiation is triggered by the physio-pathological characteristics of the cancer microenvironment (oxygen, low glucose, and pH) (Pinashi-Kimhi et al. 1986; Daniels et al. 2004). Furthermore, owing to its over-expressions in many cancerous cells, HSP rates are often not supportive at the detection stage; these are, however, potential biomarkers of tissue cancers which reflect the magnitude of modification and the aggression in different kinds of tumors (Ciocca and Stuart 2005).

9.5.12 Biochemical Biomarker

Biochemical markers play an important role in sensing tumor prognosis. Until now several biochemical markers have been reported, but neuron-specific enolase (NSE) is one of them. It is found in tumor originating from the neuroendocrine cell system. It is an isozyme of the glycolytic pathway that is found only in brain. NSE serves as an immuno-histochemical biomarker for cancers of the central nervous system and neuroblastomas. Patients evaluated with pancreatic cancer, small-cell lung tumor, skin cancers, Wilms' (nephroblastoma), kidney, and testicular tumors are identified with NSE (Isgrò et al. 2015).

9.5.13 Therapeutic Biomarker

Radiotherapy and cytotoxic drugs or cytostatics (also cytotoxic chemotherapy) remain the much effectual aids for tumor; however, these may also lead to severe side effects, due to non-expression of sufficient derivative impressions among normal and tumor cells. Progression in the molecular understanding and knowledge of clinical basis of cancer made biology promising. Through the classification and functional analysis of tumor-specific genetic changes, it has opened thrilling new prospective for designing therapeutic treatments that exclusively target the molecular pathways engaged in advancing growth of tumor cell and outsmart apoptosis like death pathways.

9.6 What Are the Potential Advantages of Using Tumor Biomarkers?

Tumor biomarkers play a significant role in monitoring and early detection of cancer prognosis. Moreover, tumor markers were first formulated to monitor for cancer in people having no symptoms, and very less tumor markers have been shown to be beneficial in such manner, because nearly all tumor markers have not been reported to sense cancer as sooner. Further, tumor markers assist in the diagnosis of tumor cells. In the majority of cases, only biopsies and biomarkers may determine the tumors that are frequently not utilized in diagnosis of malignant tumors. However, these biomarkers can help in determining if tumor is expected to be present in the patients. It may also assist in diagnosing the source of cancer in patients with progressive prevalent diseases. Additionally, it helps in determining response to therapy. One of the main usages for such biomarkers is to examine patients undergoing clinical tumor treatments. If the initial elevated tumor marker levels are falling with the treatments, it indicates the effectiveness of treatment and shows an advantageous outcome. On the contrary, if the marker level rises, then the treatment is almost certainly not feasible and changes in treatment should be carefully well thought out. Furthermore, it acts as a prognostic marker of disease prognosis and also used to sense the recurring of cancers during the initial treatment. Some tumor markers such as PSA and HCG can be useful once treatment has been done with no evidence of residual cancer left (Garg et al. 2015).

9.7 What Are the Probable Disadvantages of Using Tumor Biomarkers?

Being able to infer diagnostic patterns that are exclusive to specific tumor states is a challenging issue because of the biological variability in an individual patient's sample, as well as the wide range of biomarker concentrations in all patients compared. Differences in sample collection, handling or storage, and profiling techniques among various research sites may change the protein profile obtained from a given sample. Therefore, standardization issues regarding biological variation, preanalytical variables, and analytical variability must be tackled before standard values can be established. Most importantly, a major problem in the identification of tumor biomarkers is the very low concentrations of markers obtained from tissues with small, early-stage cancer lesions (Matsumoto et al. 1999; Garg et al. 2015). Further, there are several other probable disadvantages of using tumor biomarkers and these are as follows:

1. In various cases, tumor patients might never have abnormal blood tumor markers.
2. Lack of reliability is one of the most common problems associated with tumor markers.
3. Not frequently present in early-stage cancers.
4. Most importantly, when levels of tumor markers are higher, they are not precisely sufficient to authenticate the presence of tumor.
5. The tumor markers can also be present because of non-cancerous conditions.
6. Both the normal cells and tumor cells can produce most tumor markers.

It is to be noted that with every next people, the proteins may get varied. Similar variances may be found when it comes to types of cell or different stimuli or even when the states of the diseases alter. Under such circumstances, the accuracy of data obtained from individual patients and at the same time data of the patient indicating the problem is difficult to find (Eissa 1999; Sharma 2009).

9.8 Future for Tumor Markers and Its Relevance in Drug Development

Clinical studies and practices have shown that it is not always the most accurate indicator for cancer to evaluate a single protein or some other elements in individuals. Various other methods of the investigation may recognize good cancer indicators. It is essential to validate and centralize several factors and also to develop several techniques. Biological markers are particularly critical elements for the improvement of the pharmaceutical research cycle. The pharmacy community continues to understand that most medications actually succeed in a portion of the clinical therapy group. The sector understands that not only the medical studies would evaluate the medication smaller, faster, effective, and more affordable to a specific majority of patients, but also a market value could be placed on medicine that works for individuals that consume it more often. Some successful drug manufacturers and even small pharmaceutical companies, especially in oncology, have taken pharmacokinetic marker method to drug production.

9.9 Concluding Remarks

This chapter has extensively talked about various cancer biomarkers that are being used in monitoring cancer progression and help in diagnosis. Although they are much helpful in disease detection and diagnosis, they are still imperfect as screening tests for detection of occult cancers. The cancer biomarker level may also sense the disease stage, signifying how swiftly the cancer is likely to spread and assisting to identify the prognosis. Increased levels of cancer biomarkers on test results are not always worrisome but sometimes they can be. However, changes in biomarker levels may be the cause for alarm, and other non-cancerous abnormalities can cause test results to vary. Although conventional strategies for cancer biomarker discovery have shown promise, the expansion of medically confirmed cancer detection markers remains an unmet challenge for many common human cancers. New approaches that can complement and improve on current strategies for cancer detection are immediately needed.

References

Abelev GI (1971) Alpha-fetoprotein in ontogenesis and its association with malignant tumors. Adv Cancer Res 14:295–358

Alaoui-Jamali MA, Xu YJ (2006) Proteomic technology for biomarker profiling in cancer: an update. J Zhejiang Univ Sci B 7(6):411–420

Bao S, Wu Q, McLendon RE, Hao Y, Shi Q, Hjelmeland AB, Dewhirst MW, Bigner DD, Rich JN (2006) Glioma stem cells promote radioresistance by preferential activation of the DNA damage response. Nature 444(7120):756–760

Bhatt AN, Mathur R, Farooque A, Verma A, Dwarakanath BS (2010) Cancer biomarkers – current perspectives. Indian J Med Res 132:129–149

Bishop JM (1987) The molecular genetics of cancer. Science 235:305–311

Căinap C, Nagy V, Gherman A, Cetean S, Laszlo I, Constantin AM, Căinap S (2015) Classic tumor markers in gastric cancer. Current standards and limitations. Clujul Med 88(2):111–115

Casetta G, Piana P, Cavallini A, Vottero M, Tizzani A (1993) Urinary levels of tumor associated antigens (CA 19-9, TPA and CEA) in patients with neoplastic and non-neoplastic urothelial abnormalities. Br J Urol 72:60–64

Chatterjee SK, Zetter BR (2005) Cancer biomarkers: knowing the present and predicting the future. Future Oncol 1(1):37–50

Chen X, Ba Y, Ma L, Cai X, Yin Y, Wang K, Guo J, Zhang Y, Chen J, Guo X, Li Q, Li X, Wang W, Zhang Y, Wang J, Jiang X, Xiang Y, Xu C, Zheng P, Zhang J, Li R, Zhang H, Shang X, Gong T, Ning G, Wang J, Zen K, Zhang J, Zhang CY (2008) Characterization of microRNAs in serum: a novel class of biomarkers for diagnosis of cancer and other diseases. Cell Res 18(10):997–1006

Chen CJ, Wang LY, Yu MW (2000) Epidemiology of hepatitis B virus infection in the Asia-Pacific region. J Gastroenterol Hepatol 15(Suppl):E3–E6

Chisari FV, Isogawa M, Wieland SF (2010) Pathogenesis of hepatitis B virus infection. Pathol Biol (Paris) 58(4):258–266

Ciocca DR, Stuart K (2005) Calderwood heat shock proteins in cancer:diagnostic, prognostic, predictive, and treatment implications. Cell Stress Chaperones 10:86–103

Cole LA (1997) Immunoassay of human chorionic gonadotropin, its free subunits, and metabolites. Clin Chem 43:2233–2243

Dang CV, Semenza GL (1999) Oncogenic alterations of metabolism. Trends Biochem Sci 24:8–72

Daniels GA, Sanchez-Perez L, Diaz RM, Kottke T, Thompson J, Lia M et al (2004) A simple method to cure established tumors by inflammatory killing of normal cells. Nat Biotechnol 22:1125–1132

Dunning AM, Healey CS, Pharoah PDP, Teare DM, Ponder BAJ, Easton DF (1999) A systematic review of genetic polymorphisms and breast cancer risk. Cancer Epidemiol Biomarkers Prev 8:843–854

Dwarakanath BS, Manogaran PS, Das S, Das BS, Jain V (1994) Heterogeneity in DNA content and proliferative status of human brain tumors. Indian J Med Res 100:279–286

Eissa S (1999) Tumor markers. Lippincot Williams & Wilkins, Philadelphia

Garg A, Ahmed S, Sinha A, Singh HP (2015) Tumor markers – its advantages and limitations in diagnosis of oral cancer. Univ J Dent Sci 1:42–45

Gold P, Freeman SO (1965) Demonstration of tumor-specific antigens in human colonic carcinoma by immunological tolerance and absorption techniques. J Exp Med 121:439–462

Hall C, Valad L, Lucci A (2016) Circulating tumor cells in breast cancer patients. Crit Rev Oncog 21(1–2):125–139

Hanahan D, Weinberg RA (2000) The hallmarks of cancer. Cell 100(1):57–70

Isgrò MA, Bottoni P, Scatena R (2015) Neuron-specific enolase as a biomarker: biochemical and clinical aspects. Adv Exp Med Biol 867:125–143

Jakupciak JP, Wang W, Markowitz ME, Ally D, Coble M, Srivastava S et al (2005) Mitochondrial DNA as a cancer biomarker. J Mol Diagn 7:258–267

Khan MS, Chaouachi K, Mahmood R (2008) Hookah smoking and cancer: carcinoembryonic antigen (CEA) levels in exclusive/ever hookah smokers. Harm Reduct J 5:19

Kim JW, Tchernyshyov I, Semenza GL, Dang CV (2006) HIF-1-mediated expression of pyruvate dehydrogenase kinase: a metabolic switch required for cellular adaptation to hypoxia. Cell Metab 3:177–185

Kirk GD, Bah E, Montesano R (2006) Molecular epidemiology of human liver cancer: insights into etiology, pathogenesis and prevention from The Gambia, West Africa. Carcinogenesis 27(10):2070–2082

Koprowski H, Steplewski Z, Mitchell K, Herlyn M, Herlyn D, Fuhrer P (1979) Colorectal carcinoma antigens detected by hybridoma antibodies. Somatic Cell Genet 5:957–971

Kurtzman J, Wilson H, Rao CV (2001) A proposed role for hCG in clinical obstetrics. Semin Reprod Med 19:63–68

Maitra A, Cohen Y, Gillespie SE, Mambo E, Fukushima N, Hoque MO et al (2004) The Human MitoChip: a highthroughput sequencing microarray for mitochondrial mutation detection. Genome Res 14:812–819

Matsumoto M, Komiyama K, Okaue M, Shimoyama Y, Iwakami K, Namaki S, Tanaka H, Moro I, Sato H (1999) Predicting tumor metastasis in patients with oral cancer by means of the proliferation marker Ki67. J Oral Sci 41(2):53–56

Mazzaferri EL, Robbins RJ, Spencer CA, Braverman LE, Pacini F, Wartofsky L, Haugen BR, Sherman SI, Cooper DS, Braunstein GD, Lee S, Davies TF, Arafah BM, Ladenson PW, Pinchera A (2003) A consensus report of the role of serum thyroglobulin as a monitoring method for low-risk patients with papillary thyroid carcinoma. J Clin Endocrinol Metab 88(4):1433–1441

Mitchell PS, Parkin RK, Kroh EM, Fritz BR, Wyman SK, Pogosova-Agadjanyan EL, Peterson A, Noteboom J, O'Briant KC, Allen A, Lin DW, Urban N, Drescher CW, Knudsen BS, Stirewalt DL, Gentleman R, Vessella RL, Nelson PS, Martin DB, Tewari M (2017) Circulating microRNAs as stable blood-based markers for cancer detection. Proc Natl Acad Sci U S A 105(30):10513–10518

Nagpal M, Singh S, Singh P, Chauhan P, Zaidi MA (2016) Tumor markers: a diagnostic tool. Natl J Maxillofac Surg 7(1):17–20

Pellino G, Gallo G, Pallante P, Capasso R, De Stefano A, Maretto I, Malapelle U, Qiu S, Nikolaou S, Barina A, Clerico G, Reginelli A, Giuliani A, Sciaudone G, Kontovounisios C, Brunese L, Trompetto M, Selvaggi F (2018) Noninvasive biomarkers of colorectal cancer: role in diagnosis and personalised treatment perspectives. Gastroenterol Res Pract 2018:2397863

Pinashi-Kimhi O, Michalowitz D, Ben-Zeev A, Oren M (1986) Specific interaction between the p53 cellular tumour antigen and major heat shock proteins. Nature 320:182–185

Poveda A, Kaye SB, McCormack R, Wang S, Parekh T, Ricci D, Lebedinsky CA, Tercero JC, Zintl P, Monk BJ (2011) Circulating tumor cells predict progression free survival and overall survival in patients with relapsed/recurrent advanced ovarian cancer. Gynecol Oncol 122(3):567–572

Puglisi F, Fontanella C, Numico G, Sini V, Evangelista L, Monetti F, Gori S, Del Mastro L (2014) Follow-up of patients with early breast cancer: is it time to rewrite the story? Crit Rev Oncol Hematol 91(2):130–141

Saxena S, Sankhla B, Sundaragiri KS, Bhargava A (2017) A review of salivary biomarker: a tool for early oral cancer diagnosis. Adv Biomed Res 6:90

Schreiber TH (2007) The use of FoxP3 as a biomarker and prognostic factor for malignant human tumors. Cancer Epidemiol Biomark Prev 16(10):1931–1934

Sharma S (2009) Tumor markers in clinical practice: general principles and guidelines. Indian J Med Paediatr Oncol 30(1):1–8

Singh SK, Hawkins C, Clarke ID, Squire JA, Bayani J, Hide T, Henkelman RM, Cusimano MD, Dirks PB (2004) Identification of human brain tumour initiating cells. Nature 432(7015):396–401

Sotiriou C, Lothaire P, Dequanter D, Cardoso F, Awada A (2004) Molecular profiling of head and neck tumors. Curr Opin Oncol 16(3):211–214

Stephan C, Jung K, Diamandis EP, Rittenhouse HG, Lein M, Loening SA (2002) Prostate-specific antigen, its molecular forms, and other kallikrein markers for detection of prostate cancer. Urology 59(1):2–8

Toru H, Masaharu Y, Shinji T, Kazuaki C (2008) Genetic polymorphisms and head and neck cancer risk. Int J Oncol 32:945–973

Virji MA, Mercer DW, Herberman RB (1988) Tumor markers in cancer diagnosis and prognosis. CA Cancer J Clin 38(2):104–126

Wang JY, Lu CY, Chu KS, Ma CJ, Wu DC, Tsai HL, Yu FJ, Hsieh JS (2007) Prognostic significance of pre- and postoperative serum carcinoembryonic antigen levels in patients with colorectal cancer. Eur Surg Res 39(4):245–250

Warburg O (1956) On the origin of cancer cells. Science 123:309–314

Whitfield ML, George LK, Grant GD, Perou CM (2006) Common markers of proliferation. Nat Rev Cancer 6:99–106

Zarbo RJ, Nakhleh RE, Brown RD, Kubus JJ, Ma CK (2000) Prognostic significance of DNA ploidy and proliferation in 309 colorectal carcinomas as determined by two-color multiparametric DNA flow cytometry. Cancer 79:2073–2086

Alterations in Metabolite-Driven Gene Regulation in Cancer Metabolism

10

Saurabh Kumar Jha, Rahul Yadav, Kumari Swati, Niraj Kumar Jha, Ankur Sharma, Fahad Khan, Neeraj Kumar, Parma Nand, Prabhjot Kaur, Tanaya Gover, and Geetika Rawat

Abstract

Cancer is the leading cause of mortality among humans globally. Knowing about the etiology underlying the advancement of cancer is imperative for curtailing the monetary and social burden of cancer. In addition to genetic mutations, altered metabolism involved metabolic rewiring is needed in cancer cells to support their high nutritional demand needed for energy generation. Cancer metabolism also refers to the perturbations in biochemical pathways that are reported in tumor cells compared with most of the normal cells. Metabolic impairments in tumor cells are more frequent which include aerobic glycolysis, decreased oxidative phosphorylation, and the accelerated production of biosynthetic intermediates crucial to the proliferative cells for their growth and development. Interruptions in metabolic cascades responsible for fueling energy into the cancer cells for their growth has been observed in most of the cancer forms. These interruptions, in turn, facilitates growth in tumor cells by ceasing biochemical signals used to inhibit tumor initiation, hence eventually increase the metastatic character of the tumor cells. However, the precise mechanisms whereby metabolic pathways contribute to the cancer prognosis remain uncertain. This chapter thus consolidates recent findings regarding cross talk

S. K. Jha (✉) · K. Swati · N. K. Jha · P. Nand
Department of Biotechnology, School of Engineering & Technology, Sharda University, Greater Noida, India
email: saurabh.jha@sharda.ac.in

R. Yadav · A. Sharma · P. Kaur · T. Gover · G. Rawat
Department of Life Science, School of Basic Science and Research (SBSR), Sharda University, Greater Noida, India

F. Khan
Department of Biotechnology, Noida Institute of Engineering & Technology (NIET), Greater Noida, India

N. Kumar
Department of Chemistry, SRM University, Modi Nagar, Uttar Pradesh, India

D. Kumar (ed.), *Cancer Cell Metabolism: A Potential Target for Cancer Therapy*,
https://doi.org/10.1007/978-981-15-1991-8_10

between *metabolic alterations and cancer biology*. Further, a concrete and deep understanding of this heterogeneity may enable the advancement and optimization of potential therapeutic approaches that target biochemical pathways associated with proliferation of malignant cells.

Keywords
Cancer · Metabolism · Metabolites · Glycolysis · TCA cycle · Oncogenes · Therapeutics

10.1 Tumor Cell Metabolism: An Overview

Tumor cells have been recognized to hold strikingly different metabolic hallmarks compared with those of corresponding normal cells (Cantor and Sabatini 2012). Unlike normal cells, *tumor cells* rewire their *cellular metabolism* to *satisfy the demands* of growth and proliferation (Kerr and Martins 2018) (Fig. 10.1). The first outlined cancer-specific biochemical alteration is the Warburg effect. This is an aerobic glycolytic process reported by Otto Warburg in 1926 (Warburg 1956). In this process, tumor cells relies on glycolytic pathway for glucose metabolism even in the presence of oxygen, thus generates high levels of lactate and reducing the use of the Krebs/tricarboxylic acid (TCA) cycle (Levine and Puzio-Kuter 2010). Since

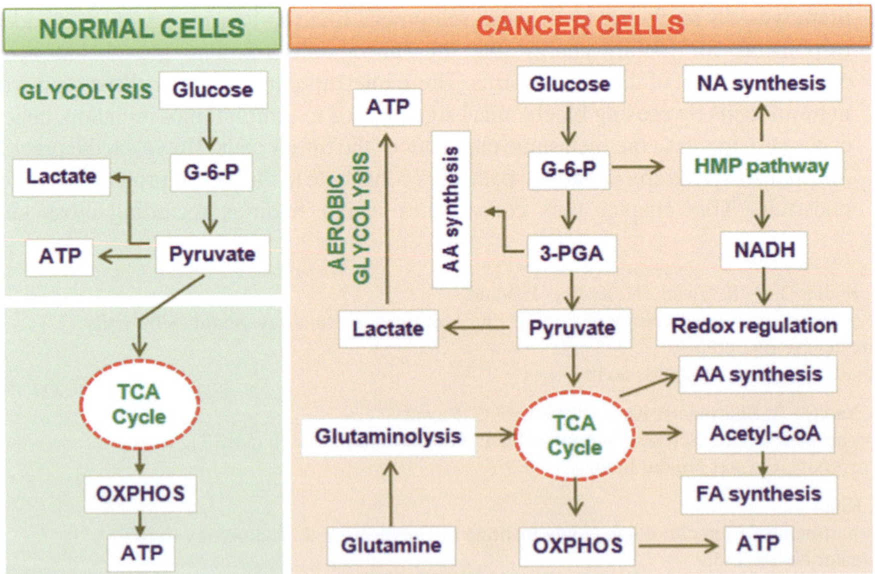

Fig. 10.1 Schematic representation of metabolic reprogramming in cancer cells compared to normal cells. *G-6-P* glucose-6-phosphate, *ATP* adenosine triphosphate, *OXPHOS* oxidative phosphorylation, *AA* amino acid, *NA* nucleic acid, *3-PGA* 3-phosphoglyceric acid, *NADH* nicotinamide adenine dinucleotide

the TCA cycle and consequent oxidative phosphorylation generate cellular energy more powerfully than glycolysis; this metabolic rearrangement has been advocated as an alternative source to compensate altered mitochondrial dynamics in tumor cells (Lee and Yoon 2015). In fact, any alterations in the TCA cycle-linked enzymes have been reported in various cancers. For instance, paraganglioma and pheochromocytoma are caused due to mutations in succinate dehydrogenase (SDH). Similarly, renal carcinoma and leiomyomatosis have reported to be associated with fumarate hydratase (FH) mutations. Likewise, isocitrate dehydrogenase mutations are accountable for acute myeloid leukemia (AML) and glioblastoma. Further, these mutations have been supposed to contribute to altered mitochondrial dynamics in tumor and tumorigenesis. However, a number of recent findings have advocated the imperative role of functional mitochondrial dynamics in tumor cells (Wallace 2012; Parker and Metallo 2015). The upregulation of oxidative phosphorylation has been observed in tumor cells and the tumorigenic potential of cancer cells has also been noticed to be considerably reduced by depletion of mitochondrial DNA (Magda et al. 2008; Whitaker-Menezes et al. 2011). For this reason, in addition to ATP synthesis, metabolic switching to aerobic glycolysis emerges to be a means of supplying tumor cells with the precursors of amino acids, proteins, sugars, lipids, and nucleic acids for their *cellular metabolism*, required for their growth and proliferation. Recent findings reveal the additional metabolic rearrangement in tumor cells and resulting impairments in cellular signaling cascades and the tumor microenvironment, including changes in glucose, lipid, and amino acid metabolisms. Additionally, regulation of the cellular redox state to bear reactive oxygen species (ROS)-induced cellular damage and remodeling of the extracellular matrix surrounding tumor cells are also recently reported (Magda et al. 2008; Whitaker-Menezes et al. 2011).

Tumor cells exhibit accelerated expression of the alternatively spliced form of pyruvate kinase (PK) and PK muscle isozyme M2 (PKM2). PK induces the conversion of phosphoenolpyruvate (PEP) to pyruvate, the major rate-limiting step of glycolysis (Dong et al. 2016). Due to the decreased enzymatic activity of PKM2, the phosphorylated metabolites in the glycolytic cascade aggregate and are finally diverted into several anabolic pathways for the biosynthesis of triglycerides, glycogen, phospholipids, amino acids, and nucleotides (Dong et al. 2016). Additionally, tumor cells introduce acetyl-CoA into a truncated TCA cycle, thereby causing export of acetyl-CoA into the cytosol, where it works as a precursor of cholesterol, fatty acids, and isoprenoids, which are used for cell growth and proliferation. Choline kinase and fatty acid synthase, which mediate phosphatidylcholines and long-chain fatty acids biosynthesis, respectively, are also known to be accelerated in cancer cells (Kroemer and Pouyssegur 2008). During amino acid metabolism, tumor cells express sensors of amino acid scarcity, including, folliculin, GATOR1, and the Ras-like small GTPase Rag complex, to confirm enough supply of amino acids to trigger mammalian target of rapamycin complex-1 (mTORC1) (Tsun and Possemato 2015). The upregulated uptake of glutamine through upregulated expression of glutamine transporters (SLC1A5 and SLC38A2) has been considered to actively play pivotal roles in the uptake of essential amino acids, the supply of nitrogen and the maintenance of mTORC1 activation in tumor cells (Wise and Thompson 2010). Tumor cells also show substantial conversion of glutamine to glutamate and elevated expression of numerous metabolic enzymes accountable for amino acid biosynthesis, including phosphoglycerate dehydrogenase (PHGDH), glutaminase (GLS), and asparagine synthetase (ASNS) (Tsun and Possemato 2015). In addition, hexose monophosphate shunt (HMP) pathway-associated nicotinamide adenine dinucleotide phosphate (NADPH) favors the defense of tumor cells against oxidative stresses and the biosynthesis of fatty acids in tumor cells (Levine and Puzio-Kuter 2010). Further, increased production of lactate through glycolytic pathway (aerobic glycolysis) assists in forming acidic tumor microenvironment, which facilitates the invasion capability of tumor cells and blood vessels through matrix remodeling and repressing anticancer immunity (Levine and Puzio-Kuter 2010). Inclusively, these complex operations permit tumor cells to endure and proliferate; however, the details are regarded to be context dependent and differentially modulated by many factors including oncogenes, tumor suppressor genes, microenvironments, and tissue of origin (Kerr and Martins 2018). Therefore, understanding the cellular or environmental impact of oncogene-mediated metabolic switches on tumor cell metabolism is crucial for the development of potential anticancer therapeutics targeting impaired metabolism in proliferating cells.

10.2 Metabolic Changes in Tumor Cells: Beyond the Warburg Effect

Perturbed metabolism is one of the characteristic features of most tumor cells. Tumor cells vary from normal cells by uncontrolled cell division. It has long been regarded that impaired metabolism in tumor cells is to ease their rapid growth and proliferation. The well-known metabolic defect in tumor cells is the Warburg effect, which exhibits an accelerated glycolysis event in the presence of oxygen. In other words, the Warburg effect has been taken for granted as a result of tumorigenesis (Liberti and Locasale 2016). However, cancer-associated metabolic defects are not restricted to impaired balance between glucose fermentation and oxidative phosphorylation. This notion is further fortified by findings that key tumor genes including c-Myc and p53 are found to be chief regulators of metabolism. However, recent progress in studying isocitrate dehydrogenase-1 and FH mutation, PKM2 alterations, and SDH mutations have shown that mutation in key metabolic enzymes alone is sufficient to set off tumors, casting doubts to previous belief. Likely, metabolic disorders are direct causes of tumor initiation. Otto Warburg's historic finding on perturbed metabolism in cancer conducted in an era of study on tumor metabolism, which was mostly centered on the relationship between glycolytic pathway and cellular bioenergetics. Although Warburg's finding is mechanistically still unknown but has been exploited clinically by 18F-deoxyglucose positron emission tomography scanning, an extensively used technology for solid tumor detection (Lu et al. 2015; Liberti and Locasale 2016).

10.3 Oncogenes: The Decisive Key Effectors in Tumor Metabolism

Transcription factors such as HIF, Myc, SREBP1, and p53 serve as a master regulator of cellular metabolism in tumor cells. These are imperative in the regulation of cell growth and proliferation and are triggered downstream of growth factor-mediated signaling. Additionally, these factors also activate the expression of several genes engaged in metabolite biosynthesis in response to growth factors. Thus, transcription factors actively participate and impart their significant role in cancer metabolism. In this section, we have discussed crucial transcription factors that are reported to be associated with biochemical pathways in various cancers.

10.3.1 Hypoxia-Inducible Factor (HIF)

Mammalian cells exposed to deprived oxygen (hypoxic condition) go through a metabolic response, where glucose utilization is increased and pyruvate is redirected to lactate to enable net adenosine triphosphate (ATP) generation via glycolytic pathway (Greer et al. 2012). This process is coordinated by the HIF1 transcription factor complex, which provokes the increased expression of genes that favor fermentative glucose metabolism, such as glycolytic enzymes, glucose transporters, pyruvate dehydrogenase kinase-1 (PDK1), and lactate dehydrogenase-A (LDHA) (Semenza 2012). HIF1 activity is reliant upon its HIF1α-subunit stabilization. Under normal conditions, HIF1α is suppressed through prolyl hydroxylation, resulting in von Hippel–Lindau (VHL) tumor suppressor-directed proteasomal degradation of HIF1. Although, mTORC1 can provoke HIF1α transcription and translation under normal conditions, and constitutive HIF1 activation can occur in cancer cells through various mechanisms, such as (1) loss of function mutations in VHL, (2) aggregation of ROS, or (3) agglomeration of the metabolites fumarate or succinate formed from loss of function mutations in the TCA cycle enzymes FH or SDH (Semenza 2010).

10.3.2 Sterol Regulatory Element-Binding Protein-1 (SREBP1)

Sterol regulatory element-binding protein-1 (SREBP1) is a member of the SREBP family of transcription factors, and provokes the expression of genes engaged in sterol and fatty acid biosynthesis in response to growth factors or intracellular sterol levels (Eberlé et al. 2004). SREBP1 also serves as a downstream effector of mTORC1, thereby affording mTORC1 with an extra mode for modulating cell growth (Düvel et al. 2010; Peterson et al. 2011). Subsequently, hyperactivation of mTORC1 further potentiates the deregulation of de novo lipid biosynthesis needed for sustained membrane production and cell proliferation (Laplante and Sabatini 2009).

10.3.3 Myc-Transcription Factor (c-Myc)

Myc in normal cells is imperative in the regulation of cell growth and proliferation and is triggered downstream of growth factor-mediated signaling (Dang 2010). In numerous tumors, though, Myc is a proto-oncogene that is aberrantly activated by gene amplification, chromosomal translocations, and single nucleotide polymorphisms or perhaps as a downstream result of mTORC1 hyperactivity (Dang et al. 2009). Like HIF1, Myc prompts enhanced expression of several genes engaged in glycolysis and the fate of glycolytic pyruvate (e.g., LDHA). Myc also targets genes that favor the proliferative utilization of glutamine, including glutamine transporters and genes engaged in both glutaminolysis and mitochondrial biogenesis (Cairns et al. 2011). Indeed, Myc-transformed cells go through apoptosis in the absence of exogenous glutamine, which is a critical carbon source for anaplerosis in these cells (Yuneva et al. 2007; Gao et al. 2009; Wise et al. 2008). In addition, Myc also activates the expression of enzymes in other anabolic pathways including, fatty acid synthase (FAS) and serine hydroxymethyltransferase (serine/glycine metabolism) (Gordan et al. 2007).

10.3.4 Tumor Suppressor—p53

p53 is an essential tumor suppressor gene, which is stimulated by cellular stress like hypoxia, ionizing radiation, carcinogens, and oxidative stress. Upon activation, p53 provokes several pathways that exert anticancer mechanisms, such as cell cycle arrest, DNA repair, and apoptosis (Vousden and Ryan 2009). Accordingly, p53 is an especially well-known tumor suppressor with an estimated 50% of all human cancers harboring either a mutation or a deletion in the TP53 encoding gene. Several lines of evidence have also revealed a multifaceted role for p53 in metabolic control as well (Gottlieb and Vousden 2010). Given the antitumor regulatory role played by p53 in a multitude of other cellular processes, it is unsurprising that p53 also guides metabolic characteristics consistent with those of normal resting cells. Namely, this influence lies in altering glucose metabolism through repression of glycolysis and concomitant stimulation of oxidative phosphorylation. Further, crucial roles of numerous other transcription factors and their corresponding clinically specific both metabolic pathways and metabolic enzymes in cancer metabolism have been addressed in Table 10.1.

10.4 Interplay Between Oncogene and Metabolic Alteration in Cancer?

There are many root causes of tumor prognosis, but oncogene-mediated biochemical alterations are one of them. This process is more prevalent and many biochemical pathways get simultaneously altered as evident even in single cancer types. In the following section, we extensively talked about alteration of numerous

Table 10.1 Cancer metabolism associated various transcription factors and their corresponding clinically specific both metabolic pathways and metabolic enzymes

Metabolism	Transcription factors	Associated metabolic enzymes	Interactions
Amino acid metabolism	Nuclear factor-κβ (NF-κβ)	Indoleamine-2,3-dioxygenase (IDO)	Associated with tumor initiation and proliferation via biosynthetic processes
	NF-κβ	Tryptophan 2,3-dioxygenase (TDO)	
	Myc	Glutamate dehydrogenase (GLUD1/2)	
	cAMP response element-binding (CREB) protein	Tryptophan hydroxylase (TPH1)	
	Myc	Phosphoglycerate dehydrogenase (PHGDH)	
	HIF-1α/Myc	Argininosuccinate synthase (ASS1)	
	Myc	Glutaminase (GLS2)	
	Myc	Serine hydroxymethyltransferase (SHMT1)	
Carbohydrate metabolism	HIF1α/Myc	Glucose transporter (GLUT1/3)	Associated with tumor initiation via aerobic glycolysis and also engaged in tumor proliferation via biosynthetic processes
	HIF1α/Myc	Hexokinase (HK2)	
	HIF1α/Myc	Phosphofructokinase (PFK1/2)	
	HIF1α/Myc	Pyruvate kinase isozymes (PKM1/2)	
	HIF1α/Myc	Lactate dehydrogenase (LDHA)	
	HIF1α	Phosphoinositide-dependent kinase (PDK1)	
	HIF1α	Isocitrate dehydrogenase (IDH1/2)	
	Specificity protein-1 (SP1)	Glucose-6-phosphate dehydrogenase (G6PDH)	
Lipid metabolism	SREBP1	ATP citrate lyase (ACLY)	Associated with tumor initiation and proliferation via biosynthetic processes
	SREBP1	Acetyl-CoA carboxylase (ACC)	
	SREBP1	Fatty acid synthase (FASN)	
	SREBP1	Acetyl-CoA synthetase (ACS)	
	SREBP1	Glycerol-3-phosphate acyltransferase (GPAT)	
	SREBP1	Stearoyl-CoA desaturase (SCD1)	

(continued)

Table 10.1 (continued)

Metabolism	Transcription factors	Associated metabolic enzymes	Interactions
Others	Myc	O-GlcNAc transferase (OGT)	Associated with tumor proliferation and metastatic spreading via altering surface glycoproteins
	Activator protein-1 (AP1)	Ceramide synthases (CerS)	

biochemical pathways that monitor the production and use of amino acids, sugars, and lipids, and also discuss how oncogenes help in regulating enzyme activity within these cascades.

10.4.1 How Does Amino Acid Metabolism Aid in Tumor Growth?

Amino acid metabolism plays a significant role in cancer metabolism since increased synthesis of proteins in tumor cells accelerates the nominal demand for amino acids. mTOR is a key signaling cascade engaged in this metabolism and this is a well-known cascade triggered by manifold oncogenic insults. AKT triggers the signaling module of mTOR whereas, liver kinase B1 (LKB1)-AMPK suppress the signaling axis (Horton et al. 2003; Hatzivassiliou et al. 2005). Moreover, cellular amino acid levels also provoke mTOR activity through brain-enriched Ras homologs and RAG GTPase signaling axis (Wullschleger et al. 2006; Bar-Peled and Sabatini 2014). Tumor cells have a high demand of glycine and serine that are needed for biogenesis of nucleotides (Amelio et al. 2014). Serine hydroxymethyltransferase 1, a crucial enzyme that gets elevated in ovarian and other tumors, pairs the 5,10-methylenetetrahydrofolate with tetrahydrofolate and serine to glycine conversions to supply carbon-deficient units for the production of purines, thymidylate, and methionine. Impaired metabolic activity of amino acid also has a decisive function in immune intolerance in tumor cells (Uyttenhove et al. 2003). For instance, T cells need adequate tryptophan for proliferation and growth. Indoleamine-2,3-dioxygenase (IDO) and tryptophan-2,3-dioxygenase degrade tryptophan that catalyzes tryptophan into kynurenines. IDO is exceedingly overproduced in tumor microenvironment and in the cancerous cells, which results in shortage of tryptophan and permits cancer cells to abstain the resistant function by restricting the T cells responses (Uyttenhove et al. 2003). Argininosuccinate synthetase-1 activity is also suppressed by tumor cells. This enzyme is helpful in catalyzing the final steps of biogenesis of arginine. Hence, numerous cancers including prostate cancer, hepatocellular carcinoma, and melanoma are auxotrophic for arginine, which is required in the production of citrulline, nitric oxide, ornithine, and urea (Dillon et al. 2004). Accordingly, bacterial arginase and arginine deiminase can inhibit the intensification of many tumor cells via reduction of arginine (Komada et al. 1997). Tumor cells are also having a high demand for asparagine and, as a result, show accelerated asparagine synthetase manifestations. A fraction of glutamine uptake by tumor cells is deflected for the biosynthesis of asparagine (Zhang et al. 2013).

10.4.2 Carbohydrate Metabolism: How Does It Benefit Tumor Cells?

Biochemical pathways associated with carbohydrate metabolism plays a pivotal role and oversee various processes during the tumor cells growth and in the tumor microenvironment. Tumor cells considerably change their metabolic energy by availing glutamine and glucose as the focal sources of energy and deflecting numerous other lipids and amino acids in the biosynthesis (Locasale and Cantley 2011). Warburg effect is well-known, however, not well identified metabolic impairment. It entails even in the presence of oxygen the tumor cells have elevated glycolytic process and lactate productions (Warburg 1956; Hsu and Sabatini 2008). Elevated productions of lactate form an acidic microenvironment around tumor cells that eases tumor invasions, extracellular matrix remodeling, angiogenesis, and immune evasions (van Horssen et al. 2013; Cardone et al. 2005; Kennedy and Dewhirst 2010; Lu et al. 2002; Colegio et al. 2014). Moreover, pyruvate deflection into lactate curtails mitochondrial pyruvate oxidations, resulting in diminishing mitochondrial activity and thus boost branching and reduces differentiation (Vega-Naredo et al. 2014). Glycolysis, the key supplier of energy in tumor cells, produces NADH, ATP, and pyruvate that is fed into the TCA pathways. The foremost regulative components in the glycolysis are LDHA, hexokinase-2, phosphofructokinase, glucose transporter-1 (GLUT1), and pyruvate dehydrogenase (PDH) (Hamanaka and Chandel 2012). Initiation of glycolysis under oncogene-mediated process occurs mostly via HIF1, which provokes the release of multiple enzymes in the glycolytic cascade (Wang et al. 1995). Oncogenic signaling, such as mitogen-activated protein kinase (MAPK) signaling downstream of RAS or BRAF helps in stabilizing HIF1 through the degradation of the VHL E3 ubiquitin ligase (Kaelin Jr and Ratcliffe 2008). The Warburg effect that results from the coordinated deregulation of several genes, initialized with the elevated expressions of GLUT1 and GLUT3 that contributes to expanded uptakes of glucose (Su et al. 1990; Yamamoto et al. 1990; Nishioka et al. 1992). GLUT1 is a well-known target of Myc and an indirect target of the RAS/RAF cascade via HIF1. Further, 2-hydroxyglutarate an onco-metabolite helps in stabilizing HIF1 by preventing release of prolyl-hydroxylase (Xu et al. 2011). The TCA pathway makes use of multiple enzymes including fumarate, pyruvate, α-ketoglutarate, succinate, and oxaloacetate received from glycolysis and amino acid metabolism (Cardaci and Ciriolo 2012). In tumor cells, the TCA pathway is driven principally by glutaminolysis, since pyruvate from glycolytic process is transferred to lactic acid formation. The pentose phosphate pathway (PPP) uses glucose-6-phosphate (G6P) produced via hexokinase enzyme and in activity assists in the production of NADPH and ribonucleotides. The PPP cascade consists of an oxidative class and a non-oxidative class. When it comes to oxidation, it is the glucose-6-phosphate dehydrogenase (G6PDH) which is catalyzing the rate-limiting steps. G6PDH is considered as well regulated enzyme and at the same time is also considered as overexpressed in tumor cells from post-translational and transcription processes (Düvel et al. 2010; Stanton et al. 1991). Transcription of G6PDH composition in an mTORC1-dependent manner is initiated by SREBP1. Further, epidermal growth factor receptor (EGFR) cascade accelerates

G6PDH function via releasing of bound G6PDH to a soluble form. Both PI3K and RAS signaling cascades are equally crucial for this process. With this biochemical pathway, 6-phosphogluconate dehydrogenase is likewise deregulated. 6-Phosphogluconate dehydrogenase guides the generation of ribulose-5-phosphate. AMPK initiation is suppressed by ribulose-5-phosphate through modifying the dynamic LKB1 complex. It further actuates acetyl-CoA carboxylase-1 and lipogenesis (Guo et al. 2019).

10.4.3 Hooked on Fat: The Role of Lipid Metabolism in Tumor Development

Although both amino acid and carbohydrate metabolisms play significant role in carcinogenesis, lipid metabolism is equally important for cancer cells growth and its proliferation. Lipids including phospholipids, cholesterol, and fatty acids are chief source of energy and serve as component for the development of cell membranes. Tumor cells having elevated fatty acid synthesis are stored as non-reactive lipids. SREBP1 is the primal transcriptional factor accountable for biosynthesis of fatty acids (Horton et al. 2003). Aberrant activation of SREBP1 can lead to fatty liver disease, obesity, insulin resistance, and could also be engaged in tumor growth (Shao and Espenshade 2012). Aberrant activation of SREBP1 and induced expression of its target genes has been found in numerous cancer types, including prostate, breast, and ovarian cancers (Ettinger et al. 2004; Swinnen et al. 2006). SREBP1 was reported to modulate the androgen receptor gene transcription and also engaged in promoting migration, invasion, and proliferation in prostate cancer (Huang et al. 2012). In addition, an activated mutant form of the EGFR reported being present in certain subtypes of glioblastoma multiforme (GBM) also exhibit high levels of nuclear SREBP1. Treatment with inhibitors of fatty acids and cholesterol biosynthesis curtailed xenograft tumor formation in GBM cells engineered to express activated EGFR (Guo et al. 2009). Collectively, these findings firmly favor the role of SREBP1 in cancer progression and tumorigenesis. It also upregulates the function of various enzymes including fatty acid synthase, ATP citrate lyase (ACLY), glycerol-3-phosphate acyltransferase, acetyl-CoA carboxylase (ACC), and stearoyl-CoA desaturase-1 during the synthesis of fatty acids. ACLY acts as a mediator for linking the TCA cycle to fatty acid biosynthesis pathway through conversion of CoA and citrate to acetyl-CoA and oxaloacetate. Thereafter, ACC converts acetyl-CoA into malonyl-CoA and recognized as the first crucial stage of fatty acid biosynthesis. It has been recently reported that targeting ACC or ACLY reduces fatty acid synthesis and suppresses tumor cell growth (Hatzivassiliou et al. 2005; Chajès et al. 2006). Malonyl-CoA and Acetyl-CoA condensation processes are catalyzed by fatty acid synthase, for the biosynthesis of long-chained fatty acids. The enzymes involved in the production of fatty acids frequently play a vital role in the cancer diagnosis. These comprise acyl-CoA synthetase, which helps in activating fatty acids before oxidative degradation, and stearoyl-CoA desaturase, which incorporates double bonds at C9 (Hatzivassiliou et al. 2005; Chajès et al. 2006).

10.4.4 Other Metabolic Pathways

In addition to the three main metabolic pathways discussed above, several other pathways are also reported to be dysregulated in cancer metabolism, resulting in tumor growth and proliferation. For instance, glycosylation pathways, attaching carbohydrate side chains (glycans) to lipids and proteins, are reported in tumor cells. Glycosylation has an effect on mobility and cell adhesion, alters cell signaling, and exerts influence on the localization, stability, and protein functions. Tumor cells show elevated levels of sialylated glycans. The increased expression of sialylated antigens provokes withdrawal of cells from the cancer clump and attachment to the endothelium, a step that is required for metastatic spreading. Further, overexpressions of heparin sulfate proteoglycans are also observed in various tumors. The glycosylated proteins serve as co-receptors for several tyrosine kinase transcription factors, suppress their thresholds for activation and change signal length (Knelson et al. 2014). The metabolic activity of sphingolipids stimulates the growth of tumor cells, mainly through an anti-apoptotic reaction. It actually happens because of the potential of this cascade to inhibit agglomeration of pro-apoptotic ceramides (Haimovitz-Friedman et al. 1997). It has been reported that overexpression of glucosyl-ceramide synthase shows resistance to doxorubicin, advocating that preventing ceramide metabolism increases chemotherapy. Additionally, numerous anticancer compounds, including cytotoxic retinoid fenretinide, elicit their effects, at least in part, by de novo synthesis of ceramide causing the agglomeration in cancer (Ponzoni et al. 1995).

10.5 Metabolic Adaptations in the Tumor Microenvironment as Promising Anticancer Therapy

Stromal cells form a complex metabolic hub plays a significant role in metabolic adaptations in tumor microenvironment. In cancer cells, cancer-associated fibroblasts (CAFs) which are metabolically activated by cytokines or oxidative stress are responsible for releasing energy-rich metabolic intermediates, such as lactate and amino acids. These metabolites are subsequently taken up via specific transporters to produce ATP. Most importantly, oxygen availability also dictates metabolic heterogeneity, as tumor cells in hypoxic vicinity utilize anaerobic glycolysis to produce lactate, which is then taken up by normoxic tumor cells and used for ATP production. Further, cancer-associated adipocytes (CAAs) also go through metabolic alterations induced by tumor cells. These alterations include heightened activity of hormone-sensitive lipases, which generates free fatty acids (FFA) that once released by CAAs, are taken up by tumor cells. Further, intracellular FFAs are chaperoned by fatty acid-binding protein-4 and fatty acids are further oxidized in mitochondria to produce ATP. This complex relationship between tumor cells and stromal cells supports cancer growth/migration/invasion and metastasis. Conversely, it also provides manifold therapeutic targets. Some of the promising approaches include targeting PDK in CAFs with dichloroacetate and preventing lactate transporters with AZD3965 (AstraZeneca) block the use of FFAs as a source of energy. Similarly provoking breakdown of non-essential amino acid asparagine with L-asparaginase and preventing induction of the CAA phenotype with Thiazolidinediones also work in the same fashion as these are accountable for blocking the use of FFAs as a source of energy. The diabetes drug Metformin may also be used to diminish oxidative stress in CAFs and prevent uptake of FFAs in tumor cells (Romero et al. 2015). Further, cross-talk between metabolic adaptations in the tumor microenvironment and associated promising therapeutic strategies have been illustrated in Fig. 10.2.

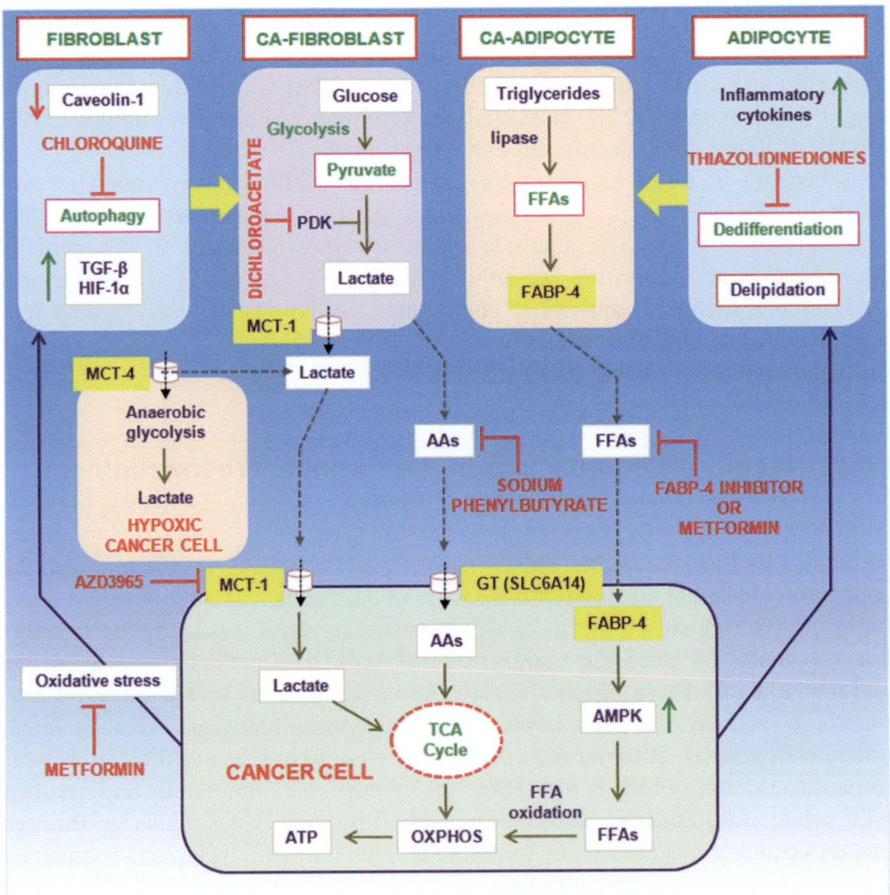

Fig. 10.2 Schematic representation depicting metabolic adaptations in the tumor microenvironment and their possible therapeutic targets. *CA* cancer associated, *TGF-β* transforming growth factor-β, *HIF-1α* hypoxia-inducible factor-1α, *PDK* pyruvate dehydrogenase kinase, *FFAs* free fatty acids, *FABP-4* fatty acid-binding protein-4, *MCT* monocarboxylate transporter, *AAs* amino acids, *GT* glutamine transporter, *AMPK* adenosine monophosphate-activated protein kinase, *OXPHOS* oxidative phosphorylation, *ATP* adenosine triphosphate

10.6 Therapeutic Approaches to Target Proliferative Metabolic Pathways

Targeting altered metabolic cascades is observed as an effective therapeutic strategy in the treatment of cancer for manifold advantages. These include (1) the reliance of tumor cells on impaired metabolism facilitates these cells susceptible to metabolic alterations, while most of these impaired cascades are not necessary in normal cells, (2) metabolic enzymes are excellent source for drug discoveries and developments, and (3) oncogene-targeted therapies permits identification of specific metabolic nodes during oncogenic activation. Most importantly, metabolic impairments are not reset completely in cancer therapies involving driver oncogenes. Moreover, targeting the signaling cascades downstream of mTOR/AMPK, individually or combined, has revealed effective role in numerous cancers (Li et al. 2015). AMPK activators found to block biosynthesis of both fatty acids and nucleotide and stimulate apoptosis and autophagy by triggering the FOXO signaling axis (Li et al. 2015; Chiacchiera and Simone 2010). The AMPK agonist Metformin has also been reported to inhibit tumor cell growth (Morales and Morris 2015). Similarly, inhibitors of mTOR, such as Rapamycin, are reportedly involved in the treatment of colon cancer and glioblastoma (Faller et al. 2015; Cloughesy et al. 2008). In fact, the management of many tumors is also permitted with Rapamycin. The anticancer effects of Rapamycin include the inhibition of nucleotide, protein, and lipid biosynthesis, the blockage of glycolytic pathway and glutaminolysis by mTOC1-induced HIF1 activation. In addition, enzymes of metabolism with selective or non-selective receptors have proved successful for managing many cancers close to attacking the signaling cascade. For instance, 2-deoxyglucose (2-DG) may serve as a non-selective regulator for different stages in glycolytic pathway as it has structural similarities to glucose and the incapability of mammalian cells in its metabolism. 2-DG functions as a competitive inhibitor for glucose receptor and regulates the activity of GLUT1 and GLUT3; it has also been regulated by the phosphorylated 2-DG (Wick et al. 1957). The AMPK cascade can be activated by the craving activity of 2-DG owing to ATP deficiency. Studies with 2-DG have also provided evidence that targeting cancer cell metabolism is viable (Pelicano et al. 2006). Many medications that block the deregulated biochemical pathways have also been documented recently. Examples include Heparin, which blocks heparin sulfate-modifying enzymes and also decreases growth factor receptor signaling by fibroblast growth factor 2 and Statins, which target cholesterol biosynthesis and also prevent RAS signaling by blocking farnesylation (Vlodavsky et al. 1994). Further, a list of drugs/bioactive agents and their indicated metabolic targets and associated cancer types is addressed in Table 10.2 (Nagarajan et al. 2016).

Table 10.2 Bioactive compounds/biomolecules-mediated targeting of cancer metabolism via metabolic enzymes/metabolites

Types of metabolism	Bioactive compounds/ biomolecules	Targeted metabolic enzymes/metabolites	Associated cancers
Amino acid metabolism	1-D-MT	Indoleamine-2,3-dioxygenase (IDO)	Metastatic solid tumors
	Indoximod		Metastatic solid tumors
	ADI-PEG20	Argininosuccinate synthase (ASS1)	Hepatocellular carcinoma
	Indole LM10	Tryptophan 2,3-dioxygenase (TDO)	Numerous TDO-expressing tumor cells
	shRNA	Serine hydroxymethyltransferase (SHMT1)	Lymphomagenesis and lung cancer
	shRNA	Phosphoglycerate dehydrogenase (PHGDH)	Melanoma and breast cancer cell lines (SkBr3, MCF7), murine mammary fat pad tumors with MDAMB-468 cells expressing PHGDH shRNA
	Acivicin	Glutamine-dependent enzymatic steps	Many cancers and high-grade astrocytoma
	L-DON		Various animal and human xenografted tumors
	Azaserin		Pancreatic cancer
Carbohydrate metabolism	3-Bromopyruvate (3-BrPA)	Hexokinase (HK)	Colon cancer, leukemia, and multiple myeloma
	Lonidamine (LND)		Lymphoma and leukemia
	2-Deoxyglucose (2-DG)		Prostate, leukemia, lymphoma, cervical, hepatocarcinoma, breast, and small lung cancer
	Ritonavir	Glucose transporter (GLUT4)	Multiple myeloma
	WZB117	Glucose transporter (GLUT1)	Lung cancer and breast cancer
	Phloretin		Colon cancer and leukemia
	TLN-232	Pyruvate kinase	Metastatic melanoma and RCC
	Dichloroacetate (DCA)	Phosphoinositide-dependent kinase (PDK1)	Colon cancer, lung cancer, squamous cell carcinoma, and prostate cancer
	Dasatinib	Isocitrate dehydrogenase (IDH1/IDH2)	Liver cancer
	Metformin	Mitochondrial complex I	Solid tumors and lymphoma
	Oxamate	Lactate dehydrogenase (LDHA)	Breast cancer

(continued)

Table 10.2 (continued)

Types of metabolism	Bioactive compounds/ biomolecules	Targeted metabolic enzymes/metabolites	Associated cancers
Lipid metabolism	Orlistat	Fatty acid synthase (FASN)	Breast and pancreatic cancer
	C75		Breast cancer
	Cerulenin		Breast cancer
	A-769662	Acetyl-CoA carboxylase (ACC)	Breast cancer
	TOFA [5-(tetradecyloxy)-2-furoic acid]		Prostate and ovarian cancer
	Soraphen-A		Breast cancer
	LY294002	ATP citrate lyase (ACLY)	Various cancer types
	SB-204990		Hematologic and solid cancers
	Thiazolidinediones (TZDs)	Acetyl-CoA synthetase (ACS)	Various cancer types
	Triascin C		Colon and breast cancer
	MN58B	Creatine kinase (CK)	Various cancer types
	TCD-717		Advanced solid tumors
	CT-32501	Glycerol-3-phosphate acyltransferase (GPAT)	Lung cancer
	Ranolazine	Carnitine palmitoyltransferase (CPT1)	Leukemia
	Etomoxir		Prostate cancer and myeloma
	FGH10019	Sterol regulatory element-binding protein (SREBP)	Various cancer types
	Fatostatin		Breast and prostate cancer
	A939572	Stearoyl-CoA desaturase (SCD)	Kidney cancer
	BZ36		Prostate cancer
	JZL184	Monoacylglycerol lipase (MAGL)	Prostate and colorectal cancer
Metabolite depletion	Arginine deiminase	Arginine	Hepatocellular carcinoma and metastatic melanoma
	Asparaginase and PEG-asparaginase	Asparagine	B cell lymphoma, T cell lymphoma and ALL
	Phenylacetate	Glutamine	Brain tumors

10.7 Concluding Remarks

The interconnected biochemical pathways of cellular metabolism are pertinent for maintaining normal homeostasis in most eukaryotic cells. In normal cells, these pathways serve as a master regulator of various key functions via supplying metabolic fuel in the form of nutrients and energy, while in tumor cells, nutrients and energy are equally needed for their growth and proliferation. Therefore, altered metabolism involved metabolic rewiring is needed in tumor cells to support their high demands on nutrients for building blocks and energy generation.

Metabolic impairments in tumor cells are numerous, which include aerobic glycolysis, decreased oxidative phosphorylation, and the accelerated production of biosynthetic intermediates crucial to proliferative cells for their growth and development. However, intricacy of biochemical pathways and redundancy in some aspects, including, the capability to generate energy via diverse sources, such as amino acids, carbohydrates, and fatty acids provide considerable flexibility. This flexibility permits the alteration of many metabolic cascades without compromising cell survival. Oncogenes (transcription factors) target these metabolic flexibilities and redundancies to stimulate tumor growth and metastatic propagation. There are now extensive facts that oncogenes are accountable for imparting their role in the impairment of cellular metabolism. Further, this chapter has addressed promising therapeutic role of various bioactive compounds/biomolecules in targeting cancer metabolism via metabolic enzymes/metabolites. Although, the advancement of immunotherapies for the treatment of various cancers needs an understanding of the connections between the tumor and associated microenvironment and the way in which oncogene-directed metabolic aberrations contribute to immune evasion. This understanding will facilitate the more effectual use of immunotherapies and help in the advancement of other potential cancer therapies. In a nutshell, however, this chapter has elucidated considerable progress toward understanding the interlink between metabolic alterations and cancer metabolism, there is much to gain knowledge of. An in-depth knowledge of impaired cellular metabolism and carcinogenesis is still required to better understand tumor biology and enrich therapeutic outcomes.

References

Amelio I, Cutruzzolá F, Antonov A, Agostini M, Melino G (2014) Serine and glycine metabolism in cancer. Trends Biochem Sci 39(4):191–198

Bar-Peled L, Sabatini DM (2014) Regulation of mTORC1 by amino acids. Trends Cell Biol 24(7):400–406

Cairns RA, Harris IS, Mak TW (2011) Regulation of cancer cell metabolism. Nat Rev Cancer 11:85–95

Cantor JR, Sabatini DM (2012) Cancer cell metabolism: one hallmark, many faces. Cancer Discov 2(10):881–898

Cardaci S, Ciriolo MR (2012) TCA cycle defects and cancer: when metabolism tunes redox state. Int J Cell Biol 2012:161837

Cardone RA, Casavola V, Reshkin SJ (2005) The role of disturbed pH dynamics and the Na+/H+ exchanger in metastasis. Nat Rev Cancer 5(10):786–795

Chajès V, Cambot M, Moreau K, Lenoir GM, Joulin V (2006) Acetyl-CoA carboxylase alpha is essential to breast cancer cell survival. Cancer Res 66(10):5287–5294

Chiacchiera F, Simone C (2010) The AMPK-FoxO3A axis as a target for cancer treatment. Cell Cycle 9(6):1091–1096

Cloughesy TF, Yoshimoto K, Nghiemphu P, Brown K, Dang J, Zhu S, Hsueh T, Chen Y, Wang W, Youngkin D, Liau L, Martin N, Becker D, Bergsneider M, Lai A, Green R, Oglesby T, Koleto M, Trent J, Horvath S, Mischel PS, Mellinghoff IK, Sawyers CL (2008) Antitumor activity of rapamycin in a Phase I trial for patients with recurrent PTEN-deficient glioblastoma. PLoS Med 5(1):e8

Colegio OR, Chu NQ, Szabo AL, Chu T, Rhebergen AM, Jairam V, Cyrus N, Brokowski CE, Eisenbarth SC, Phillips GM, Cline GW, Phillips AJ, Medzhitov R (2014) Functional polarization of tumor-associated macrophages by tumour-derived lactic acid. Nature 513(7519):559–563

Dang CV (2010) Rethinking the Warburg effect with Myc micromanaging glutamine metabolism. Cancer Res 70:859–862

Dang CV, Le A, Gao P (2009) MYC-induced cancer cell energy metabolism and therapeutic opportunities. Clin Cancer Res 15:6479–6483

Dillon BJ, Prieto VG, Curley SA, Ensor CM, Holtsberg FW, Bomalaski JS, Clark MA (2004) Incidence and distribution of argininosuccinate synthetase deficiency in human cancers:a method for identifying cancers sensitive to arginine deprivation. Cancer 100(4):826–833

Dong G, Mao Q, Xia W, Xu Y, Wang J, Xu L, Jiang F (2016) PKM2 and cancer: the function of PKM2 beyond glycolysis. Oncol Lett 11(3):1980–1986

Düvel K, Yecies JL, Menon S, Raman P, Lipovsky AI, Souza AL, Triantafellow E, Ma Q, Gorski R, Cleaver S, Vander Heiden MG, MacKeigan JP, Finan PM, Clish CB, Murphy LO, Manning BD (2010) Activation of a metabolic gene regulatory network downstream of mTOR complex 1. Mol Cell 39(2):171–183

Eberlé D, Hegarty B, Bossard P, Ferré P, Foufelle F (2004) SREBP transcription factors: master regulators of lipid homeostasis. Biochimie 86:839–848

Ettinger SL, Sobel R, Whitmore TG, Akbari M, Bradley DR, Gleave ME, Nelson CC (2004) Dysregulation of sterol response element-binding proteins and downstream effectors in prostate cancer during progression to androgen independence. Cancer Res 64(6):2212–2221

Faller WJ, Jackson TJ, Knight JR, Ridgway RA, Jamieson T, Karim SA, Jones C, Radulescu S, Huels DJ, Myant KB, Dudek KM, Casey HA, Scopelliti A, Cordero JB, Vidal M, Pende M, Ryazanov AG, Sonenberg N, Meyuhas O, Hall MN, Bushell M, Willis AE, Sansom OJ (2015) mTORC1-mediated translational elongation limits intestinal tumour initiation and growth. Nature 517(7535):497–500

Gao P, Tchernyshyov I, Chang TC, Lee YS, Kita K, Ochi T et al (2009) c-Myc suppression of miR-23a/b enhances mitochondrial glutaminase expression and glutamine metabolism. Nature 458:762–765

Gordan JD, Thompson CB, Simon MC (2007) HIF and c-Myc: sibling rivals for control of cancer cell metabolism and proliferation. Cancer Cell 12:108–113

Gottlieb E, Vousden KH (2010) p53 regulation of metabolic pathways. Cold Spring Harb Perspect Biol 2:a001040

Greer SN, Metcalf JL, Wang Y, Ohh M (2012) The updated biology of hypoxia-inducible factor. EMBO J 31:2448–2460

Guo D, Prins RM, Dang J, Kuga D, Iwanami A, Soto H, Lin KY, Huang TT, Akhavan D, Hock MB, Zhu S, Kofman AA, Bensinger SJ, Yong WH, Vinters HV, Horvath S, Watson AD, Kuhn JG, Robins HI, Mehta MP, Wen PY, DeAngelis LM, Prados MD, Mellinghoff IK, Cloughesy TF, Mischel PS (2009) EGFR signaling through an Akt-SREBP-1-dependent, rapamycin-resistant pathway sensitizes glioblastomas to antilipogenic therapy. Sci Signal 2(101):ra82

Guo H, Xiang Z, Zhang Y, Sun D (2019) Inhibiting 6-phosphogluconate dehydrogenase enhances chemotherapy efficacy in cervical cancer via AMPK-independent inhibition of RhoA and Rac1. Clin Transl Oncol 21(4):404–411

Haimovitz-Friedman A, Kolesnick RN, Fuks Z (1997) Ceramide signaling in apoptosis. Br Med Bull 53(3):539–553

Hamanaka RB, Chandel NS (2012) Targeting glucose metabolism for cancer therapy. J Exp Med 209(2):211–215

Hatzivassiliou G, Zhao F, Bauer DE, Andreadis C, Shaw AN, Dhanak D, Hingorani SR, Tuveson DA, Thompson CB (2005) ATP citrate lyase inhibition can suppress tumor cell growth. Cancer Cell 8(4):311–321

Horton JD, Shah NA, Warrington JA, Anderson NN, Park SW, Brown MS, Goldstein JL (2003) Combined analysis of oligonucleotide microarray data from transgenic and knockout mice identifies direct SREBP target genes. Proc Natl Acad Sci U S A 100(21):12027–12032

Hsu PP, Sabatini DM (2008) Cancer cell metabolism: Warburg and beyond. Cell 134(5):703–707

Huang WC, Li X, Liu J, Lin J, Chung LW (2012) Activation of androgen receptor, lipogenesis, and oxidative stress converged by SREBP-1 is responsible for regulating growth and progression of prostate cancer cells. Mol Cancer Res 10(1):133–142

Kaelin WG Jr, Ratcliffe PJ (2008) Oxygen sensing by metazoans: the central role of the HIF hydroxylase pathway. Mol Cell 30(4):393–402
Kennedy KM, Dewhirst MW (2010) Tumor metabolism of lactate: the influence and therapeutic potential for MCT and CD147 regulation. Future Oncol 6(1):127–148
Kerr EM, Martins CP (2018) Metabolic rewiring in mutant Kras lung cancer. FEBS J 285(1):28–41
Knelson EH, Nee JC, Blobe GC (2014) Heparan sulfate signaling in cancer. Trends Biochem Sci 39(6):277–288
Komada Y, Zhang XL, Zhou YW, Ido M, Azuma E (1997) Apoptotic cell death of human T lymphoblastoid cells induced by arginine deiminase. Int J Hematol 65(2):129–141
Kroemer G, Pouyssegur J (2008) Tumor cell metabolism: cancer's Achilles' heel. Cancer Cell 13(6):472–482
Laplante M, Sabatini DM (2009) An emerging role of mTOR in lipid biosynthesis. Curr Biol 19(22):R1046–R1052
Lee M, Yoon JH (2015) Metabolic interplay between glycolysis and mitochondrial oxidation: the reverse Warburg effect and its therapeutic implication. World J Biol Chem 6(3):148–161
Levine AJ, Puzio-Kuter AM (2010) The control of the metabolic switch in cancers by oncogenes and tumor suppressor genes. Science 330(6009):1340–1344
Li W, Saud SM, Young MR, Chen G, Hua B (2015) Targeting AMPK for cancer prevention and treatment. Oncotarget 6(10):7365–7378
Liberti MV, Locasale JW (2016) The Warburg effect: how does it benefit cancer cells? Trends Biochem Sci 41(3):211–218
Locasale JW, Cantley LC (2011) Metabolic flux and the regulation of mammalian cell growth. Cell Metab 14(4):443–451
Lu H, Forbes RA, Verma A (2002) Hypoxia-inducible factor 1activation by aerobic glycolysis implicates the Warburg effect in carcinogenesis. J Biol Chem 277(26):23111–23115
Lu J, Tan M, Cai Q (2015) The Warburg effect in tumor progression: mitochondrial oxidative metabolism as an anti-metastasis mechanism. Cancer Lett 356(2 Pt A):156–164
Magda D, Lecane P, Prescott J, Thiemann P, Ma X, Dranchak PK, Toleno DM, Ramaswamy K, Siegmund KD, Hacia JG (2008) mtDNA depletion confers specific gene expression profiles in human cells grown in culture and in xenograft. BMC Genomics 3(9):521
Morales DR, Morris AD (2015) Metformin in cancer treatment and prevention. Annu Rev Med 66:17–29
Nagarajan A, Malvi P, Wajapeyee N (2016) Oncogene-directed alterations in cancer cell metabolism. Trends Cancer 2(7):365–377
Nishioka T, Oda Y, Seino Y, Yamamoto T, Inagaki N, Yano H, Imura H, Shigemoto R, Kikuchi H (1992) Distribution of the glucose transporters in human brain tumors. Cancer Res 52(14):3972–3979
Parker SJ, Metallo CM (2015) Metabolic consequences of oncogenic IDH mutations. Pharmacol Ther 152:54–62
Pelicano H, Martin DS, Xu RH, Huang P (2006) Glycolysis inhibition for anticancer treatment. Oncogene 25(34):4633–4646
Peterson TR, Sengupta SS, Harris TE, Carmack AE, Kang SA, Balderas E et al (2011) mTOR complex 1 regulates lipin 1 localization to control the SREBP pathway. Cell 146:408–420
Ponzoni M, Bocca P, Chiesa V, Decensi A, Pistoia V, Raffaghello L, Rozzo C, Montaldo PG (1995) Differential effects of N-(4-hydroxyphenyl)retinamide and retinoic acid on neuroblastoma cells: apoptosis versus differentiation. Cancer Res 55(4):853–861
Romero IL, Mukherjee A, Kenny HA, Litchfield LM, Lengyel E (2015) Molecular pathways: trafficking of metabolic resources in the tumor microenvironment. Clin Cancer Res 21(4):680–686
Semenza GL (2010) HIF-1: upstream and downstream of cancer metabolism. Curr Opin Genet Dev 20:51–56
Semenza GL (2012) Regulation of metabolism by hypoxia-inducible factor 1. Cold Spring Harb Symp Quant Biol 76:347–353
Shao W, Espenshade PJ (2012) Expanding roles for SREBP in metabolism. Cell Metab 16(4):414–419

Stanton RC, Seifter JL, Boxer DC, Zimmerman E, Cantley LC (1991) Rapid release of bound glucose-6-phosphate dehydrogenase by growth factors. Correlation with increased enzymatic activity. J Biol Chem 266(19):12442–12448

Su TS, Tsai TF, Chi CW, Han SH, Chou CK (1990) Elevation of facilitated glucose-transporter messenger RNA in human hepatocellular carcinoma. Hepatology 11(1):118–122

Swinnen JV, Brusselmans K, Verhoeven G (2006) Increased lipogenesis in cancer cells: new players, novel targets. Curr Opin Clin Nutr Metab Care 9(4):358–365

Tsun ZY, Possemato R (2015) Amino acid management in cancer. Semin Cell Dev Biol 43:22–32

Uyttenhove C, Pilotte L, Théate I, Stroobant V, Colau D, Parmentier N, Boon T, Van den Eynde BJ (2003) Evidence for a tumoral immune resistance mechanism based on tryptophan degradation by indoleamine 2,3-dioxygenase. Nat Med 9(10):1269–1274

van Horssen R, Buccione R, Willemse M, Cingir S, Wieringa B, Attanasio F (2013) Cancer cell metabolism regulates extracellular matrix degradation by invadopodia. Eur J Cell Biol 92(3):113–121

Vega-Naredo I, Loureiro R, Mesquita KA, Barbosa IA, Tavares LC, Branco AF, Erickson JR, Holy J, Perkins EL, Carvalho RA, Oliveira PJ (2014) Mitochondrial metabolism directs stemness and differentiation in P19 embryonal carcinoma stem cells. Cell Death Differ 21(10):1560–1574

Vlodavsky I, Mohsen M, Lider O, Svahn CM, Ekre HP, Vigoda M, Ishai-Michaeli R, Peretz T (1994) Inhibition of tumor metastasis by heparanase inhibiting species of heparin. Invasion Metastasis 14(1–6):290–302

Vousden KH, Ryan KM (2009) p53 and metabolism. Nat Rev Cancer 9:691–700

Wallace DC (2012) Mitochondria and cancer. Nat Rev Cancer 12(10):685–698

Wang GL, Jiang BH, Rue EA, Semenza GL (1995) Hypoxia-inducible factor 1 is a basic-helix-loop-helix-PAS heterodimer regulated by cellular O_2 tension. Proc Natl Acad Sci U S A 92(12):5510–5514

Warburg O (1956) On the origin of cancer cells. Science 123(3191):309–314

Whitaker-Menezes D, Martinez-Outschoorn UE, Flomenberg N, Birbe RC, Witkiewicz AK, Howell A, Pavlides S, Tsirigos A, Ertel A, Pestell RG, Broda P, Minetti C, Lisanti MP, Sotgia F (2011) Hyperactivation of oxidative mitochondrial metabolism in epithelial cancer cells in situ: visualizing the therapeutic effects of metformin in tumor tissue. Cell Cycle 10(23):4047–4064

Wick AN, Drury DR, Nakada HI, Wolfe JB (1957) Localization of the primary metabolic block produced by 2-deoxyglucose. J Biol Chem 224(2):963–969

Wise DR, DeBeradinis RJ, Mancuso A, Sayed N, Zhang XY, Pfeiffer HK et al (2008) Myc regulates a transcriptional program that stimulates mitochondrial glutaminolysis and leads to glutamine addiction. Proc Natl Acad Sci U S A 105:18782–18787

Wise DR, Thompson CB (2010) Glutamine addiction: a new therapeutic target in cancer. Trends Biochem Sci 35(8):427–433

Wullschleger S, Loewith R, Hall MN (2006) TOR signaling in growth and metabolism. Cell 124(3):471–484

Xu W, Yang H, Liu Y, Yang Y, Wang P, Kim SH, Ito S, Yang C, Wang P, Xiao MT, Liu LX, Jiang WQ, Liu J, Zhang JY, Wang B, Frye S, Zhang Y, Xu YH, Lei QY, Guan KL, Zhao SM, Xiong Y (2011) Oncometabolite 2-hydroxyglutarate is a competitive inhibitor of α-ketoglutarate-dependent dioxygenases. Cancer Cell 19(1):17–30

Yamamoto T, Seino Y, Fukumoto H, Koh G, Yano H, Inagaki N, Yamada Y, Inoue K, Manabe T, Imura H (1990) Over-expression of facilitative glucose transporter genes in human cancer. Biochem Biophys Res Commun 170(1):223–230

Yuneva M, Zamboni N, Oefner P, Sachidanandam R, Lazebnik Y (2007) Deficiency in glutamine but not glucose induces MYC-dependent apoptosis in human cells. J Cell Biol 178:93–105

Zhang B, Dong LW, Tan YX, Zhang J, Pan YF, Yang C, Li MH, Ding ZW, Liu LJ, Jiang TY, Yang JH, Wang HY (2013) Asparagine synthetase is an independent predictor of surgical survival and a potential therapeutic target in hepatocellular carcinoma. Br J Cancer 109(1):14–23

Role of Phytochemicals in Cancer Cell Metabolism Regulation

11

Abhijeet Kumar, Anil Kumar Singh, Mukul Kumar Gautam, and Garima Tripathi

Abstract

The alteration in cellular metabolism whereby cancer cell meets the demand of bioenergetics, biosynthesis, and redox status to support their uncontrolled cell proliferation, growth, tumor progression, and metastasis is considered as a prominent hallmark of cancer. Warburg effect is the most commonly noticed consequence of these metabolic reprogramming which aggravate cancer cell to opt for glycolytic pathway over more efficient oxidative phosphorylation even under normoxic condition to generate lactate, as well as intermediates for lipid, nucleotide, amino acids synthesis, which are essential to maintain tumorigenesis and cancer progression. In order to develop efficient chemotherapeutic drug, various enzymes and proteins involved or associated with glycolytic pathways such as PMK2, LDHA and signaling pathways such as PKI3-Akt-mTOR are being targeted to inhibit various stages of cancer progression. In that direction, phytochemicals that are bioactive compounds obtained from plant sources have displayed promising results in hampering the growth of various cancer cell lines. Compounds of flavonoid class such as quercetin and fisetin along with other polyphenols and non-flavonoids such as resveratrol, isothiocyanates, and curcumin have displayed remarkable inhibitory effect on cancer cell metabolism. Overall, this chapter will highlight the effect of different phytochemicals on the metabolic pathways of cancer cells to inhibit various stages of cancer progression.

A. Kumar · A. K. Singh
Department of Chemistry, School of Physical Sciences, Mahatma Gandhi Central University, Motihari, Bihar, India

M. K. Gautam
Buddha Institute of Dental Sciences and Hospital, Patna, Bihar, India

G. Tripathi (✉)
Department of Chemistry, T.N.B. College, TMBU, Bhagalpur, Bihar, India

D. Kumar (ed.), *Cancer Cell Metabolism: A Potential Target for Cancer Therapy*,
https://doi.org/10.1007/978-981-15-1991-8_11

Keywords
Phytochemicals · Polyphenol · Metabolism

11.1 Introduction

Cancer has been emerging as one of the principal causes of death across the world. As per the data available with World Health Organization (WHO), a total of 18,078,957 new cases of different types of cancer were reported only in 2018 across the world and out of which more than 95 lakh deaths were reported in the same year. In developing countries like India, more than 9 lakh new reports of cancer have been registered and out of which approximately 70% death occurred. With the development of science and technology, most of the diseases which were considered incurable few decades back, no more remain so as the identification of the specific pathogens or targets responsible for them were successfully identified, which helped in design and development of suitable medicines. In drug discovery, the identification of the prime target that is chiefly responsible for altering the usual physiological activities is a crucial point and based on that identification of lead molecule along with different phases of drug development lead to the discovery of a new drug molecule.

Cancer which is a general term used to describe a group of diseases in which the aberration/alterations in normal signaling pathways responsible for controlled metabolic activities and cellular proliferation leads to uncontrolled and atypical cell proliferation and growth (Cairns et al. 2011; Snyder et al. 2018). For proper growth and functioning of an organ, the balance between the rate of division of cells and their loss due to death and differentiation along with their survival and maintenance are essential. This balance gets altered leading to unchecked proliferation of cells, which gives rise to the formation of a tumor. It is basically a lump of cells that could be benign, malignant (cancerous), and precancerous in nature (Sarkar et al. 2013). The uncontrolled cell proliferation disrupts the normal functioning and metabolic activity of a cell. The alternation or reprogramming of normal metabolic pathways is a consequence of several intrinsic as well as extrinsic changes and is mandatory to meet the augmented demands of energy in the form of ATP, biosynthesis of macromolecules, maintenance of cellular redox status, and homeostasis, which are essential to support uncontrolled cell proliferation. For example, the excessive uptake of glucose in a specified region is a consequence of abnormal variation in the core cellular metabolism which helps in the detection of tumor. Abnormally high glucose uptake at a particular part of the body helps in the detection of region of uncontrolled cell proliferation by positron emission tomography (PET) imaging where [^{18}F] fluorodeoxyglucose is used as tracer to locate the tumor cells. Therefore, this technique is also known as [^{18}F] fluorodeoxyglucose positron emission tomography (FDG-PET) (Cairns et al. 2011). Warburg effect is also one of the consequences of altered metabolic activity wherein the cancerous cell favors glycolysis over oxidative phosphorylation even in presence of sufficient amount of oxygen to generate ATP (Ngo et al. 2015; Vaupel et al. 2019). In general, in normal cells, the pyruvate produced at the end of glycolysis step is carried to the mitochondria where following citric acid cycle or Krebs cycle and electron transport chain (ETC), ATP production occurs through the process of oxidative phosphorylation. Whereas in case of cancer cells, due to the alternation in the signaling pathway, larger amount of pyruvate converts into lactate (Hay 2016) which gets transported to the extracellular medium using monocarboxylate transporters (MCTs) and skips two efficient catalytic cycles (TCA and ETC) which are essential for the maximum production of ATP. Therefore, in order to fulfill the soaring demand of energy and material, the conversion of glucose into lactate occurs very fast which gets reflected in the very high uptake and consumption of glucose in the region of uncontrolled cell proliferation. Otto Heinrich Warburg in 1956 observed this phenomenon for the first time in case of cancer cells and found this as the most common metabolic phenotype so this effect is known as Warburg effect (Granchi and Minutolo 2012; Liberti and Locasale 2016).

In order to develop an effective drug for the treatment of various types of cancer, different strategies are being employed by targeting the different molecules involved in either in signaling pathways such as PKI3-Akt-mTOR, oncogenes such as MYC, RAS, p53, and PTEN or enzymes involved in metabolic pathways etc. (Sever and Brugge 2015). As it is a well-established fact that only single target is not there in case of cancer and this is why it is being difficult to design and develop an effective drug which could cure this disease at any stage of its development.

11.2 Effect of Phytochemicals on Cancer Cell Metabolic Pathways

Phytochemicals that are bioactive compounds obtained from plant sources have displayed promising results in hampering the growth of various cancer cell lines (Hosseini and Ghorbani 2015; Wang et al. 2012). Compounds of flavonoid class such as quercetin and fisetin along with other polyphenols (Estrela et al. 2017) and non-flavonoids such as resveratrol, isothiocyanates, and curcumin have displayed remarkable inhibitory effect on cancer cell metabolism (Chirumbolo et al. 2018; Russo et al. 2010). Phytochemicals have always been an active component of herbal medicines. The core skeleton of some of the most common phytochemicals with huge therapeutic values has been depicted in Fig. 11.1 (Estrela et al. 2017).

Among the several phytochemicals, polyphenols which are defined as compounds having more than one phenolic group are important class of phytochemicals which have been found to exhibit wide range of biological activities such as anti-inflammatory, antibacterial, antimalarial, and anticancerous (Pandey and Rizvi 2009). Few examples of naturally occurring flavones and isoflavones with anticancerous properties have been demonstrated in Fig. 11.2.

Similarly, non-flavonoids (Fig. 11.3) such as curcumin, resveratrol, and caffeic acid have also been reported to affect signaling pathways leading to alteration in cancer cell metabolism.

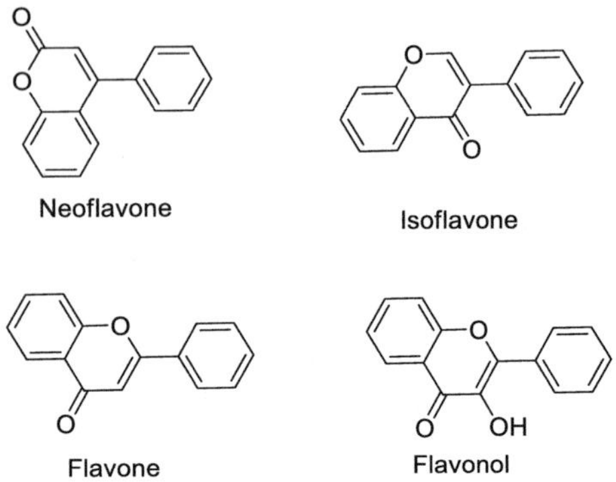

Fig. 11.1 Structure of the common core scaffolds present in therapeutically important phytochemicals

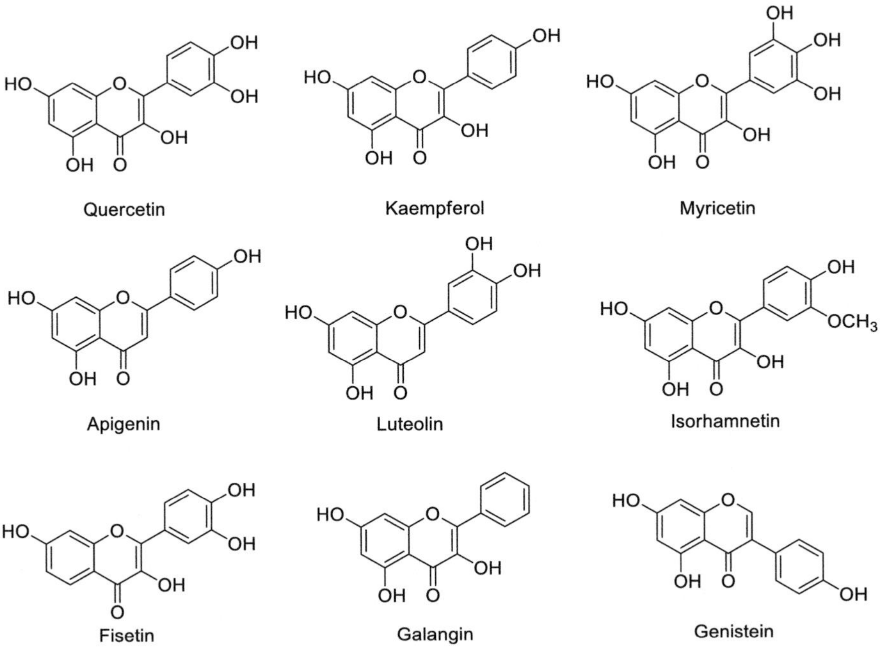

Fig. 11.2 Examples of naturally occurring flavones and isoflavones with anticancerous properties

In order to devise an efficient therapeutic strategy and develop efficient chemotherapeutic agent to manage uncontrolled cell proliferation, tumorigenesis and other such alteration leading to metastasis, the role of these phytochemicals in cancer cell metabolism regulation are being investigated on different cell lines either alone or in combination with other anticancer drugs to understand the synergistic effect of these phytochemicals. In succeeding sections, the roles of these phytochemicals have been described separately.

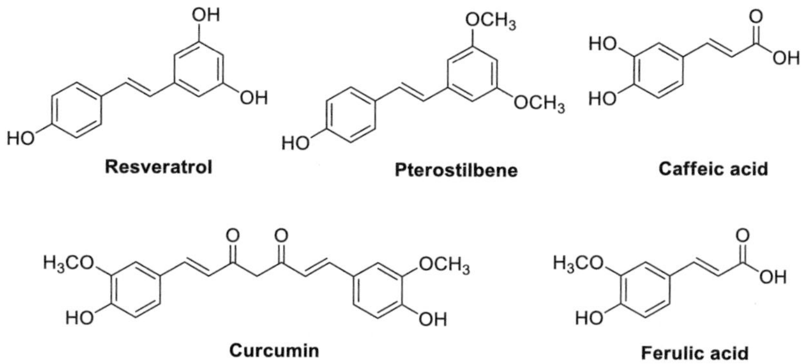

Fig. 11.3 Examples of naturally occurring non-flavonoids with anticancerous properties

11.3 Effect of Flavonoids on Cancer Cell Metabolism

Flavones and isoflavones that are chromone derivatives with aryl substitution at second and third position respectively (Fig. 11.2) and their derivatives such as flavonols are among few bioactive phytochemicals which have displayed enormous biological activities such as anticancerous, anti-inflammatory, anti-alzheimer and these were also found to be effective against various other such neurodegenerative disorders (Gaspar et al. 2014; Abotaleb et al. 2018). More specifically, the anticancerous effects of these classes of compounds are being studied to exploit their anticancerous effect and develop an anticancer drug with high efficacy and low toxicity (Abotaleb et al. 2018).

Quercetin (2-(3,4-dihydroxyphenyl)-3,5,7-trihydroxy-4*H*-chromen-4-one) (Fig. 11.2) that remains attached with sugar moiety as glycosides in the plant is an example of phytochemicals which is also used as dietary supplement and is present in various vegetables and fruits such as kale, grapes, onion, strawberries, garlic, and apple (Srivastava et al. 2016). It is mainly obtained from onion in which the amount varies from 0.03 to 1.31 mg/100 g of their fresh weights. It is estimated that on an average a human consumes almost 25 mg of quercetin every day. Both in vitro and in vivo investigations using it have revealed its potential therapeutic applicability as antioxidant, anticancerous, antimalarial, and anti-inflammatory as well as neuroprotective agent. In particular, it has been found to affect various stages of development and growth of cancer cells by affecting different signaling as well as metabolic pathways in which the alteration leads to cancer (Kashyap et al. 2019; Reyes-Farias and Carrasco-Pozo 2019). It has also been found that this flavonol exhibits dose-dependent effect resulting in antioxidant and prooxidant at low and high concentrations respectively. It has already been mentioned earlier that in contrast to normal cell, cancer cell prefers glycolysis over oxidative phosphorylation process even under normoxic condition. Therefore, targeting various enzymes and signaling molecules involved in the glycolysis pathways to inhibit it, is considered as a promising therapeutic strategy toward controlling the cancer progression. Quercetin has been found to inhibit glucose transporter 1 (GLUT1) which is responsible for transportation of glucose across the plasma membrane (Hamilton et al. 2018). Apart from inhibiting the action of GLUT1, quercetin also impedes the glycolysis process by downregulating the expression of various other glycolytic enzymes and proteins such as lactate dehydrogenase A (LDHA) and protein pyruvate kinase M2 (PMK2) involved in it as was observed in case of breast cancer cell lines MCF-7 and MDA-MB-231 (Srivastava et al. 2016). Consequently, these effects of quercetin on glycolysis in case of breast cancer cells were reflected as reduction in glucose efflux and lactate production. As the glycolysis step and acidic environment are two essential requirements for the survival, mobility, and progression of cancer cells, the quercetin inhibits the metastasis in breast cancer cell by blocking glycolysis, which consequently reduces lactic acid production. Quercetin is also known to exert antitumor activity through inactivation of Akt-mTOR pathways which were also found to induce autophagy leading to inhibition of metastasis (Rivera Rivera et al. 2016).

Fisetin (2-(3,4-dihydroxyphenyl)-3,7-dihydroxy-4*H*-chromen-4-one) (Fig. 11.2) which is also a member of flavonol group is the most common flavonol found in a variety of fruits and vegetables such as apple, Kiwi, grapes, onion, strawberry, black tea, and green tea in varying concentrations ranging from 0.1 to 539 μg/g. It has exhibited broad range of biological activities such as anticancerous, neuroprotective, and antioxidant. The constructive effect of fisetin in affecting the cancer cell metabolism has also been found on different variety of cancer cells which indicates that it also primarily targets the PKI3–Akt–Mtor signaling pathways and reduces their expression in cancer cell which consequently also affect the metabolic pathways (Sundarraj et al. 2018).

11.4 Effect of Non-flavonoids on Cancer Cell Metabolism

Like flavonoids, other compounds that are polyphenols and no-flavonoids have also displayed interesting anticancerous effects by reorienting the cancer cell metabolism toward the metabolic activity of normal cells. Resveratrol, pterostilbene, and isothiocyanates are examples of few such non-flavonoids that have been extensively used to explore their effect on metabolic and signaling pathways.

Resveratrol ((*E*)-5-(4-hydroxystyryl)benzene-1,3-diol) (Fig. 11.3) is another medicinally important phytoalexin which is mainly found in red grapes and red wine. It is known to display a broad range of pharmacological activities and also known to impart beneficial effect especially in case of diabetes, cardiovascular diseases, cancer, etc. The effect of resveratrol on cancer cell metabolism has also been investigated by several research groups. In human ovarian cancer cells, resveratrol is found to hamper glucose metabolism by lessening the glucose uptake and reducing the production of lactate by reducing the level of Akt and mTOR which are important members of PI3K pathways. In human breast cancer cell, MCF-7, resveratrol is known to targets and inhibits the activity of 6-phosphofructo-1-kinase (PFK) which results in the decrease in cancer cell viability along with the consumption of glucose and ATP production which are essential for the survival and cell proliferation. In human diffuse large B-Cell Lymphomas (DLBCLs), resveratrol is known to affect the glycolysis process by hampering PI3K pathway (Faber et al. 2006). In a normal cell, this phosphatidylonisitol 3-kinase (PKI3) receives stimulation from growth factors and transfer it to downstream pathways AKT followed by mammalian target of Rapamycin (mTOR) and this is highly ordered pathway which is essential for to support the growth of cancer cell. Resveratrol is also known to inhibit mTOR which plays a crucial role in the biosynthesis of macromolecules such as proteins and lipid which are essential for tumoregenesis. In colon cancer cells, resveratrol is found to shift the aerobic glycolytic pathway toward oxidative phosphorylation which was observed to increase ATP production by 20%. Apart from that it also significantly suppresses the formation of lipid through pentose phosphate pathway by utilizing glucose in human colon cell, Caco2. In addition to that resveratrol is also found to affect lipid metabolism. In colon cancer cells, the exposure to resveratrol causes a decrease in the unsaturated fatty acids compared to saturated fatty acids. Although in human leukemic cell lines U-937 and HL-60, the resveratrol was found to hamper glucose uptake by interaction with GLUT1, but in colon cancer cell line, Caco2, it is not found to modulate the level of important transporter protein and enzymes such as GLUT1, pyruvate kinase M2 (PMK2), and lactate dehydrogenase A (LADH) (Saunier et al. 2017). Instead of that resveratrol was found to enhance the activity of pyruvate dehydrogenase (PDH) complex, which is composed of three enzymes, is found in mitochondria and catalyzes the oxidation of pyruvate inside it. Therefore, it plays a crucial role in connecting glycolysis and TCA cycle. Therefore, resveratrol was found to reorient the preferred glycolysis pathway of the cancer cell to oxidative phosphorylation by enhancing the activity of PDH complex in colon cancer cell line Caco2 (Saunier et al. 2017).

11.4.1 Isothiocyanates

Vegetables and fruits are the important sources of secondary metabolites which have an immense need in human health beyond basic nutrition. Sulforaphane is one such product of the compound glucosinolate. Glucosinolates are a large group of sulfur-containing secondary metabolites which occur in the members of Brassicaceae family. They belong to the class glucosides and are water-soluble anions. Plants use these compounds for their defense against herbivores due to its bitter taste. The glucosinolates are biologically inactive and chemically stable compounds in their native structure. They possess β-D-thioglucose group and a sulfonated oxime moiety attached to the variable side-chains derived from methionine, tryptophan, phenylalanine, and some branched-chain amino acids. The plant enzyme myrosinase (β-thioglucoside glycohydrolase) hydrolyzes glucosinolates and form glucose and some unstable intermediates that degrades into thiocyanates, isothiocyanates (ITCs), and nitriles (Fig. 11.4) Isocyanates are the active ingredients which plant employ them against parasites.

Isothiocyanates are the group of organic compounds having -N=C=S functional group as common structural features. These are biologically active and electrophilic in nature. Several studies have revealed that isothiocyanates are able to

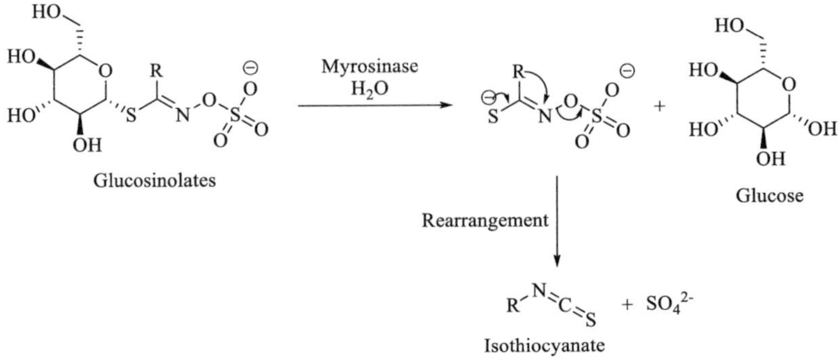

Fig. 11.4 The enzyme myrosinase hydrolyzes the glucosinolate to yield glucose and an unstable intermediate aglycone. This product then spontaneously rearranges to form an isothiocyanate and sulfate group

inhibit cancer development in animals (Xu and Thornalley 2000; Kuroiwa et al. 2006). The pioneer works regarding anticarcinogenic activities of isothiocyanates have been established in rats as animal models administrating various chemical carcinogens, such as ethionine, fluorenyl acetamide, aromatic hydrocarbons, azo dyes, and several nitrosamines. Studies advocate that the effect of these carcinogens on target organs including the lungs, liver, esophagus, stomach, mammary gland, small intestine, colon, and bladder are diminished (Zhang and Talalay 1994; Hecht 1995).

7,12-Dimethylbenz[a]anthracene (DMBA) is a carcinogen responsible for mammary cancer in female rats. ITC, when administrated 4 h prior to DMBA administration, inhibited the tumor formation. Benzyl-ITC is reported to inhibit benz(a)pyrene-induced mouse forestomach cancer (Wattenberg 1977, 1987). 4-(Methylnitrosamino)-1-(3-pyridyl)-1-butanone (NNK) is responsible for tobacco-induced lung tumors, and it is assumed to be inducer of lung cancer in smokers. Phenylethyl-ITC (PEITC), BITC, and phenyl isothiocyanate (PITC) were found to inhibit lung tumorigenesis and O^6-methylguanine formation (DNA-adduct formation in the NNK-induced tumors) in the DNA of lung cells from A/J mice treated with NNK (Morse et al. 1989, b, Morse et al. 1991, 1993). PEITC is also reported to inhibit N-nitrosomethylbenzylamine (NMBA)-induced esophageal carcinogenesis and DNA methylation in rodents. ITCs can regulate the events linked to cell division in leukemia transformed cells, like cell cycle progression, differentiation, and apoptosis. ITCs have been established to exhibit antiproliferative activities against fungi and bacteria (Virtanen et al. 1963). PEITC, Allyl-ITC (AITC), and their cysteine conjugates have been reported to inhibit in vitro growth and induced the apoptosis of human leukemia HL-60 (p53+) and myeloblastic leukemia-1 cells (p53-) (Xu and Thornalley 2001). Inhibitory action of PEITC and BITC on the growth of human non-small cell lung carcinoma A549 cells was reported by Kuang and Chen (Kuang and Chen 2004). Both PEITC and BITC inhibited the growth of A549 cells in a dose-dependent manner.

11.4.2 Mode of Action of ITCs

By depression of the activation of carcinogens, most of the isothiocyanates may exhibit chemoprotective activity in protocols involving administration of the isothiocyanate either before or during exposure to the carcinogen. ITCs can inhibit phase I enzymes that are responsible for activation of several carcinogens, for example, Cytochrome P-450 is an important enzyme which is required for normal metabolic processing of numerous endogenous and exogenous compounds but may also activate certain carcinogens. ITCs are very potent inhibitors of several members of Cyt. P-450. Sulforaphane (SFN) has been found to inhibit the catalytic activity of several cytochrome enzymes, including Cyt. 1A1, 1A2, 2B1/2, 2E1, and 3A4 (Fimognari et al. 2008a, b). Several factors may play role in the potency of isothiocyanate to inhibit or enhance tumorigenesis. This may comprise the alkyl chain length, substituents, and other structural features of the isothiocyanates, the animal species, target tissues, and the specific carcinogen employed (Jiao et al. 1994; Conaway et al. 1996).

Enhanced disposal of carcinogens: Phase 2 enzymes are the important family of enzymes involved in metabolism of a variety of reactive carcinogens, mutagens, and other toxins (Fimognari et al. 2008a, b). Isothiocyanates are inducers of phase 2 enzymes. ITCs can induce quinone reductase (QR) and glutathione S-transferase (GST, known for the metabolism which results in detoxification) activity in various rodent tissues. For example, aromatic isothiocyanates, α- or β-naphthyl isothiocyanate, allyl isothiocyanate (AITC), sulforanes, and exo-2-acetyl-exo-6-isothiocyanato-norbornane are the inducers of QR and GST in various organs of the body. These compounds when administrated leads to enhanced specific activities of GST and QR in the cytosol by 1.2- to 9.4-times over those of control animals (Zhang and Talalay 1994). GSH levels were increased in the esophagus and small bowel by 63–75% when BITC was administrated to ICR/Ha mice (Talalay and Zhang 1996).

Apoptosis Induction: The pioneering work regarding the study of apoptotic induction by ITCs was demonstrated by Yu et al. (1998). They reported induced apoptosis in HeLa cells by PEITC and other structurally related ITCs, phenylmethyl isothiocyanate (PMITC), phenyl butyl isothiocyanate (PBITC), and phenyl hexyl isothiocyanate (PHITC) in time- and dose-dependent manner. Proteolytic cleavage of poly-(ADP-ribose) polymerase is found to be activated by these ITCs, which leads to the caspase activation and DNA fragmentation. Isothiocyanates induce apoptosis through a caspase-3-dependent mechanism. Recent studies advocate the induction of apoptosis in prostate cancer cell lines by sulforaphane. SFN promotes induction of caspases, ERK1/2, Akt, and increasing p53 and Bax protein levels. Also, sulforaphane is reported to induce apoptosis in glioblastoma cell lines (Fimognari et al. 2008a, 2008b). ITCs induced mitochondria which is directly involved in apoptotic activities. PEITC and Ally ITC are the inhibitors of leukemic cell growth through apoptosis. They enhance the activity of caspase 3 and caspase 8 which leads to breakdown of p22 BID protein to p11, p13, and p15 fragments, activation of c-Jun N-terminal kinase (JNK), and tyrosine phosphorylation (Xu and Thornalley 2001). MAPK (mitogen-activated protein kinases)/extracellular signal-regulated protein kinase (ERKs) are the chain of proteins in cell which communicates signal from cell surface to the DNA inside the nucleus and invoke some changes like cell division. Recent findings of Satyan et al. (2006) on ovarian cancer cells, OVCAR-3, suggest that PEITC inhibits Akt- and ERK1/2-mediated survival signaling and activates pro-apoptotic p38 and JNK1/2 signaling.

The activator protein-1 (AP-1) along with MAPK signaling pathways directly involved in tumor cell growth, its proliferation, apoptosis, and survival. Xu et al. (2005) demonstrated the effects of three ITCs, SFN, PEITC, and AITC on AP-1 activation and investigated the roles of ERK and JNK signaling pathways in the regulation of AP-1 activation and cell death on human prostate cancer cells (PC-3). Their study proved that SFN, PEITC, and AITC each induced AP-1 activity significantly and caused a substantial elevation in the phosphorylation of ERK1/2, JNK1/2, Elk-1, and c-Jun. The transfection with ERK2 and upstream kinase DNEE-MEK1 activated AP-1 activity, and transfection with dominant-negative mutant ERK2 (dnERK2) prominently decreased AP-1 activation induced by SFN, PEITC, and AITC. Transfection with JNK1 and upstream kinase MKK7 activated AP-1 activity, and transfection with dominant-negative mutant JNK1-APF significantly suppresses AP-1 activation induced by SFN, PEITC, and AITC. Pre-treatment with MEK1-ERK inhibitor U0126 and JNK inhibitor SP600125 substantially attenuated the decrease in cell viability induced by SFN, PEITC, and AITC. Transfection with dnERK2 and JNK1-APF significantly reversed the decrease of Bcl-2 expression elicited by these ITCs. Furthermore, transfection with dnERK2 and JNK1-APF blocked the apoptosis induced by these ITCs in PC-3 cells. The results of Xu et al. suggest the activation of the ERK and JNK signaling pathways play a significant role in the transcriptional activity of AP-1 and is involved in the regulation of cell death elicited by ITCs in PC-3 cells.

Cell death by oxidative stress: Reactive oxygen species (ROS) are well known to stimulate cell proliferation and induce genetic instability. Accumulation of ROS in the cancerous cell could be exploited to selectively kill them by depleting the antioxidant level (GSH) inside the cell. PEITC effectively disables the glutathione (GSH) antioxidant system and causes ROS accumulation preferentially in the cancer cells due to their active ROS output. Excessive ROS in the transformed cell leads to oxidative mitochondrial damage, cytochrome c release, inactivation of redox-sensitive molecules (GXP), and massive cell death. Trachootham et al. exploited the above strategy to treat the chronic lymphocytic leukemia (CLL) (the most common adult leukemia, and resistance to fludarabine-based therapies which is a major challenge in CLL treatment) cells with PEITC which induced severe GSH reduction, ROS accumulation, and oxidation of mitochondrial cardiolipin and hence leads to the massive cell death. Their study demonstrated that PEITC is effective in eliminating fludarabine-resistant CLL cells through a redox-mediated mechanism (Trachootham et al. 2008).

Inhibition of cell cycle progression: Hasegawa and co-workers in 1993 first reported the induction of cell cycle arrest by isothiocyanates (Hasegawa et al. 1993). Their results suggest that isothiocyanates (such as AITC, BITC, and PEITC) arrest the cell in G2/M phase and delay the cell cycle progression of HeLa cells, resulting in the inhibition of cell growth. Also, the treatment with SFN in 20 μmol/L caused G2/M-phase arrest and completely inhibited the growth of LM8 cells. Matsui et al. (2007) reported that SFN induced the expression of p21(WAF1/CIP1) protein, which caused cell cycle arrest in a dose-dependent manner. Liang et al. (2008) showed that SFN inhibited human lung adenocarcinoma LTEP-A2 cell growth by causing G2/M-phase arrest. Isothiocyanates may promote cell cycle arrest in different phases in different cell lines and with various mechanisms (Zhang et al. 2003, 2006; Miyoshi et al. 2004; Xiao et al. 2003).

Inhibition of Glycolysis: Singh et al. (2018) studied the role of PEITC in c-Myc-regulated glycolysis in prostate cancer cells. Treatment of PEITC to human prostate cancer cell; LNCaP (androgen-responsive) and 22Rv1 (castration-resistant) decreases the expression as well as transcriptional activity of c-Myc. Prostate cancer cell growth inhibition by PEITC was significantly attenuated by stable overexpression of c-Myc. Myc expression and gene expression of many glycolysis-related genes, including hexokinase II and lactate dehydrogenase A are closely associated. Upon exposure to PEITC, these enzyme proteins and lactate levels were suppressed in prostate cancer cells, and these effects were significantly attenuated by ectopic expression of c-Myc. Their studies revealed that there was a significant decrease in plasma lactate and pyruvate levels in prostate cancer cells of TRAMP mice when treated with PEITC. It is because chemoprevention by PEITC leads to inhibition of glycolysis pathways in the cell.

Angiogenesis is the new growth in the vascular network and is important for the proliferation and metastatic spread of cancer cells because it provides an adequate supply of oxygen and nutrients to the growing cell. Inhibition of angiogenesis may be an important mechanism shown by PEITC to decrease the survival of human umbilical vein endothelial cells (HUVEC) in a concentration- and time-dependent manner (Xiao and Singh 2007). Also, isothiocyanates are known to inhibit the activity of histone deacetylase (Dashwood and Ho 2008). SFN was first reported to inhibit HDAC activity in human colon cancer cells.

Several in vitro and in vivo studies advocate the candidature of isothiocyanates as future drug. The chemopreventive ability of isothiocyanate to inhibit tumorigenesis depended on the structure of the isothiocyanates, the animal species, target tissues, and the specific carcinogen employed. Isothiocyanates also exhibit antitumor activity. There is adequate number of evidences that they target multiple pathways including apoptosis, the MAPK pathway, oxidative stress, and the cell cycle machinery. Despite the substantial progress in the understanding of chemopreventive action of isothiocyanates there are limited clinical trials have been reported.

11.4.3 Curcumin

Curcumin is a polyphenol (diferuloylmethane, bis-α,β-unsaturated β-diketone) extracted from the rhizome of *Curcuma longa* (Fig. 11.5). *Curcuma longa* commonly known as turmeric belongs to the family, Zingiberaceae. This is a herb

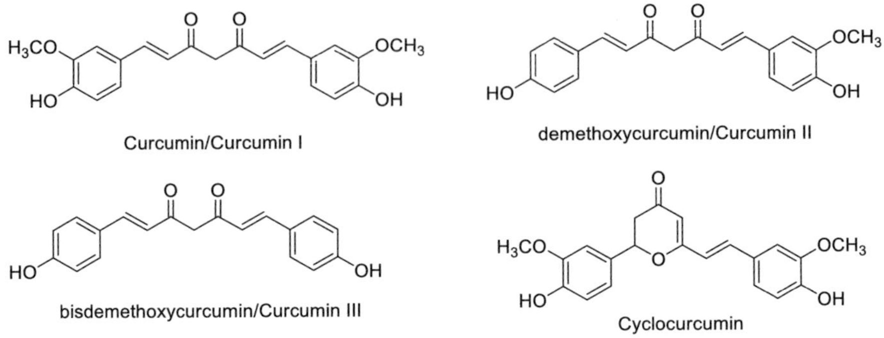

Fig. 11.5 Structure of various curcuminoids

cultivated in Southern Asiatic regions like India and China as a major component of spices. The yellow-pigmented part of turmeric contains curcuminoids: curcumin I (the main component), demethoxycurcumin (curcumin II), bisdemethoxycurcumin (curcumin III), and cyclocurcumin (Fig. 11.5).

Curcuminoids are structurally similar and represent 3–5% of the total mass of turmeric powder. Various literature revealed that natural curcuminoids have several therapeutic effects, such as antioxidant, anticancer, antimicrobial, anti-inflammatory, antiarthritic, hepatoprotective, thrombosuppressive, and hypoglycemic (Maheshwari et al. 2006; Aggarwal and Harikumar 2009). Further, curcumin and its related compounds have been reported to induce apoptosis and regulate several cellular mechanisms in diverse human cancer cells (Collett and Campbell 2004; Chaudhary and Hruska 2003; Martín-Cordero et al. 2003; Mukhopadhyay et al. 2001). In a nutshell, curcumin and its congeners can modulate several important molecular targets, including cell cycle proteins, cytokines, transcription factors, various enzymes, receptors, and cell surface adhesion molecules (Sharma et al. 2005; Shishodia et al. 2005).

Regarding anticancer potential of curcumin, it has been referred by several studies that its congeners can inhibit proliferation and induce apoptosis of cancer cells of different tissues with varying origin, such as epidermis, prostate, B and T cells, colon, breast and head and neck squamous cell carcinoma, by arresting the cell progression in the G2/M phase of the cell cycle. It is shown that curcumin derivatives can inhibit transformation, suppress tumor initiation and invasion, inhibit angiogenesis, and metastasis; and induce the suppression of carcinogenesis of the skin, stomach, colon, and liver in rodents.

11.4.4 Mode of Action of Curcumin

Warburg effect: The metabolic route of cancer cells differs remarkably from normal cells as the cancer cell opt glycolysis pathway rather than oxidative phosphorylation even in the presence of abundant oxygen and produce a large quantity of lactate.

Also, it is established that pyruvate kinase M2 (PKM2) is one of the critical regulators of Warburg effect (Prakasam et al. 2018; Chaneton and Gottlieb 2012). Recently, Siddiqui et al. (2018) reported that curcumin inhibits glucose uptake and lactate production in a variety of cancer cell lines by downregulating PKM2 expression, via inhibition of mTOR-HIF1α axis. Further, they showed that PKM2 overexpression suppressed the effects of curcumin, which can be concluded that inhibition of Warburg effect by curcumin is PKM2 mediated. Their study showed the PKM2-mediated inhibitory effect of curcumin on metabolic path of cancer cells.

Induction of Apoptosis: Adams et al. (2005) reported that curcumin like EF24 (Fig. 11.6) induces the cell cycle arrest and apoptosis by means of a redox-dependent mechanism on different cancer cell lines, MDA-MB-231 human breast cancer cells and DU-145 human prostate cancer cells. Investigation of cell cycle demonstrated that EF24 arrests the cell cycle in the G2/M phase in both cell lines which is followed by the induction of apoptosis. Their findings were evidenced by caspase-3 activation, phosphatidylserine externalization, and cells with a sub-G1 DNA cleavage. They also reported that EF24 induces apoptosis by altering mitochondrial function and reacts glutathione (GSH) and thioredoxin 1. Reaction with these agents in vivo leads to reduction in intracellular GSH as well as oxidized GSH in both the wild-type and Bcl-xL overexpressing HT29 human colon cancer cells. He et al. (2016) have similar findings on colon cancer cell lines. They demonstrated that EF24 induced apoptosis by enhancing intracellular accumulation of ROS in both HCT-116 and SW-620 cells, but with moderate effects in HT-29 cells. They also reported the decrease in mitochondrial membrane potential in the colon cancer cells, results in release of mitochondrial cytochrome c. EF24 induced activation of caspases 9 and 3, causing decreased Bcl-2 protein expression and Bcl-2/Bax ratio.

Nuclear factor-κB (NF-κβ) is an inducible transcription factor that is involved in the modulation of several cell processes, including cell growth and apoptosis (Schmitz et al. 2004). LoTempio et al. (2005) tested curcumin in head and neck squamous carcinoma (HNSCC) cell lines, CCL 23, CAL 27, and UM-SCC1 in a dose-dependent manner, which resulted in reduced nuclear expression of NF-κβ. This leads to decrease in the expression of phospho-Iκβ-α and cyclin D1 protein and hence inhibition of tumor growth was observed in xenograft mice. There are several literature advocated different metabolic pathways which lead to apoptosis-like inhibition of telomerase activity (Chakraborty et al. 2006), downregulation of Notch-1 signaling, caspase-9 and caspase-3 activation, and suppression of antiapoptotic proteins such as Bcl-2, Bcl-XL, and Myc. The decrease in GSH tends to curcumin-induced apoptosis in carcinoma cells (Syng-ai et al. 2004).

ROS metabolic pathway: Larasati et al. (2018) studied the anti-tumorigenic effects of curcumin on CML-derived leukemic cells in xenograft mouse model and in vitro culture system. Their studies revealed that curcumin increases the ROS

Fig. 11.6 Structure of curcumin analogue, EF24

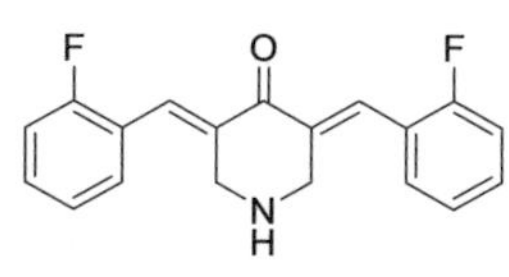

levels over the threshold in cancerous cells through the miscellaneous inhibition of ROS metabolic enzymes (carbonyl reductase, glutathione-S-transferase, glyoxalase) and hence modulate the Glutathione (GSH) level. Curcumin has potential to regulate ROS levels in tumor cells, thereby controlling tumor growth. Kocyigit and Guler (2017) demonstrated that ROS plays a key role in curcumin-induced DNA damage, apoptosis, and cell death. They investigated the effect of curcumin on cytotoxicity, genotoxicity, apoptotic, ROS generation, and mitochondrial membrane potential (MMP) on mouse melanoma cancer cells (B16-F10) and fibroblastic normal cells (L-929). Their results advocated that curcumin decreased cell viability and MMP and increased DNA damage, apoptosis, and ROS levels higher in melanoma cancer cells than in normal cells in a dose-dependent manner.

11.5 Conclusion

Overall phytochemicals including the members of flavonoids and non-flavonoids along with other polyphenols have been found to exhibit anticancerous activity by remodulating the cancer cell metabolism toward the normal cell. These phytochemicals have been found to target various enzymes and proteins involved in the metabolic and signaling pathways and consequently hampers the uncontrolled cell proliferation, viability, tumorigenesis, and other stages in cancer progression. Considering the potential anticancerous activities, one of these phytochemicals could be developed as chemotherapeutic drugs in future to combat cancer.

References

Abotaleb M, Samuel SM, Varghese E, Varghese S, Kubatka P, Liskova A, Busselberg D (2018) Flavonoids in cancer and apoptosis. Cancers 11(1):28

Adams BK, Cai J, Armstrong J, Herold M, Lu YJ, Sun A, Snyder JP, Liotta DC, Jones DP, Shoji M (2005) EF24, a novel synthetic curcumin analog, induces apoptosis in cancer cells via a redox-dependent mechanism. Anticancer Drugs 16(3):263

Aggarwal BB, Harikumar KB (2009) Potential therapeutic effects of curcumin, the anti-inflammatory agent, against neurodegenerative, cardiovascular, pulmonary, metabolic, autoimmune and neoplastic diseases. Int J Biochem Cell Biol 41(1):40–59

Cairns RA, Harris IS, Mak TW (2011) Regulation of cancer cell metabolism. Nat Rev Cancer 11(2):85–95

Chakraborty S, Ghosh U, Bhattacharyya NP, Bhattacharya RK, Roy M (2006) Inhibition of telomerase activity and induction of apoptosis by curcumin in K-562 cells. Mutat Res 596(1):81–90

Chaneton B, Gottlieb E (2012) Rocking cell metabolism: revised functions of the key glycolytic regulator PKM2 in cancer. Trends Biochem Sci 37:309–316

Chaudhary LR, Hruska KA (2003) Inhibition of cell survival signal protein kinase B/Akt by curcumin in human prostate cancer cells. J Cell Biochem 89(1):1–5

Chirumbolo S, Bjørklund G, Lysiuk R, Vella A, Lenchyk L, Upyr T (2018) Targeting cancer with phytochemicals via their fine tuning of the cell survival signaling pathways. Int J Mol Sci 19(11):3568

Collett GP, Campbell FC (2004) Curcumin induces c-jun N-terminal kinase-dependent apoptosis in HCT116 human colon cancer cells. Carcinogenesis 25(11):2183–2189

Conaway CC, Jiao D, Chung FL (1996) Inhibition of rat liver cytochrome P450 isozymes by isothiocyanates and their conjugates: a structure-activity relationship study. Carcinogenesis 17(11):2423–2427

Dashwood RH, Ho E (2008) Dietary agents as histone deacetylase inhibitors: sulforaphane and structurally related isothiocyanates. Nutr Rev 66(Suppl 1):S36–S38

Estrela JM, Mena S, Obrador E, Benlloch M, Castellano G, Salvador R, Dellinger RW (2017) Polyphenolic phytochemicals in cancer prevention and therapy: bioavailability versus bioefficacy. J Med Chem 60(23):9413–9436

Faber AC, Dufort FJ, Blair D, Wagner D, Roberts MF, Chiles TC (2006) Inhibition of phosphatidylinositol 3-kinase-mediated glucose metabolism coincides with resveratrol-induced cell cycle arrest in human diffuse large B-cell lymphomas. Biochem Pharmacol 72(10):1246–1256

Fimognari C, Lenzi M, Hrelia P (2008a) Chemoprevention of cancer by isothiocyanates and anthocyanins: mechanisms of action and structure-activity relationship. Curr Med Chem 15(5):440–447

Fimognari C, Lenzi M, Hrelia P (2008b) Interaction of the isothiocyanate sulforaphane with drug disposition and metabolism: pharmacological and toxicological implications. Curr Drug Metab 9(7):668–678

Gaspar A, Matos MJ, Garrido J, Uriarte E, Borges F (2014) Chromone: a valid scaffold in medicinal chemistry. Chem Rev 114(9):4960–4992

Granchi C, Minutolo F (2012) Anticancer agents that counteract tumor glycolysis. ChemMedChem 7(8):1318–1350

Hamilton KE, Rekman JF, Gunnink LK, Busscher BM, Scott JL, Tidball AM, Stehouwer NR, Johnecheck GN, Looyenga BD, Louters LL (2018) Quercetin inhibits glucose transport by binding to an exofacial site on GLUT1. Biochimie 151:107–114

Hasegawa T, Nishino H, Iwashima A (1993) Isothiocyanates inhibit cell cycle progression of HeLa cells at G2/M phase. Anticancer Drugs 4(2):273–279

Hay N (2016) Reprogramming glucose metabolism in cancer: can it be exploited for cancer therapy? Nat Rev Cancer 16(10):635–649

He G, Feng C, Vinothkumar R, Chen W, Dai X, Chen X, Ye Q, Qiu C, Zhou H, Wang Y, Liang G, Xie Y, Wu W (2016) Curcumin analog EF24 induces apoptosis via ROS-dependent mitochondrial dysfunction in human colorectal cancer cells. Cancer Chemother Pharmacol 78(6):1151–1161

Hecht SS (1995) Chemoprevention by isothiocyanates. J Cell Biochem 59(S22):195–209

Hosseini A, Ghorbani A (2015) Cancer therapy with phytochemicals: evidence from clinical studies. Avicenna J Phytomed 5(2):84–97

Jiao D, Eklind KI, Choi CI, Desai DH, Amin SG, Chung FL (1994) Structure-activity relationships of isothiocyanates as mechanism-based inhibitors of 4-(methylnitrosamino)-1-(3-pyridyl)-1-butanone-induced lung tumorigenesis in A/J mice. Cancer Res 54(16):4327–4333

Kashyap D, Garg VK, Tuli HS, Yerer MB, Sak K, Sharma AK, Kumar M, Aggarwal V, Sandhu SS (2019) Fisetin and quercetin: promising flavonoids with chemopreventive potential. Biomol Ther 9(5):174

Kocyigit A, Guler E (2017) Curcumin induce DNA damage and apoptosis through generation of reactive oxygen species and reducing mitochondrial membrane potential in melanoma cancer cells. Cell Mol Biol 63:97

Kuang YF, Chen YH (2004) Induction of apoptosis in a non-small cell human lung cancer cell line by isothiocyanates is associated with P53 and P21. Food Chem Toxicol 42(10):1711–1718

Kuroiwa Y, Nishikawa A, Kitamura Y, Kanki K, Ishii Y, Umemura T, Hirose M (2006) Protective effects of benzyl isothiocyanate and sulforaphane but not resveratrol against initiation of pancreatic carcinogenesis in hamsters. Cancer Lett 241(2):275–280

Larasati YA, Yoneda-Kato N, Nakamae I, Yokoyama T, Meiyanto E, Kato JY (2018) Curcumin targets multiple enzymes involved in the ROS metabolic pathway to suppress tumor cell growth. Sci Rep 8(1):2039

Liang H, Lai B, Yuan Q (2008) Sulforaphane induces cell-cycle arrest and apoptosis in cultured human lung adenocarcinoma LTEP-A2 cells and retards growth of LTEP-A2 xenografts in vivo. J Nat Prod 71(11):1911–1914

Liberti MV, Locasale JW (2016) The Warburg effect: how does it benefit cancer cells? Trends Biochem Sci 41(3):211–218
LoTempio MM, Veena MS, Steele HL, Ramamurthy B, Ramalingam TS, Cohen AN, Chakrabarti R, Srivatsan ES, Wang MB (2005) Curcumin suppresses growth of head and neck squamous cell carcinoma. Clin Cancer Res 11(19):6994
Maheshwari RK, Singh AK, Gaddipati J, Srimal RC (2006) Multiple biological activities of curcumin: a short review. Life Sci 78(18):2081–2087
Martín-Cordero C, López-Lázaro M, Gálvez M, Ayuso MJ (2003) Curcumin as a DNA topoisomerase II poison. J Enzyme Inhib Med Chem 18(6):505–509
Matsui TA, Murata H, Sakabe T, Sowa Y, Horie N, Nakanishi R, Sakai T, Kubo T (2007) Sulforaphane induces cell cycle arrest and apoptosis in murine osteosarcoma cells in vitro and inhibits tumor growth in vivo. Oncol Rep 18:1263–1268
Miyoshi N, Uchida K, Osawa T, Nakamura Y (2004) Benzyl isothiocyanate modifies expression of the G2/M arrest-related genes. Biofactors 21(1GÇÉ4):23–26
Morse MA, Amin SG, Hecht SS, Chung FL (1989) Effects of aromatic isothiocyanates on tumorigenicity, O6-methylguanine formation, and metabolism of the tobacco-specific nitrosamine 4-(methylnitrosamino)-1-(3-pyridyl)-1-butanone in A/J mouse lung. Cancer Res 49(11):2894
Morse MA, Eklind KI, Amin SG, Hecht SS, Chung FL (1989) Effects of alkyl chain length on the inhibition of NNK-induced lung neoplasia in A/J mice by arylalkyl isothiocyanates. Carcinogenesis 10(9):1757–1759
Morse MA, Eklind KI, Hecht SS, Jordan KG, Choi CI, Desai DH, Amin SG, Chung FL (1991) Structure-activity relationships for inhibition of 4-(methylnitrosamino)-1-(3-pyridyl)-1-butanone lung tumorigenesis by arylalkyl isothiocyanates in A/J mice. Cancer Res 51(7):1846
Morse MA, Zu H, Galati AJ, Schmidt CJ, Stoner GD (1993) Dose-related inhibition by dietary phenethyl isothiocyanate of esophageal tumorigenesis and DNA methylation induced by N-nitrosomethylbenzylamine in rats. Cancer Lett 72(1):103–110
Mukhopadhyay A, Bueso-Ramos C, Chatterjee D, Pantazis P, Aggarwal BB (2001) Curcumin downregulates cell survival mechanisms in human prostate cancer cell lines. Oncogene 20(52):7597–7609
Ngo H, Tortorella SM, Ververis K, Karagiannis TC (2015) The Warburg effect: molecular aspects and therapeutic possibilities. Mol Biol Rep 42(4):825–834
Pandey KB, Rizvi SI (2009) Plant polyphenols as dietary antioxidants in human health and disease. Oxidative Med Cell Longev 2(5):270–278
Prakasam G, Iqbal MA, Bamezai RNK, Mazurek S (2018) Posttranslational modifications of pyruvate kinase M2: tweaks that benefit cancer. Front Oncol 8:22
Reyes-Farias M, Carrasco-Pozo C (2019) The anti-cancer effect of quercetin: molecular implications in cancer metabolism. Int JMol Sci 20(13):3177
Rivera Rivera A, Castillo-Pichardo L, Gerena Y, Dharmawardhane S (2016) Anti-breast cancer potential of quercetin via the Akt/AMPK/mammalian target of rapamycin (mTOR) signaling cascade. PLoS One 11(6):e0157251
Russo M, Spagnuolo C, Tedesco I, Russo GL (2010) Phytochemicals in cancer prevention and therapy: truth or dare? Toxins 2(4):517–551
Sarkar S, Horn G, Moulton K, Oza A, Byler S, Kokolus S, Longacre M (2013) Cancer development, progression, and therapy: an epigenetic overview. Int J Mol Sci 14(10):21087–21113
Satyan KS, Swamy N, Dizon DS, Singh R, Granai CO, Brard L (2006) Phenethyl isothiocyanate (PEITC) inhibits growth of ovarian cancer cells by inducing apoptosis: role of caspase and MAPK activation. Gynecol Oncol 103(1):261–270
Saunier E, Antonio S, Regazzetti A, Auzeil N, Laprévote O, Shay JW, Coumoul X, Barouki R, Benelli C, Huc L, Bortoli S (2017) Resveratrol reverses the Warburg effect by targeting the pyruvate dehydrogenase complex in colon cancer cells. Sci Rep 7(1):6945
Schmitz ML, Mattioli I, Buss H, Kracht M (2004) NF-κB: a multifaceted transcription factor regulated at several levels. Chembiochem 5(10):1348–1358
Sever R, Brugge JS (2015) Signal transduction in cancer. Cold Spring Harb Perspect Med 5(4):a006098

Sharma RA, Gescher AJ, Steward WP (2005) Curcumin: the story so far. Eur J Cancer 41(13):1955–1968

Shishodia S, Sethi G, Aggarwal BB (2005) Curcumin: getting back to the roots. Ann N Y Acad Sci 1056(1):206–217

Siddiqui FA, Prakasam G, Chattopadhyay S, Rehman AU, Padder RA, Ansari MA, Irshad R, Mangalhara K, Bamezai RNK, Husain M, Ali SM, Iqbal MA (2018) Curcumin decreases Warburg effect in cancer cells by down-regulating pyruvate kinase M2 via mTOR-HIF1α inhibition. Sci Rep 8(1):8323

Singh KB, Hahm ER, Rigatti LH, Normolle DP, Yuan JM, Singh SV (2018) Inhibition of glycolysis in prostate cancer chemoprevention by phenethyl isothiocyanate. Cancer Prev Res (Phila) 11(6):337–346

Snyder V, Reed-Newman TC, Arnold L, Thomas SM, Anant S (2018) Cancer stem cell metabolism and potential therapeutic targets. Front Oncol 8:203

Srivastava S, Somasagara RR, Hegde M, Nishana M, Tadi SK, Srivastava M, Choudhary B, Raghavan SC (2016) Quercetin, a natural flavonoid interacts with DNA, arrests cell cycle and causes tumor regression by activating mitochondrial pathway of apoptosis. Sci Rep 6(1):24049

Sundarraj K, Raghunath A, Perumal E (2018) A review on the chemotherapeutic potential of fisetin: in vitro evidences. Biomed Pharmacother 97:928–940

Syng-ai C, Kumari AL, Khar A (2004) Effect of curcumin on normal and tumor cells: role of glutathione and bcl-2. Mol Cancer Ther 3(9):1101

Talalay P, Zhang Y (1996) Chemoprotection against cancer by isothiocyanates and glucosinolates. Biochem Soc Trans 24(3):806–810

Trachootham D, Zhang H, Zhang W, Feng L, Du M, Zhou Y, Chen Z, Pelicano H, Plunkett W, Wierda WG, Keating MJ, Huang P (2008) Effective elimination of fludarabine-resistant CLL cells by PEITC through a redox-mediated mechanism. Blood 112(5):1912–1922

Vaupel P, Schmidberger H, Mayer A (2019) The Warburg effect: essential part of metabolic reprogramming and central contributor to cancer progression. Int J Radiat Biol 95(7):912–919

Virtanen AI, Kreula M, Kies-vaara M (1963) Investigations on the alleged goitrogenic properties of milk. Z Ernahrungswiss 3:23–37

Wang H, Khor TO, Shu L, Su ZY, Fuentes F, Lee JH, Kong ANT (2012) Plants against cancer: a review on natural phytochemicals in preventing and treating cancers and their druggability. Anti Cancer Agents Med Chem 12(10):1281–1305

Wattenberg LW (1977) Inhibition of carcinogenic effects of polycyclic hydrocarbons by benzyl isothiocyanate and related compounds. J Natl Cancer Inst 58(2):395–398

Wattenberg LW (1987) Inhibitory effects of benzyl isothiocyanate administered shortly before diethylnitrosamine or benzo[a]pyrene on pulmonary and forestomach neoplasia in A/J mice. Carcinogenesis 8(12):1971–1973

Xiao D, Singh SV (2007) Phenethyl isothiocyanate inhibits angiogenesis in vitro and ex vivo. Cancer Res 67(5):2239–2246

Xiao D, Srivastava SK, Lew KL, Zeng Y, Hershberger P, Johnson CS, Trump DL, Singh SV (2003) Allyl isothiocyanate, a constituent of cruciferous vegetables, inhibits proliferation of human prostate cancer cells by causing G2/M arrest and inducing apoptosis. Carcinogenesis 24(5):891–897

Xu C, Shen G, Yuan X, Kim JH, Gopalkrishnan A, Keum YS, Nair S, Kong ANT (2005) ERK and JNK signaling pathways are involved in the regulation of activator protein 1 and cell death elicited by three isothiocyanates in human prostate cancer PC-3 cells. Carcinogenesis 27(3):437–445

Xu K, Thornalley PJ (2001) Signal transduction activated by the cancer chemopreventive isothiocyanates: cleavage of BID protein, tyrosine phosphorylation and activation of JNK. Br J Cancer 84(5):670–673

Xu K, Thornalley PJ (2000) Studies on the mechanism of the inhibition of human leukaemia cell growth by dietary isothiocyanates and their cysteine adducts in vitro. Biochem Pharmacol 60(2):221–231

Yu R, Mandlekar S, Harvey KJ, Ucker DS, Kong ANT (1998) Chemopreventive isothiocyanates induce apoptosis and caspase-3-like protease activity. Cancer Res 58(3):402
Zhang R, Loganathan S, Humphreys I, Srivastava SK (2006) Benzyl isothiocyanate-induced DNA damage causes G2/M cell cycle arrest and apoptosis in human pancreatic cancer cells. J Nutr 136(11):2728–2734
Zhang Y, Talalay P (1994) Anticarcinogenic activities of organic isothiocyanates: chemistry and mechanisms. Cancer Res 54(7 Suppl):1976s
Zhang Y, Tang L, Gonzalez V (2003) Selected isothiocyanates rapidly induce growth inhibition of cancer cells. Mol Cancer Ther 2(10):1045

Correction to: Cancer Cell Metabolism: A Potential Target for Cancer Therapy

Dhruv Kumar

Correction to:
D. Kumar (ed.), *Cancer Cell Metabolism: A Potential Target for Cancer Therapy*, https://doi.org/10.1007/978-981-15-1991-8

The following late corrections have been carried out in the updated version of chapters 6 and 7:

1. In chapter 6, the following affiliation has been added to author Ramesh Choudhari:

   Shri B. M. Patil Medical College, Hospital and Research Centre, BLDE (Deemed to be University), Vijayapur, India
2. In chapter 7, author's family name has been corrected to "Choudhari" from "Choudhary" and also the following affiliation has been added to author Ramesh Choudhari:

   Center of Emphasis in Cancer Research, Department of Molecular and Translational Medicine, Paul L. Foster School of Medicine, Texas Tech University Health Sciences Center El Paso, El Paso, TX, USA

The updated online version of these chapters can be found at
https://doi.org/10.1007/978-981-15-1991-8_6
https://doi.org/10.1007/978-981-15-1991-8_7

D. Kumar (ed.), *Cancer Cell Metabolism: A Potential Target for Cancer Therapy*,
https://doi.org/10.1007/978-981-15-1991-8_12

MIX
Papier aus verantwortungsvollen Quellen
Paper from responsible sources
FSC® C105338

If you have any concerns about our products,
you can contact us on
ProductSafety@springernature.com

In case Publisher is established outside the EU,
the EU authorized representative is:
Springer Nature Customer Service Center GmbH
Europaplatz 3, 69115 Heidelberg, Germany

Printed by Libri Plureos GmbH
in Hamburg, Germany